PROGRESS IN CLINICAL MEDICINE

PROGRESS IN CLINICAL MEDICINE

Volume Eight

EDITED BY

A. R. HORLER MD FRCP

Consultant Physician, Royal Victoria Infirmary,
Newcastle upon Tyne

J. B. FOSTER MD FRCP

Consultant Neurologist, Newcastle University Hospitals;
Honorary Reader in Neurology, University of
Newcastle upon Tyne

CHURCHILL LIVINGSTONE
EDINBURGH LONDON MELBOURNE AND NEW YORK 1983

CHURCHILL LIVINGSTONE
Medical Division of Longman Group Limited

Distributed in the United States of America by
Churchill Livingstone Inc., 1560 Broadway, New York,
N.Y. 10036, and by associated companies,
branches and representatives throughout
the world.

First published 1983

ISBN 0 443 02541 X

British Library Cataloguing in Publication Data
Progress in clinical medicine.—(Progress; v.8)
1. Diseases—Periodicals
616'.005 RB111

Library of Congress Cataloging in Publication Data
Progress in clinical medicine.
"Volume eight."
Includes index.
1. Internal medicine. I. Horler, A. R. II. Foster.
J. B. (John Barnes) [DNLM: 1. Medicine. WB 100 P9625]
RC46.P898 1983 61682-19884

Printed in Great Britain by Butler & Tanner Ltd, Frome, Somerset.

PREFACE

Our previous volume in this series appeared in 1978 after an interval of 6 years, the first under our joint editorship. Our intention was to continue the style and composition that had been followed so successfully by our predecessors, and we included contributions from most of the medical specialities as well as from other disciplines which regularly impinge upon the sphere of the general physician.

In this present volume we have confined our contributions entirely to the field of clinical medicine, comprising a shorter list of chapters, and we have endeavoured to include advances in subjects of direct relevance to those for whom the book is primarily intended. It is necessary, therefore, to consider this volume as a continuation of the last, rather than as a completely new venture. Medical progress is a continuing phenomenon and a book such as this can be only selective. We hope our present selection will continue to attract the interest of practising physicians and postgraduate students.

We are grateful to Mrs Heather Russell for her invaluable assistance with script reading and to those authors and publishers whose material we have been permitted to reproduce. We also appreciate the continuing interest and encouragement of Dr Raymond Daley who for so long shared the responsibility of editorship.

Newcastle upon Tyne, 1983

A.R.H.
J.B.F.

CONTRIBUTORS

P. L. Amlot MB BS MRCP
Senior Lecturer, Department of Medicine, Guy's Hospital Medical School, London

John Anderson MB BS FRCP
Academic Sub-Dean and Senior Lecturer in Medicine, The Medical School, University of Newcastle upon Tyne; Honorary Consultant Physician, Royal Victoria Infirmary, Newcastle upon Tyne

J. B. Foster MD FRCP
Consultant Neurologist, Newcastle University Hospitals; Honorary Reader in Neurology, University of Newcastle upon Tyne

Reginald Hall BSc MD FRCP
Professor of Medicine, Welsh National School of Medicine, Cardiff

Alan R. Horler MD FRCP
Consultant Physician, Royal Victoria Infirmary, Newcastle upon Tyne

Graham R. V. Hughes MD FRCP
Reader in Medicine and Head of Rheumatology Unit, Royal Postgraduate Medical School, Hammersmith Hospital, London

O. F. W. James MA FRCP
Reader in Medicine (Geriatrics) and Consultant Physician, University of Newcastle upon Tyne, Freeman Hospital, Newcastle upon Tyne

D. G. Julian MA MD FRCP FRCPE FRACP
Professor of Cardiology, University of Newcastle upon Tyne, Freeman Hospital, Newcastle upon Tyne

Maurice H. Lessof MA MD FRCP
Professor of Medicine, Guy's Hospital Medical School, London

B. E. C. Nordin MD FRCP DSc
Senior Research Fellow and Clinical Professor, Royal Adelaide Hospital, Adelaide, South Australia

M. Peacock MB FRCP
Assistant Director of Mineral Metabolism Unit and Honorary Consultant Physician, Leeds General Infirmary, Leeds

T. B. Stretton MB FRCP
Consultant Physician, Manchester Royal Infirmary, Manchester

Mark J. Walport MA MRCP
Registrar in General Medicine and Rheumatology, Department of Medicine, Royal Postgraduate Medical School, Hammersmith Hospital, London

J. M. A. Whitehouse MA MD FRCP

Professor of Medical Oncology, Southampton University; Director, Wessex Regional Oncology Service, Southampton General Hospital, Southampton

Robert Wilkinson BSc MD FRCP

Senior Lecturer in Medicine, University of Newcastle upon Tyne; Consultant Physician, Department of Nephrology, Freeman Hospital, Newcastle upon Tyne

Christopher J. Williams DM MRCP

Senior Lecturer in Medical Oncology and Honorary Consultant Physician, University of Southampton CRC Medical Oncology Unit, Southampton General Hospital, Southampton

CONTENTS

1.	**Endocrinology** R. Hall	1
2.	**Diabetes mellitus** J. Anderson	17
3.	**Clinical immunology** P. L. Amlot and M. H. Lessof	62
4.	**Cardiology** D. G. Julian	79
5.	**Respiratory disease** T. B. Stretton	100
6.	**Neurology** J. B. Foster	122
7.	**Haematology** A. R. Horler	141
8.	**Developments in medical oncology** C. J. Williams and J. M. A. Whitehouse	165
9.	**Renal disease** R. Wilkinson	197
10.	**Gastroenterology** O. James	222
11.	**Connective tissue diseases** M. J. Walport and G. R. V. Hughes	257
12.	**Calcium and bone metabolism** B. E. C. Nordin and M. Peacock	287
Index		317

1

Endocrinology

R. Hall

DISEASES OF THE HYPOTHALAMUS

Hypothalamic disease is rare and its clinical manifestations are often non-specific; hence it is easily overlooked when a diagnosis is being sought. A wide variety of diseases may affect the hypothalamus either directly or indirectly (Table 1.1).

Table 1.1 Diseases of the hypothalamus

Congenital GH deficiency with or without other deficiencies LH and/or FSH deficiency with anosmia (Kallman's syndrome) or without anosmia Isolated deficiencies of TSH or ACTH Laurence-Moon-Biedl syndrome (polydactyly, mental retardation, retinitis pigmentosa and hypogonadism)	*Granulomatous diseases* Sarcoidosis Histiocytosis X Multi-system granulomas *Vascular disease* Post-partum hypopituitarism Carotid and other aneurysms Subarachnoid haemorrhage Pituitary apoplexy
Tumours Hypothalamic Craniopharyngiomas Germinomas Sphenoidal ridge meningiomas Gliomas of the optic chiasm Other cerebral tumours Secondary deposits Lymphomas Pituitary Suprasellar extension of pituitary tumours	*Structural* Secondary to internal hydrocephalus from any cause, e.g. aqueduct stenosis in neurofibromatosis, colloid cysts, ependymomas *Iatrogenic* Radiation or neurosurgical treatment of pituitary lesions Nasopharyngeal irradiation After prolonged steroid or thyroid hormone medication *Trauma* After head injury (usually with fractured base of skull)
Infectious diseases Encephalitis Meningitis (tuberculous or bacterial) Syphilis	*Functional* Anorexia nervosa, starvation, emotional deprivation syndromes

Clinical features

Hypothalamic disease presents either as a result of the effects of the local lesion or as hypopituitarism.

Local effects

Infiltrative or expanding local lesions may cause headaches and field defects differing from those of a primary pituitary lesion, because pressure on the chiasm from above usually causes an initial inferior quadrantic temporal hemianopia. Behavioural, functional and autonomic abnormalities may mimic a wide variety of psychiatric disorders.

Appetite disorders are common, usually leading to obesity or, more rarely, profound weight loss. However, the great majority of obese patients are not suffering from any detectable organic disease of the hypothalamus, although an 'endocrine cause' is often suspected. The most gross example of 'hypothalamic obesity' is seen in the Prader Willi syndrome of voracious appetite, gross obesity, mental retardation, hypogonadism, diabetes mellitus, and small hands and feet. In the equally rare Laurence–Moon–Biedl syndrome, obesity and mental retardation are associated with retinitis pigmentosa and extra digits. Sleep disorders are not uncommon, with hypersomnia or altered sleep rhythm. Sexual behaviour may be disturbed, with loss of libido or promiscuity, and puberty may be either precocious or delayed. Precocious puberty in boys is usually organic and points to a lesion in the region of the pineal. Loss of thirst sensation is common in patients with expanding hypothalamic lesions and is particularly dangerous if the patient has already developed diabetes insipidus. Gross hypernatraemia, sometimes fatal, can occur because of uncompensated water loss, and plasma sodium values up to 200 mmol/l may be recorded. Disorders of temperature control are easily overlooked. The patient may develop hypothermia or hyperthermia, or poikilothermia in which the body temperature fluctuates with that of the environment. Emotional behaviour may be immature, inappropriate, aggressive or retarded and is often a cause of great distress to the relatives. Motor activity may be grossly decreased and the inactivity contributes to the development of obesity. Memory defects may be profound: defects of short-term memory result from involvement of the mamillary bodies.

Endocrine effects

Hypothalamic disease may reduce the synthesis or transport of the prolactin-inhibiting factor dopamine and lead to hyperprolactinaemia and its various sequelae (*see* p. **6**). Apart from prolactin deficiency, hypothalamic lesions cause hypopituitarism of varying severity. Diabetes insipidus could be better classified as a local effect, as it results from damage either to the magnocellular neurones of the supraoptic nucleus in the hypothalamus or to the supraoptico-hypophysial tract. The commonest clinical presentation of hypothalamic disease is diabetes insipidus associated with hypogonadism in a patient with a normal pituitary fossa. It should be stressed that primary pituitary disease does not itself cause diabetes insipidus unless there is suprasellar spread or there has been surgical or radiotherapeutic intervention.

Diagnosis

Diagnosis consists of defining the local lesion or syndrome and characterising the extent, if any, of hormone deficiency. Formal visual-field charting may suggest hypothalamic disease and indicate its location and rate of extension. Skull X-rays may be normal, or show distortion or erosion of the posterior clinoids, pineal or aberrant calcification. CT scans with and without intravenous contrast medium may outline a tumour. Metrizamide cisternography can be helpful in delineating the extent of a lesion (Hall K et al 1980) and a combination of CT scanning after intrathecal administration of the contrast medium is also useful. Air encephalography is less pleasant for the patient but can provide valuable information. Cerebral arteriography is now less often required but may demonstrate tumour extension or vascular blushes and exclude aneurysms.

The search for extracranial evidence of a systemic disease may yield clues to the diagnosis. For example, a pneumothorax occurring in a patient with a hypothalamic disorder suggests an underlying eosinophilic granuloma. Pulmonary infiltration may be seen in eosinophilic granulomas or sarcoidosis. Chromosomal anomalies can occur in some patients with germinomas. Cutaneous manifestations of neurofibromatosis may suggest a diagnosis of hydrocephalus from aqueduct stenosis.

Sometimes all diagnostic manoeuvres fail and, if there is evidence of an expanding hypothalamic lesion, neurosurgical exploration may be required with biopsy of any suspicious tissue or correction of internal hydrocephalus by shunting.

Treatment

Obviously, treatment of the disease will depend on the cause. Hormonal deficiencies are corrected as in hypopituitarism. Some tumours, such as craniopharyngiomas, may be amenable to excision or decompression; others, such as germinomas, may be radiosensitive. Chemotherapy may be of use in lymphomas and histiocytosis X. Sarcoidosis may respond to corticosteroid medication in some cases.

PITUITARY ADENOMAS

Pathology

Modern techniques of electron microscopy and immunocytochemistry have allowed eight distinct types of anterior pituitary cell adenomas to be defined (Table 1.2).

Table 1.2 Types of pituitary adenoma (Kovacs & Horvath 1979)

Cell type	Frequency (%)
Growth hormone	21
Prolactin	32
Mixed growth hormone, prolactin	6
Acidophil stem cell	3.5
Corticotroph	13
Thyrotroph	0.5
Gonadotroph	1.0
Undifferentiated	23

Clinical features

Pituitary tumours may present as a result of hypersecretion of one or more hormones, as hypopituitarism from compression of the normal pituitary tissue or pituitary stalk by the adenoma, or as a result of local expansion within the fossa or into the infra-, para- or suprasellar regions. A detailed discussion of the clinical features and routine endocrine investigations is provided in Hall R et al (1980).

Radiological investigation of pituitary tumours

Lateral and anteroposterior views of the fossa demonstrate the size and extent of the tumour. Intrasellar lesions produce enlargement of the fossa with erosions of its bony outlines. A double contour of the floor of the fossa may be caused by uneven downward expansion but is more often attributable to an inadequate radiological technique ('a poor lateral') or to a normal variant in the shape of the fossa. It is now apparent that many so-called minor abnormalities of the fossa are, in fact, normal variants and do not signify the presence of a pituitary tumour. Many radiologists doubt the advantage of detailed sellar tomography which involves a significant dose of radiation.

Computerised tomography (CT scanning) is of great value in the neuroradiological investigation of pituitary lesions. Axial (horizontal) plane scans can demonstrate a suprasellar extension which may show enhancement after intravenous contrast medium (Conray). Coronal or semicoronal scans give an even better demonstration of the extent of the lesion. The water-soluble contrast medium, metrizamide, can be run into the basal subarachnoid cisternae and around the brain after introduction by the lumbar route. The suprasellar cisterna can be identified easily and lateral radiographs of this area will demonstrate all the structures shown by pneumoencephalography. The technique is simpler than others and the side effects fewer and less severe so that serial examinations are possible. An empty sella is clearly shown by this technique. A metrizamide cisternogram can be combined with a CT scan — a metrizamide CT cisternogram in both the axial and coronal planes provides a three-dimensional appreciation of the extent of the lesion. Using the new generation of CT scanners it is now possible to demonstrate microadenomas a few millimetres in diameter within the pituitary fossa.

Angiography is not often required in the investigation of pituitary tumours although some surgeons prefer to know the precise location of the carotid arteries before embarking on pituitary surgery.

Growth-hormone-secreting adenomas

GH-secreting adenomas produce a wide variety of clinical manifestations leading to acromegaly in adults and gigantism (with some features of acromegaly) if the condition develops before fusion of the epiphyses. Gigantism is now very rare, making up less than 1% of the syndromes of GH excess. Estimates of the incidence and prevalence of acromegaly have been presented in a study from the north-east of England (Alexander et al 1980). The annual incidence appears to be close to three cases per million and the prevalence of diagnosed cases up to 40 per million. The study showed that in men there was a significant increase in the risk of death from cardiovascular, cerebrovascular and malignant diseases whereas in women there was excess mortality from cerebrovascular disease only; these findings are similar to those reported by Wright et al (1970).

Diagnosis

Even when the clinical features are obvious, GH oversecretion must be confirmed by measurements of GH during a standard glucose tolerance test. In normal subjects GH levels should fall to <4 mU/litre (<2 ng/ml). Radiological enlargement of the pituitary fossa is detectable in at least 90% of cases. If surgical ablation or yttrium-90 implantation is contemplated the upper level of the tumour should be defined by CT scanning or pneumoencephalography. When active therapy is not contemplated and the visual fields are normal, invasive neuroradiological procedures may be withheld. Secretion of other pituitary hormones should be tested. The combination of thyrotrophin-releasing hormone (200 μg), plus gonadotrophin-releasing hormone (100 μg) is convenient to use, bearing in mind that active acromegaly is insulin-resistant. Basal levels of prolactin (PRL) should be measured because there is often associated oversecretion of this hormone: there is some evidence that patients with concomitant GH and PRL hypersecretion respond better to bromocriptine.

The diagnostic problem is usually to decide which patients with rugged features and large hands and feet justify further investigation. Patients who complain of a change in their appearance, especially if this is confirmed by inspection of previous photographs, are worthy of investigation. Other causes of enlargement of the hands include manual work, obesity, hypothyroidism and primary amyloidosis. Enlargement of the feet usually affects their width rather than their length. Enlargement of the tongue may also be complained of in hypochondriasis, hypothyroidism and primary amyloidosis.

Treatment

No treatment can as yet be guaranteed to restore GH levels to normal, to prevent further tumour growth and to avoid hypopituitarism or other local complications. For patients up to the age of 60 years or so with active disease and a tumour confined to the fossa, or with only a small suprasellar extension, the treatment of choice is now trans-sphenoidal hypophysectomy, if a sufficiently experienced surgeon is available. Hypopituitarism is produced in only about one-quarter of the patients because some normal tissue is usually left around the stalk. Cure rates of about 80% can be achieved, as judged by the return of GH levels to normal (Richards & Thomas 1980). If GH levels remain high postoperatively, residual tumour growth can usually be prevented by external radiation in a total dose of up to 4500 rad. Treatment with bromocriptine can then be used to reduce GH levels and to bring about symptomatic improvement until radiation becomes effective.

In specialised centres yttrium-90 implantation can be effective. A dose of 50000 rad is used if the GH level is <100 mU/l and 150000 rad if the level exceeds 100 mU/l. Further implants can be inserted if GH levels are not sufficiently reduced, and small suprasellar extensions can also be treated.

When there is a large suprasellar extension which is inaccessible from the trans-sphenoidal route, transfrontal decompression of the chiasm is performed, followed by external radiation of the residual tumour. Again, bromocriptine can be given to achieve further symptomatic improvement.

When invasive therapy is considered to be inappropriate because of a patient's wishes, age or concomitant disease, medical treatment with bromocriptine, a long-acting dopamine agonist, produces a worthwhile clinical response in at least 75% of cases. Treatment is built up gradually to an average dose of 5 mg four times daily. It has now been shown that, as well as lowering GH levels, bromocriptine can reduce the size of some GH-secreting tumours, although its effect on prolactinomas is more obvious.

It is essential to treat the associated hypopituitarism which can complicate untreated acromegaly or may be an early or late effect of such treatment.

Prolactin-secreting adenomas

Prolactin-secreting pituitary adenomas now appear to be the commonest of the pituitary tumours, although it is still uncertain whether this is attributable to a true increase in frequency, an increased index of suspicion, the ready availability of PRL immunoassays, the advent of an effective therapy such as bromocriptine, or to a combination of these factors. Although PRL-secreting adenomas can be induced by oestrogen medication in animals, there is still no clear evidence that oral contraceptive medication induces prolactinomas, despite the clinical suspicion of this possibility.

Clinical features

Hyperprolactinaemia in women causes a combination of amenorrhoea or oligomenorrhoea, galactorrhoea, infertility, loss of libido and, very occasionally, hirsutism. In men the clinical features may be less obvious: they include impotence, loss of libido, galactorrhoea, oligospermia or azoospermia, reduced prostatic size and semen volume, infertility and a female distribution of body fat. The hypogonadism seen in either sex may be caused partly by pressure of the adenoma on normal pituitary tissue or by PRL blocking the action of gonadotrophins. Galactorrhoea may be detected only by careful expression of the breasts but can be absent even in the presence of very high PRL levels.

Diagnosis

Many drugs and diseases can cause hyperprolactinaemia and the serum PRL level may also be raised in a variety of physiological situations (Table 1.3). Serum for PRL estimation should be taken after 11:00 hours to avoid the effects of the nocturnal increase which can persist into the earlier morning. Although PRL levels rise in response to stress, the effects of stress in routine blood sampling have probably been overestimated. In the appropriate clinical context, if PRL levels are raised ($>$400 mU/l) the problem is to decide the cause. The higher the PRL level, the more likely is the patient to have a pituitary tumour, although tumours can be found in some patients who have only a modest increase in PRL levels. A lateral skull X-ray should be performed: if this shows a definitely enlarged fossa, the diagnosis is established and the extent of the tumour and secretion of other pituitary hormones must be determined. If the PRL level is raised and the pituitary fossa normal or only 'suspicious', one is faced with what has been termed 'the prolactinoma problem'. Is the hyperprolactinaemia functional or does the pituitary fossa harbour a microadenoma? It has been shown that patients with prolactinomas have an impaired PRL response both to TRH and to dopamine-receptor blockade with metoclopramide or domperidone. Patients with functional hyperprolactinaemia show a normal (several hundred per cent) increase in PRL in response to these stimuli. Patients with macro- or microadenomas secreting PRL also tend to show an exaggerated TSH response to dopamine-receptor blockade. Modern CT scans can sometimes reveal the presence of a microadenoma within the fossa.

Table 1.3 Causes of hyperprolactinaemia

Physiological
Neonatal period
Puberty in girls
Coitus and orgasm
Nipple stimulation
Pregnancy and suckling
Sleep
Stress
Drugs
Dopamine-receptor-blocking agents:
Phenothiazines, e.g. chlorpromazine
Haloperidol
Metoclopramide, sulpiride, pimozide, domperidone
CNS-dopamine depleting agents:
Reserpine
Methyl dopa
Others:
Oestrogens
TRH
Hypothalamic or pituitary stalk lesions
Craniopharyngiomas, gliomas, 'pinealomas'
Granulomas — sarcoidosis, eosinophilic granuloma, TB meningitis
Stalk section following trauma, pituitary surgery, or pressure from a tumour
Pituitary tumours
Prolactin cell
Mixed growth hormone cell/prolactin cell
Acidophil stem cell
Mixed corticotrophin cell/prolactin cell
Miscellaneous
Idiopathic/functional
Hypothyroidism
Chronic renal failure
Ectopic, e.g. from bronchogenic carcinoma or hypernephroma

Treatment

The optimal treatment of prolactinomas has yet to be decided. The problem is to decide whether to employ trans-sphenoidal hypophysectomy, external radiation or bromocriptine, or a combination of these.

It is unlikely that large tumours in association with a markedly enlarged pituitary fossa and very high PRL levels (> 2000 mU/l) can be removed completely by any surgical procedure. In this situation, bromocriptine is the treatment of choice, supplemented by external radiation in some centres. If the tumour is large enough to cause definite but not gross enlargement of the fossa, trans-sphenoidal hypophysectomy is performed in some centres, again supplemented by radiation and bromocriptine if PRL levels remain high postoperatively.

If the pituitary fossa is not enlarged, but neuroendocrine tests indicate the presence of a microadenoma, there is still debate as to whether bromocriptine alone should be used, particularly if the patient's complaint is primarily of infertility, or whether an attempt should be made to remove the lesion trans-sphenoidally. In patients with suprasellar extensions of the tumour, or recurrence after previous surgery and/or external radiation, bromocriptine is the treatment of choice because there is now clear evidence of shrinkage of the tumour with this drug. The duration of therapy required is uncertain but it is probably wise to check the hormonal activity and extent of the tumour every year.

Bromocriptine has a major role in the management of prolactinomas and there is much to be said for treating all patients with this drug alone. Early side effects consist of nausea, vomiting and syncope; later effects are constipation, nasal stuffiness and Raynaud's phenomenon. It is usual gradually to increase the dose to 2.5 mg 8-hourly over the course of a week or two, to minimise side effects. Initially, half a tablet (1.25 mg) is given in bed at night after a meal, for a few nights; the dose is gradually increased after meals, with the patient sitting or lying at first. Once a dose of 7.5 mg daily has been established, the initial side effects usually resolve and the later ones are rarely troublesome at this dose level. A few patients require doses of up to 20 mg daily but, in general, patients with hyperprolactinaemia are more sensitive to bromocriptine than those with acromegaly.

If pregnancy results from bromocriptine therapy the drug is usually discontinued, although there is no evidence that it causes any damage to the fetus. Because of the small risk (probably about 5%) of tumour extension during the pregnancy, the patient should be seen at monthly intervals for review and visual-field testing, and should be warned to report immediately if she develops headaches or nausea. If tumour expansion does occur during pregnancy it is seldom necessary to resort to surgery: tumour shrinkage can be produced effectively and safely by recommencing bromocriptine.

Corticotroph adenomas

These were discussed in the last edition (Horler & Foster 1978, p. 43) and no further comment is required here.

Thyrotroph adenomas

Raised TSH levels are usually the result of primary thyroid failure. In rare instances, if thyroid failure is prolonged, a feedback thyrotrophin-secreting adenoma may arise and cause enlargement of the pituitary fossa.

Very occasionally, hyperthyroidism, with increased circulating thyroid hormone levels, is associated with a raised serum TSH level. The pituitary fossa is usually enlarged and the disease can be cured by removal of the tumour. A characteristic finding is the presence of raised levels of α-subunits, presumably of TSH, but neither these nor the TSH level rise after thyrotrophin-releasing hormone (TRH).

In the less frequent syndrome of non-tumour TSH-induced hyperthyroidism the α-subunit cannot be detected in the circulation. Most of these patients have had previous destructive therapy to the thyroid. They show a partial TSH response to TRH and some suppression of TSH induced thyroidal radioiodine uptake by triiodothyronine. It is possible that they result from an altered set point for thyroid hormone–TSH interaction and may reflect partial resistance of the thyrotroph to thyroid hormone feedback.

Gonadotroph adenomas

These tumours can also arise from long-standing gonadal failure such as that which occurs in Klinefelter's syndrome or Turner's syndrome. Here, low levels of sex steroids are associated with raised FSH and either raised, normal or low LH levels and enlargement of the pituitary fossa. The tumours are normally responsive to gonadal steroid replacement therapy.

Very occasionally, gonadotrophin-secreting tumours, usually secreting FSH, may arise de novo. In such cases sexual function is often well maintained and the presence of normal-sized testes in a patient with an apparently non-functioning pituitary tumour should lead to measurement of gonadotrophin levels. Some patients may have reduced libido, potency and sexual function and this may, on occasion, result from concomitant hyperprolactinaemia. An attempt should be made to remove the tumour whenever possible.

Multiple endocrine adenoma syndromes

The MEA syndromes consist of associations of endocrine hyperplasia, adenomas or carcinomas which are often familial and inherited in a Mendelian dominant manner, although sporadic cases can occur.

MEA type 1

The tumours and their frequency are shown in Table 1.4. Associations of parathyroid, pituitary and pancreatic adenomas are by far the commonest. Growth hormone cell adenomas are the most frequent pituitary tumour, although probably less than 5% of acromegalics show evidence of MEA 1. Prolactinomas, corticotroph cell adenomas and apparently non-secretory tumours may also be associated. Pancreatic tumours are usually islet-cell adenomas secreting insulin or, less often, gastrin or other pancreatic hormones, but may be non-secretory. It is uncertain whether the association of thyroid adenomas is a real one, for these tumours are common in the general population.

Table 1.4 Multiple endocrine adenoma Type 1

Lesion	% Affected
Parathyroid adenomas and hyperplasia	90
Pancreatic islet adenomas (β and non-ß cells)	80
Pituitary adenomas (functioning and non-functioning)	65
Adrenocortical adenomas	38
Thyroid adenomas	18

The clinical relevance of the MEA 1 syndrome is that any patient with one of the more commonly associated tumours should be asked about other such disease in the family and other relevant clinical manifestations should be sought. A few simple screening tests should be performed: for example, in a patient with hyperparathyroidism, a skull X-ray should be taken to exclude a pituitary tumour, and fasting blood glucose and insulin measured to exclude an insulinoma. Certainly, whenever lesions in more than one gland are discovered in a patient, all of his first-degree relatives should be screened.

MEA type 2a

This syndrome comprises medullary carcinoma of the thyroid, phaeochromocytomas, commonly bilateral and, more rarely, parathyroid adenomas or hyperplasia. As a result of family screening it has been possible to detect the earliest manifestations of the syndrome, which consist of hyperplasia of the 'C cells' and of adrenal medullary tissue. All patients with medullary carcinoma of the thyroid should be screened for phaeochromocytoma by urinary 4-hydroxy-3-methoxy mandelic acid (HMMA) measurements, although this test is not always sufficiently sensitive to detect small phaeochromocytomas. Similarly, all patients with phaeochromocytomas should be screened, by measurement of basal and stimulated calcitonin, for medullary carcinoma of the thyroid. In families with this type of carcinoma it has also been found necessary to use provocative tests to detect early cases. Calcium infusion tests are helpful: 15 mg Ca^{2+}/kg is given over 4 hours, with basal and 4-hour calcitonin measurements. Injections of pentagastrin (0.5 μg/kg over 5 seconds) causes rapid release of calcitonin within 2 minutes. This is a useful outpatient screening procedure, although the injection may cause faintness and it is best to keep the patient recumbent. Administration of alcohol (50 ml orally in adults and 30 ml in children over the age of five years) leads to release of calcitonin which is detectable at 15 minutes. The patient must be fasting and warned to avoid driving afterwards.

It should be stressed that the majority of patients in most centres, with either medullary carcinoma of the thyroid or phaeochromocytoma, do not suffer from the MEA syndrome and the diseases usually appear to occur sporadically. However, a single family with MEA may produce a large number of affected subjects in a given area.

MEA type 2b

This syndrome consists of medullary carcinoma of the thyroid associated with a variety of somatic abnormalities, which is more often sporadic and less frequently combined with parathyroid or adrenal medullary disease. The somatic changes include a 'Marfanoid appearance', a proximal myopathy, thickened lips, neuromas of the tongue, cornea and eyelids, ganglioneuromatosis of the bowel and pigmentation of the skin. The facial appearance and tongue neuromas are characteristic.

Mixed syndromes

Mixed MEA syndromes can occur, albeit rarely. Patients with acromegaly may have a phaechromocytoma or aldosteronoma. Similarly, a patient with the MEA 2 syndrome who developed the Zollinger-Ellison syndrome has been described.

Tumours of the APUD system

The term APUD indicates 'amine precursor uptake and decarboxylation' — properties common to most peptide-hormone-producing cells. Tumours arising from the APUD system can occur in many different sites because of the wide distribution of such cells. Insulinomas, gastrinomas, vipomas, glucagonomas, somatostatinomas and pancreatic polypeptide-producing tumours (PP-omas) are all examples of tumours of the APUD system.

Gastrinomas (Zollinger-Ellison syndrome)

The clinical features include attacks of severe abdominal pain, vomiting, intractable peptic and even jejunal ulceration with episodes of gastrointestinal haemorrhage and perforation. More recently, examples have been described in which the symptoms are mild and long-standing. Although gastrin-secreting pancreatic adenomas are usually responsible, hyperplasia of islet cells may be found without a discrete tumour.

Diagnosis. When ulcer symptoms are severe or long-standing, when there are multiple ulcers and when there is hypertrophy of the gastric mucosa, this diagnosis should be considered. With the advent of cimetidine therapy it is likely that a number of cases will be overlooked until local effects of the tumour, 60% of which are malignant, become apparent. Again, a gastrinoma should be suspected in MEA type 1 families.

Basal acid secretion is high and there is little increase on stimulation with pentagastrin. Plasma gastrin levels are raised but this can also be seen in patients with pernicious anaemia and other causes of achlorhydria. The output of gastrin can be stimulated by calcium or by secretin, whereas it is suppressed in normal subjects.

When a diagnosis of inappropriate gastrin secretion has been made it is important to localise the tumour (for they can occur outside the pancreas) and to ascertain whether there are secondary deposits in the liver. Ultrasonography, CT scanning, coeliac-axis arteriography and selective venous sampling may be required.

Treatment. The gastric acid hypersecretion can be readily controlled by cimetidine, which renders total gastrectomy unnecessary; nevertheless, early removal of the tumour is desirable.

Vipomas (Verner-Morrison syndrome)

This syndrome results from excessive secretion of vasoactive intestinal peptide (VIP) by tumours of the pancreas, phaeochromocytomas, ganglioneuroblastomas and bronchogenic carcinomas or from islet cell hyperplasia. The clinical features comprise profuse watery diarrhoea, facial flushing, hypotension, hypokalaemia and achlorhydria or hypochlorhydria.

Diagnosis. High levels of VIP can be detected by radioimmunoassay.

Treatment. Early removal of the tumour is desirable to control the symptoms and because of the frequency of malignancy.

Glucagonomas

Glucagon-secreting tumours produce a striking clinical syndrome, usually in postmenopausal women. The skin rash is characteristic and consists of migrating erythema, ulceration and crusting affecting the legs, genital region, trunk and sometimes the face. There is also a painful glossitis, a normocytic normochromic anaemia, mild diabetes, weight loss and sometimes intermittent diarrhoea and hypokalaemia.

Diagnosis. The unusual clinical features are diagnostic and can be confirmed by high circulating glucagon levels.

Therapy. The tumour should be removed after a functional and anatomical diagnosis has been made.

Somatostatinomas

The somatostatinoma syndrome has been comprehensively reviewed by Krejs et al (1979). The clinical features of the syndrome are summarised in Table 1.5. Gallstones probably result from decreased gall-bladder contractility following suppression of cholecystokinin; diabetes mellitus from suppression of insulin; steatorrhoea and diarrhoea from suppression of pancreatic exocrine function; hypochlorhydria from suppression of gastrin; weight loss from the general gastrointestinal disturbance.

Table 1.5 Clinical manifestations in six patients with somatostatinoma* (modified from Krejs et al 1979)

Age	55	46	54	NR	70	52
Sex	F	F	M	NR	F	M
Home country	Sweden	USA	Canada	Belgium	France	Canada
Cholelithiasis	+	+	–	+	+	+
Diabetes mellitus	+	+	+	+	+	+
Steatorrhoa	+	NS	NS	+	+	+
Diarrhoea	+	–	–	—	+	+
Hypochlorhydria	+	–	NS	NS	+	+
Anaemia	NR	+	NR	NR	NR	+
Weight loss	+	+	+	+	+	+
Liver metastases	+	–	+	+	+	+
Localisation of primary pancreatic tumour	Head	Head	Tail	NR	NR	Head
Additional features	None	None	ACTH production	None	Calcitonin production	Calcitonin production
Treatment	Whipple's procedure	Whipple's procedure	Exploratory laparotomy	Chemotherapy with streptozocin	Whipple's procedure	Whipple's procedure, chemotherapy†
Outcome	Died after operation	Asymptomatic 4 years later	Died after operation	Not known	Died after operation	Not known

*+denotes present, – absent, NR not reported and NS not studied
†Streptozocin, doxorubicin and 5-fluorouracil

Diagnosis. A diagnosis of somatostatinoma should be considered from the clinical features and on the finding of increased plasma levels of somatostatin, and of calcitonin which is also present in the tumour. Localisation of the tumour in the pancreas is determined as for other pancreatic endocrine tumours. Early diagnosis is unlikely, however, because the initial symptoms of dyspepsia, mild diabetes and cholelithiasis are common and non-specific.

Therapy. Removal of the tumour is desirable but the outlook is not good. In the reported cases, five of the six patients had malignant disease with metastases in the liver at the time of diagnosis; chemotherapy is only palliative.

Pancreatic polypeptide-producing tumours (PP-omas)

Circulating levels of pancreatic polypeptide are raised in virtually all varieties of pancreatic endocrine tumours.

GRAVES' DISEASE AND THE RECEPTOR ANTIBODY DISEASES

There is now good evidence that the hyperthyroidism and goitre of Graves' disease result from the action of antibodies to the TSH receptor. Evidence that Graves'

Table 1.6 Evidence that Graves' immunoglobulins are antibodies to the TSH receptor

Inhibition of labelled TSH-binding using thyroid membrane preparations
Inhibition of labelled TSH-binding using solubilised thyroid membranes
Activation of adenylate cyclase
Increase of thyroid hormone production
Correlation of titre with some indices of thyroid stimulation
TSH interferes with binding of labelled Graves' IgG to the thyroid
Analogy with other receptor-antibody diseases

immunoglobulins are antibodies to the TSH receptor is summarised in Table 1.6.

Evidence has recently accumulated for the recognition of a new group of diseases, the so-called receptor-antibody diseases (Table 1.7). There is no doubt that the factor responsible for the fatiguability and weakness in myasthenia gravis is an antibody to the acetylcholine receptor on the muscle surface. These antibodies interact with the ACh receptor in such a way as to interfere with neuromuscular transmission. In most cases they probably do not merely block the action of ACh on the receptor but increase the shedding or turnover of the receptor, reducing its availability to ACh. In one rare form of insulin-resistant diabetes mellitus associated with acanthosis nigricans, antibodies can be detected which bind to the insulin receptor. These antibodies interfere with the binding of exogenous and endogenous insulin and are a rare cause of severe insulin resistance. In some instances the antibodies may bind and activate the insulin receptor, causing profound hypoglycaemia, which was the cause of death in one such patient.

Antibodies have been demonstrated to the β_2-adrenergic receptor in a few patients with allergic rhinitis and/or asthma. Further studies are required to elucidate the frequency and relevance of this observation but if such antibodies are present they could block the receptor in a manner analogous to the β-adrenergic blockers and exacerbate rhinitis or asthma. Patients with chronic renal failure have been described in whom antibodies to the parathyroid hormone (PTH) receptor could be detected. This could be a factor in the PTH resistance seen in some such patients and further studies are awaited to confirm these observations.

Table 1.7 The receptor-antibody diseases

Disease	Antigen	Antibody
Graves' disease	TSH receptor	Antibodies to TSH receptor
Myasthenia gravis	Acetylcholine receptor	Antibodies to ACh receptor
Diabetes mellitus with acanthosis nigricans	Insulin receptor	Antibodies to insulin receptor
Allergic rhinitis and asthma	β_2-adrenergic receptor	Antibodies to the β_2-adrenergic receptor
Uraemia with parathormone resistance	Parathormone (PTH) receptor	Antibodies to the PTH receptor

Prediction of relapse of hyperthyroidism after antithyroid therapy in Graves' disease

The frequency of a prolonged remission after a conventional course of antithyroid drugs varies from 70 to 14% in different reported series. The reasons for this wide variation are unknown but they could reflect geographic differences related to ethnic origin or iodine intake, selection of patients, the severity and type of hyperthyroidism and the nature and duration of drug therapy. If it were possible to select patients with a high chance of relapse after antithyroid drugs and, conversely, those with a high remission rate, a more rational regimen of therapy could be developed.

Many clinical and laboratory features of this disease have been studied in an effort to predict relapse. Clinical features have not proved very helpful, although patients with severe disease or large goitres which do not shrink during the course of treatment are more prone to relapse. Biochemical indices which tend to predict relapse include lack of thyroid suppressibility by tri-iodothyronine, high levels of circulating thyroglobulin or of Graves' immunoglobulins and HLA typing. There is no doubt that lack of suppressibility of thyroidal radio-isotope uptake by tri-iodothyronine, 6 months or more after the start of antithyroid drug treatment, is associated with a greater frequency of relapse, although the chance of relapse in the non-suppressible group varies from 46 to 98%. Relapse is more likely in patients with high pretreatment serum thyroglobulin levels which persist during treatment and probably reflect persistent thyroid stimulation. Again, relapse after medical treatment is commoner in patients who are HLA-B8- or Dw3-positive. Several studies assaying Graves' immunoglobulins by different methods have all shown that patients with raised levels at the end of a course of treatment relapse more frequently, although some patients without antibodies may also relapse.

McGregor et al (1980) have combined analysis of HLA-DRw3 status and measurement of Graves' immunoglobulins using their receptor assay at the time of drug withdrawal. They were able to predict the course of the disease in 95% of 65 patients with Graves' disease. More than 90% of DRw3-positive patients relapsed within 12 months of a 6-month course of carbimazole. Of the 55% of DRw3 negative patients, relapse was characterised by the presence of readily detectable antibody at the time of drug withdrawal.

These findings suggest that patients who are HLA-DRw3-positive might be considered for destructive therapy to the thyroid as primary treatment. Patients who are DRw3-negative could then be treated with a 6-month course of antithyroid drugs, reserving partial thyroidectomy or radio-iodine for those with persistently increased antibody levels. Further extensive studies are now required from other centres with different ethnic groups and iodine intake to confirm or refute these results.

SCREENING FOR NEONATAL HYPOTHYROIDISM

It is difficult to make a clinical diagnosis of neonatal hypothyroidism in the first month or two of life; it has therefore been necessary to develop screening tests to allow early diagnosis. Clinical features which suggest neonatal hypothyroidism include prolonged neonatal jaundice, the classic cretinous facial appearance, feeding difficulties, a protruding tongue, umbilical hernia, constipation, delayed closure of the posterior fontanelle and delayed growth, although some of these features are commonly absent in children recognised early by screening. The case for screening has been extensively reviewed recently (Report of the Joint Standing Subcommittee on Screening in Medical Care 1980)

Prevalence

Surveys of several million children in Europe and North America have indicated that the prevalence of neonatal hypothyroidism is between 1/3000 and 1/4000 live births, at least twice that of phenylketonuria, suggesting that about 150 affected children are born in England and Wales each year.

Pathogenesis

The hypothyroidism results from primary thyroid disease (86%), hypothalamic–pituitary disease (<4%) and transient causes (10%) (Fisher et al 1979). The commonest cause of primary hypothyroidism is an ectopic thyroid, but hypoplasia, aplasia, dyshormonogenesis and goitrogens may all be responsible. Secondary hypothyroidism, which is rarer than previously believed, probably makes little impact on the problem and other features of hypothalamic–pituitary disease may be associated. Transient neonatal hypothyroidism is more liable to occur in preterm infants or in those whose mothers have received thyroid hormone medication.

Screening procedure

It is now generally agreed that the screening method of choice is measurement of TSH on the Guthrie paper used for PKU screening, 5–10 days after birth, because TSH methods are now sufficiently sensitive and cheap to be widely available. The recall rate for false positives is lower than that with any other method and false-negative results are extremely rare. Values of less than 25 mU/l can be regarded as normal and those greater than 80 mU/l as positive; those in between require further assessment.

Treatment

As soon as the diagnosis is established by a positive screening test, repeat venous blood samples are taken for confirmation by T_4 and TSH measurements. Whenever possible, a thyroid scan using ^{123}I should be performed to locate any functioning thyroid tissue. Therapy with thyroxine is then started. The optimum dose schedule has yet to be ascertained but 50 ug T_4 daily is usually adequate. Treatment should not be monitored by TSH measurements alone because abnormalities of the T_4/TSH set point can occur over the first year of life and the TSH level may remain raised despite high T_4 doses and clinical hyperthyroidism. Treatment is monitored clinically, by growth charts and serum T_4 estimations, aiming to keep the T_4 level in the mid-normal range.

Prognosis

Although conclusive evidence is not yet available, preliminary studies suggest that early, effective treatment does improve the outlook for mental development, although minor defects of brain function, such as cerebellar dysfunction, may persist. Carefully co-ordinated long-term studies are required to assess the real cost-benefit of screening.

REFERENCES

Alexander L, Appleton D, Hall R, Ross W M, Wilkinson R 1980 Epidemiology of acromegaly in the Newcastle region. Clinical Endocrinology 12: 71–79

Fisher D A, Dussault J H, Foley T P R et al 1979 Screening for congenital hypothyroidism: results of screening one million North American infants. Journal of Pediatrics 94: 700

Hall K, McGregor A M, Scanlon M F, Hall R 1980 Metrizamide cisternography in the assessment of pituitary tumour size, with special reference to the demonstration of tumour (prolactinoma) shrinkage on bromocriptine therapy. In: Hubinont P O (ed) Progress in reproductive biology. Karger, Basel, vol 6, p 232–243

Hall R, Anderson J, Smart G A, Besser M 1980 Fundamentals of clinical endocrinology, 3rd edn. Pitman Medical, Tunbridge Wells

Horler A R, Foster J B 1978 Progress in clinical medicine, 7th edn. Churchill Livingstone, Edinburgh, p 43

Joint Standing Subcommittee on Screening in Medical Care 1980, Report on screening for congenital hypothyroidism. Recommendations to Standing Medical Advisory Committee and Scottish Health Services Planning Council. Appendix HN(81) 20 1st May 1980

Kovacs K, Horvath E 1979 Pituitary adenomas. In: Tolis G, Labrie F, Martin J B, Naftolin F (eds) Pathologic aspects in clinical neuroendocrinology: a pathophysiological approach. Raven Press, New York, p 367–384

Krejs G J, Orci L, Conlon M, Ravazzola M, Davis G. R, Ruskin P et al 1979 Somatostatinoma syndrome. Biochemical, morphologic and clinical features. New England Journal of Medicine 301: 285–292

McGregor A M, Rees Smith B, Hall R, Petersen M M, Miller M, Dewar P J 1980 Prediction of relapse in hyperthyroid Graves' disease. Lancet 1: 1101–1103

Richards S H, Thomas J P 1980 Treatment of acromegaly by transethmoidal hypophysectomy. Quarterly Journal of Medicine (NS) 49: 21–31

Wright A D, Hill D M, Lowy C, Fraser T R 1970 Mortality in acromegaly. Quarterly Journal of Medicine (NS) 39:1–16

2

Diabetes mellitus

J. Anderson

DIAGNOSTIC CRITERIA FOR DIABETES MELLITUS

The term 'diabetic' carries both social and clinical implications. No diagnostic criteria can help in the decision as to when the label should be attached and specific treatment advised in 'borderline' cases. Jarrett & Keen (1976) pointed out that none of the criteria in use at that time for diagnosing diabetes was derived from long-term observations of the further development and consequences of different degrees of glucose intolerance, although all published criteria included a 'borderline' or 'suspicious' range. It became increasingly apparent that the British Diabetic Association criteria (Fitzgerald & Keen 1964) were too rigid and were set too low: if the 2 h blood glucose during the glucose tolerance test was in excess of 6.7 mmol/l the test was regarded as abnormal. A number of studies have suggested that the risk of diabetic complications attributable to small vessel disease becomes important only in subjects with capillary whole blood glucose concentrations exceeding 11.1 mmol/l 2 h after a 50 g oral glucose load. Among those with lesser degrees of glucose intolerance, a variable percentage show further sustained deterioration.

The WHO Expert Committee on Diabetes Mellitus (1980) has proposed raising the degrees of hyperglycaemia necessary for a diagnosis of diabetes, and the creation of a new category of 'impaired glucose tolerance' (IGT), which is not regarded as diabetic. These proposals state that in patients with symptoms, a fasting venous plasma glucose concentration of 8 mmol/l or more is diagnostic of diabetes. If the concentration is below 6 mmol/l, the diagnosis is excluded. Patients with results in the intermediate zone should be given a 75 g oral glucose load. If the 2 h venous plasma concentration is greater than 11 mmol/l, the test is diagnostic of diabetes. If it is below 11 mmol/l but greater than 8 mmol/l the diagnosis is impaired glucose tolerance. In patients without symptoms the criteria require an additional abnormal value after a 75 g oral glucose load: for example, a 1 h value of 11 mmol/l or greater. If subsequent tests confirm that either the fasting or 2 h value is raised, these patients, too, may be reclassified as diabetic. A diagnosis of diabetes should not be made on the basis of a single abnormal glucose value in an asymptomatic patient. The 75 g glucose load is a compromise: the North American 100 g load often produces nausea and the 50 g European load may not be a sufficiently rigorous stimulus. These new criteria are arbitrary, although they have been derived from epidemiological studies on both sides of the Atlantic. Although the rate of progression from IGT to diabetes is low, it cannot be ignored (especially in pregnancy) and may be amenable to intervention.

Without advice or treatment the rate is about 3% a year; with dietary advice this may be reduced to about 1.3%. One study has claimed that with the further addition of tolbutamide the rate may be cut to zero (Sartor et al 1980). It has also been suggested that mild diabetes in children may be reversed by the use of chlorpropamide (Mutch & Stowers 1980).

CLASSIFICATION

The traditional classification of clinical diabetes mellitus is based on the age of onset and recognises 'juvenile-onset' (JOD) and 'maturity-onset' (MOD) varieties. A further presentation of diabetes in the young has been described — 'maturity-onset diabetes of young people' (MODY) (Tattersall & Fajans 1975). This condition may be more common than we realise. The onset is early in life, serious ketosis does not occur and long-term complications are infrequent — although not absent. Obesity is a characteristic feature and insulin is probably not required in treatment. The MODY variant is inherited as an autosomal dominant trait, whereas inheritance of the 'classic' varieties of diabetes is multifactorial. A few rare syndromes have been described in which a JOD type of disease associated with other conditions is inherited as an autosomal recessive trait (Page et al 1976a). The 'DIDMOAD' syndrome is one example of this group and comprises diabetes insipidus, diabetes mellitus, optic atrophy and deafness. Another is the association of diabetes mellitus with Friedreich's ataxia, where the inheritance is again recessive. These syndromes are of considerable interest because they provide an opportunity to study patients with diabetes in whom heredity seems to be the sole aetiological factor. However, the pathogenesis of these disorders remains unknown.

The terms 'juvenile' and 'maturity' onset are now regarded as unsatisfactory and misleading. Some patients, mature in years, may develop diabetes that is insulin-dependent, and the presentation of a 'maturity' onset in the young is referred to above. Cudworth & Woodrow (1976) have pointed out that insulin-dependent diabetics over the age of 30 years at the time of diagnosis are genetically similar to insulin-dependent diabetics diagnosed before that age, at least in respect of HLA haplotype (see below). New information on genetic and immunological mechanisms in diabetes mellitus have led to the need for a revised classification. Furthermore, the terms previously used to describe the various types of 'subclinical' diabetes (prediabetes, potential diabetes, latent diabetes) need to be more clearly defined. Cudworth (1976) proposed the term 'type I' to describe all insulin-dependent patients, regardless of age. Bottazzo & Doniach (1976) have further subdivided type I diabetes into types IA and IB. Both of these subgroups show the presence of circulating pancreatic islet cell antibodies (PICA) immediately after the onset of the disease, but in type IA they are transient. In type IB, PICA may be detected long before the onset and may persist for many years afterwards. Autoimmune antibodies to other endocrine tissues are also found in type IB diabetes and it seems certain that, although insulinopenia is present in both subtypes, their pathogenesis is entirely different.

Type II diabetes (Cudworth 1976) includes those patients previously classified as MOD. These patients are not insulin-dependent and may be controlled by diet alone or with the aid of oral hypoglycaemic agents. Type II diabetes, in general a disease of later life, is usually associated with obesity and has no association with any HLA antigens. Insulinopenia is not present (except in the later stages) although there is a blunted or delayed insulin response to a glucose stimulus. The insulin response to arginine and to tolbutamide is normal in these individuals, so the inherited deficiency of the β-cell receptor may be specific for glucose. Another major defect seems to be in the biological effectiveness of circulating insulin. This cellular insensitivity is caused mainly by a change in the insulin receptor sites associated with obesity, but may also be related to premature cellular ageing.

With all these considerations in mind, a revised classification of diabetes mellitus has been proposed by the Medical and Scientific section of the British Diabetic Association (1978). This classification was produced by a Workshop of European and North American contributors and is presented in Table 2.1.

Table 2.1 Classification of diabetes mellitus

A.	*Primary diabetes mellitus*	
	Defined by the criteria described earlier	
	Type I	Insulin-dependent (I.D.D.)
		Can be further subdivided into:
		Type IA — transient PICA; no autoimmune features
		Type IB — persistent PICA; other autoimmune features
	Type II	Non-insulin dependent (N.I.D.D.)
		Can be further subdivided into:
		Obese
		Non-obese
B.	*Impaired glucose tolerance*	
	Defined by the criteria described earlier	
C.	*Gestational diabetes mellitus*	
	First recognised during pregnancy and remitting afterwards	
D.	*Previous abnormality (latent diabetes)*	
E.	*Potential abnormality*	
F.	*Diabetes mellitus or IGT associated with certain conditions and syndromes*	
	1. Hormonal	4. Genetic and chromosomal syndromes
	2. Drug-induced	5. Insulin receptor abnormalities
	3. Pancreatic disease	6. Other types

Primary diabetes mellitus

The typical features of the two main clinical syndromes are listed in Table 2.2.

It should be remembered that type I diabetics may not always require insulin from the outset but, by definition, will inevitably need this treatment eventually. Similarly, type II diabetics may require insulin on a temporary basis as, for instance, during a severe infection or to cover a surgical operation. In the early stages of type I diabetes, insulin requirements may fluctuate markedly, and it is not unusual for the daily insulin requirements to fall to very low levels for some weeks or months after the initial acute hyperglycaemic episode has been corrected. This 'honeymoon' period reflects in part a reduction of glucagon secretion (high during the initial metabolic crisis) and some recovery of endogenous insulin secretion (conceivably, in some patients, a latent period following recovery from viral isletitis before permanent islet cell damage occurs). There is also some evidence that acute insulin release is

Table 2.2 Typical clinical features of primary diabetes mellitus

Type I (I.D.D.)	Type II (N.I.D.D.)
Underweight	Overweight or of normal weight
Young (usually < 30 years)	Older age groups
Peak age onset 12–14 years	Incidence rises with age — peak age onset > 50 years
Onset usually rapid	Onset insidious
Peak incidence autumn and winter	No seasonal incidence
Ketosis-prone	Ketotic only if acute or severe infection, trauma etc., is present
Low or absent endogenous insulin secretion	Normal or increased endogenous insulin secretion in earliest stages; in the more advanced stages insulin secretion low
β-cell mass $< 10\%$	β-cell mass moderately reduced
Treatment with insulin necessary	Treatment with diet alone or diet and oral drugs. Insulin required only temporarily to cover infection, trauma, surgery etc.
Insulin-sensitive	Tendency to insulin resistance — increases with increasing obesity
Antipancreatic cell-mediated immunity frequent at onset. Antibodies to islet cells frequent at onset.	No autoimmune features
HLA association	No HLA association

improved when the chronic glucose stimulus (hyperglycaemia) is reduced by exogenous insulin. Finally, cell receptor affinity for insulin may increase. However, as time goes on there is progressive loss of β-cell function and a continuing reduction of β-cell mass leading to increased requirements of exogenous insulin.

Type II is the commonest form of diabetes, although it is by no means certain that this is a completely homogeneous group. There is no evidence of seasonal incidence or of any HLA association, and no correlation with islet cell antibodies. Patients with the type II syndrome can be divided clinically into those who are obese and who require and respond to dietary treatment alone, and those without significant obesity who fail to respond completely to dietary measures and who often require treatment with a sulphonylurea to achieve and maintain adequate control. These sulphonylurea-responsive patients seem to be a distinct clinical subgroup of the type II syndrome. Such patients tend to present at a younger age, are of average weight, do not respond completely to carbohydrate restriction alone and, although usually sulphonylurea-responsive at first (those who are not would automatically be classified as type I patients) may, after a variable period of good control, deteriorate and require insulin. This intermediate-onset or subacute variety seems to occupy a place in the clinical spectrum somewhere between the characteristic type I and type II varieties and this probably reflects the fact that there is an overlap in middle age between these two major clinical syndromes. Such patients do not seem to represent a discrete third type of diabetes but are presumably either 'late-onset' type I or 'early-onset' type II diabetics in whom pancreatic β-cell failure supervenes. Time will usually tell which group such patients fall into, if this is not apparent at the outset: patients who begin as type II may sooner or later become insulin-dependent, whereas genuine type II patients (typically obese) will remain non-insulin-dependent under normal circumstances. A study of the family history may help in determining the prognosis for these patients; a family history of type I will suggest that the patient is likely to become insulin-dependent in due course, whereas a family history of type II suggests that the patient also will fall into this group. However, this is by no means an absolute rule, because type II diabetes is such a common disease. The MODY presentation is best regarded as type II diabetes occurring at a particularly early age and showing a dominant mode of inheritance.

Impaired glucose tolerance

Such individuals, although not unequivocally diabetic, have an increased chance of becoming so. Patients who present with associated symptoms should be treated by appropriate methods (usually dietary), and for purposes of follow-up are best regarded as being mildly diabetic; further deterioration of glucose tolerance is likely to occur. Asymptomatic patients may not require specific treatment other than weight reduction, but should nevertheless remain under periodic review. The physician must use his own judgement, but IGT can never be ignored. These patients are at risk in a number of other respects, notably for large vessel disease. The physician should therefore identify, and, where possible, correct, other 'risk factors' such as hypertension, hyperlipidaemia, obesity and cigarette smoking. If drugs are responsible for IGT they should, if possible, be discontinued or changed. During pregnancy the identification and management of IGT is of particular importance.

Gestational diabetes and impaired glucose tolerance

It is important to detect disturbances of glucose tolerance during pregnancy at as early a stage as possible. A normal range for random blood glucose estimations during pregnancy has been established (Lind & McDougall 1981), and a standard oral glucose tolerance test (using the same criteria for interpretation as in the non-pregnant individual) is indicated in women whose random values lie above the upper limit of normal. Normoglycaemia must be restored and maintained as this will improve fetal outcome. Although the condition (by definition) reverts to normal after delivery, it may recur during future pregnancies and there is a high risk of the subsequent development of diabetes later in life.

Previous abnormality (latent diabetes)

This diagnostic category refers to those persons currently with normal glucose tolerance who have previously demonstrated diabetes mellitus or IGT occurring either spontaneously or in response to some identifiable stimulus (myocardial infarction, trauma, infection, drugs).

Potential abnormality

This is the state of those individuals who may eventually develop the overt syndrome but in whom no abnormality of glucose tolerance is demonstrable. Situations in which the potential diabetic state may be suspected include:

1. The identical non-diabetic twin of a diabetic
2. An individual, both of whose parents are diabetic
3. An individual with one diabetic parent and whose other parent has a diabetic parent, sibling or offspring, or a sibling with a diabetic child

4. A woman who has given birth to a live or stillborn child weighing 4.5 kg or more at birth, or to a stillborn child showing islet cell hyperplasia not related to rhesus incompatibility

5. Individuals with histocompatibility haplotypes identical to those of a diabetic sibling

6. Individuals with circulating pancreatic islet cell antibodies.

Prediabetes

This term can only be applied retrospectively and should be reserved for the period of life of a diabetic before glucose tolerance becomes abnormal.

Diabetes mellitus or IGT associated with certain conditions and syndromes

Some of the commoner causes of 'secondary' diabetes are listed below.

1. *Hormonal*
   Cushing's syndrome
   Acromegaly
   Primary aldosteronism
   Phaeochromocytoma
   Apudomas
2. *Drug-induced* (see Anderson 1981)
   Corticosteroids
   Thiazide diuretics
   Oral contraceptives (combined)
   Frusemide and other loop diuretics
   Diazoxide
3. *Pancreatic disease*
   Chronic pancreatitis
   Haemochromatosis
   Pancreatectomy
   Cystic fibrosis
   Pancreatic calcification ('tropical' DM)
   Carcinoma of pancreas
4. *Genetic and chromosomal syndromes*
   DIDMOAD syndrome
   Friedreich's ataxia
   Muscular dystrophy
   Down's syndrome
   Turner's syndrome
   Klinefelter's syndrome
   Refsum's syndrome
5. *Insulin receptor abnormalities* (see Flier et al 1979)
   Type A: females only age 8–16 years, ovarian dysfunction, lipodystrophy. Defect in insulin receptors.
   Type B: Mostly females, age 12–60 years, pseudoacanthosis nigricans, autoimmune disorders. Antibody to insulin receptor.

6. *Other types*
   Hyperlipoproteinaemia (Types III, IV and V)
   Type I glycogenosis
   Chronic renal failure
   Hepatic cirrhosis

AETIOLOGY OF TYPE I DIABETES MELLITUS

It is now generally accepted that diabetes mellitus is not one but several diseases, with different causes and, possibly, different modes of transmission. Until the late 1970s, most studies on the inheritance of diabetes regarded it as a single entity, but the multifactorial nature and genetic heterogeneity of the disorder are now widely accepted. Studies currently focus on the β cells as the final common denominator, whether they fail under apparently normal conditions of day-to-day life or because peripheral demands for insulin place a burden on the islets that they are unable to meet. Both hereditary and environmental factors are concerned in the aetiology of type I diabetes mellitus. Probably the major genetic susceptibility to diabetes is determined by one or more genes in the HLA regions of chromosome 6. Other factors, including immunological processes and viral and other environmental stimuli to islet cell damage, appear to contribute to the pathogenesis of type I diabetes. These factors will be considered under separate headings.

Histocompatibility antigens

For some years attention has been focussed on associations between type I diabetes and the major histocompatibility complex. On the short arm of chromosome 6 is a region which codes for three products—class I antigens, known as HLA-A, B and C; class II, known as D and DR in man; and class III, which are complement components (C2, C4 and factor B). Except for the complement components, the products of these genes are expressed in the cell membranes of lymphocytes and other cells, the distribution of the class II antigens being more limited than that of class I. Several of these antigens have an increased prevalence in patients with type I diabetes. The first links between the HLA system and this disorder were found for the antigens HLA-B8, B15, B18 and Cw3 (Nerup et al 1974, Cudworth 1976, Cudworth & Woodrow 1976). Later, a strong association was found with HLA Dw3, Dw4, DR3 and DR4 (Thomsen et al 1975). Raum et al (1979) reported a strong association between type I diabetes and the rare genetic type BfF1 of properdin factor B, and claimed that BfF1 is a marker for nearly one out of four diabetic patients. This association has not been universally confirmed, but the discrepancies might be due to differences in the ethnic backgrounds of the populations studied.

These associations, although suggestive, do not point unequivocally to the existence of one or more genes determining the development of type I diabetes. They can be interpreted as a reflection either of linkage disequilibrium with immune response (Ir) genes directly involved in the development of type I diabetes or of differences in immune responsiveness in relation to different HLA haplotypes. The associations between type I diabetes and certain complement allotypes, and the possibility that these allotypes and the HLA alleles influence immune activity, favour the second possibility, but they are by no means mutually exclusive.

As regards the full HLA haplotype, several combinations appear to indicate genetic susceptibility to type I diabetes. The first combination, termed the S_1 axis, includes HLA-B8, Dw3 and DR3. The second (the S_2 axis) includes HLA-B15, Cw3, Dw4 and DR4. A third haplotype has been described which comprises HLA-B18, BfF1 and DR3 (Rittner & Bertrams 1981); this haplotype seems particularly to be associated with type I diabetes which presents at the age of 10 years or earlier. The S_2 axis predominantly occurs in those diabetics whose disease presents when they are at least 20 years old, whereas the S_1 axis is found in type I diabetics of any age. It seems, therefore, that various genes may be involved, perhaps with different modes of inheritance and even with additive effects, as observed by the higher frequency of type I diabetes in individuals heterozygous for DR3/DR4. The different HLA haplotypes associated with insulin-dependent diabetes at different ages of onset support the idea of a polygenic aetiology. The additive effect of the presence of both S_1 and S_2 axes (first observed with B8 and B15) also suggests the existence of different immune response genes on the sixth chromosome, each conferring susceptibility to type I diabetes — one in linkage disequilibrium with the S_1 axis and another in linkage disequilibrium with the S_2 axis. The third axis (B18) suggests the possible presence of a third Ir gene. A study in identical twins, one or both of whom had type I diabetes (Nelson et al 1975), has shown that the frequency of the B15 antigen (S_2 axis) was equally increased in the concordant and discordant pairs, whereas HLA-B8 (S_1 axis) was increased only in the concordant pairs. This suggests that B8 and B15 might represent different risk factors in the genetic susceptibility to type I diabetes. This concept has important implications, for if two or more genes predisposing to diabetes happen to be located in linkage disequilibrium with the HLA genes, inheritance might falsely simulate an autosomal recessive pattern. These findings have also been interpreted in terms of a dominant inheritance with incomplete penetrance and of intermediate inheritance (Editorial, Lancet 1982). The picture is further complicated by the observation that another region, not HLA-linked, is involved in the development of type I diabetes. Hodge and her colleagues (1981) have reported an association with the Kidd blood-group locus. Thus, what might appear at first sight to be a simple Mendelian mode of inheritance, must be regarded as polygenic.

Several diseases, particularly the autoimmune endocrinopathies, are also associated with HLA-B8 and there is an increased prevalence both of these diseases and of organ-specific humoral autoimmunity in type IB diabetics and their relatives, suggesting an autoimmune pathogenesis for this subgroup. In these patients, circulating islet cell antibodies persist for many years (see below), whereas in type IA patients islet cell antibodies are a transient phenomenon. Type IB diabetes is associated with the S_1 HLA axis (B8, etc.) and type IA with the S_2 axis (B15, etc). This suggests a possible autoimmune aetiology for type IB diabetes and a different aetiology (possibly viral) for type IA diabetes.

Immunological factors

The association between type IB diabetes and many organ-specific autoimmune diseases has been referred to earlier and is well recognised. There is also a relationship between type IB diabetes and autoimmune associations such as vitiligo and alopecia areata.

Serological studies in type IB patients have shown a high prevalence of various circulating organ-specific antibodies (Irvine et al 1977); the common association with HLA-B8 has been mentioned above. There is also a recognised association between type IB diabetes and gluten-sensitive enteropathy (coeliac disease) (Walsh et al 1978) — the latter condition is associated with the B8 antigen. Human antibodies to pancreatic islet cells (PICA) are commonly found in newly diagnosed type I patients. Lendrum et al (1976) detected PICA in 38% of insulin-dependent patients, in 5% of type II patients and in 1.7% of non-diabetic individuals. In the insulin-dependent group, PICA were found in 85% of patients immediately after the onset of symptoms and they became less common as the duration of the disease increased — after 3 years only about 20% of type I diabetics possess detectable circulating PICA. These 'classic' islet cell antibodies are IgG in nature (ICA-IgG) and are directed against cytoplasmic components of islet cells. They are not directed against insulin itself and the appearance of these antibodies probably follows cell damage occurring before the onset of symptoms — they are simply 'markers' for the autoimmune response and are not necessarily the cause of cell destruction. The presence of ICA-IgG may precede the onset of clinical diabetes by several years and Irvine et al (1976) have suggested that their presence might serve as a marker for type I diabetes.

Type IA diabetics show only temporary ICA-IgG positivity (perhaps secondary to viral isletitis), whereas in type IB patients there is greater permanence of these antibodies. Lendrum and his colleagues (1976) found that although ICA-IgG were equally common in both sexes, associated thyroid and gastric autoantibodies were more common in older patients and in females. They found no correlation between the presence of these antibodies and ICA-IgG in patients with diabetes either of recent onset or long-standing disease. Morris et al (1976) have found that the frequency of HLA-B8 was significantly increased in ICA-IgG-positive patients (61%) compared with ICA-IgG-negative patients (35%) and a control population (28%). Among type IB patients the frequency of HLA-B8 was even higher — 71%.

Bottazzo et al (1980) have presented evidence for the existence of a separate species of islet cell antibodies which fix complement. Their studies showed that these complement-fixing islet cell antibodies (ICA-CF) are more closely related to the onset of clinical disease than the 'classic' IgG antibodies and that they tend to disappear more rapidly. These ICA-CF may reflect damage of pancreatic β cells more selectively and are preferable to the ICA-IgG as a serological marker for studying the natural history of type I diabetes. In a recent prospective investigation of the prediabetic period before the onset of type I diabetes, Gorsuch et al (1980) determined HLA genotypes in the healthy parents and siblings of 160 affected children. Islet cell antibodies both of the ICA-IgG and the ICA-CF types were sought during regular prospective investigation over a mean period of 2 years. Out of the group of 582 parents and siblings, four siblings and two parents became diabetic: the interval before detection of any biochemical abnormality exceeded a year in four of these, and in all of these ICA-IgG was positive from the outset, ICA-CF being positive in five. These observations suggest that the initiation of pathogenesis may precede the abrupt clinical onset of diabetes by several years, even in children. HLA haplotype, taken in association with a search for ICA-CF, can be used accurately to predict the development of type I diabetes in first-degree relatives of patients with the disease.

Lernmark et al (1978) have demonstrated an islet cell membrane antibody in the serum of patients with newly diagnosed disease. The relationship of this antibody to ICA-IgG and ICA-CF is not known. Evidence of cell-mediated immune responses has also been found in type I diabetes (Nerup et al 1971, MacCuish et al 1975).

Immunological factors therefore seem to play a major part in the pathogenesis of insulin-dependent diabetes: in some patients (type IB) a primary autoimmune reaction may be the major factor causing diabetes in susceptible individuals, whereas in other patients (type IA) the autoimmune response seems to be triggered by some environmental stimulus such as a virus infection and is only transient.

Viral infection

There is extensive evidence from animal studies that diabetes may follow virus infection. Reovirus type 3 and Coxsackie virus infection can damage islet cells in mice, causing a diabetes-like syndrome. The M variant of the encephalomyocarditis virus (EMC), a picornavirus unrelated to Coxsackie virus, infects and destroys β cells in certain strains of mice, producing a syndrome analogous to type I diabetes. Observations on the onset of type I diabetes in various seasons of the year offer some evidence that viruses may also be involved in the pathogenesis of diabetes in man. A number of studies have documented an increased prevalence of diabetes in either the winter or early autumn months and a relative paucity in late spring and early summer (Bloom et al 1975) and it has been suggested that these seasonal trends correspond to the prevalence of common viral infections in the community. There is evidence that diabetes starting in childhood may result, in a small proportion of cases, from recent mumps infection (Gamble 1980). There is an increased prevalence of diabetes in cases of congenital rubella (Menser et al, 1978). A report of a case of childhood diabetes directly attributed to Coxsackie B4 virus infection (Yoon et al 1979) provides definitive evidence of viral diabetogenesis in man.

Of particular interest is the observation that type I diabetics in the UK with HLA-B8 and B15 tend to cluster during the winter peak of incidence of diabetes (Cudworth et al 1977). Subjects with B15, and in particular those who were both B8- and B15-positive, had higher neutralising antibody titres to Coxsackie virus types B1–B4. Of the cases studied, 58% had ICA-IgG, but their presence was not correlated with HLA haplotypes or viral antibody titres. In 37 per cent of subjects who gave a definite history of antecedent illness, evidence indicated that this was a precipitating infection and not the initiating event producing islet cell damage. Barbosa (1977) also found a similar correlation between histocompatibility profile and the development of diabetes in the winter months. These findings were the first epidemiological link between the possession of certain HLA haplotypes and a particular virus that might be associated with the development of diabetes.

It is therefore possible that a viral 'trigger' might be a key factor leading to islet cell damage in patients with type IA diabetes (S_2 axis — B15, Dw4, DR4), and other external factors apart from viruses might also serve as precipitants of β-cell damage in susceptible individuals. Helgason & Jonasson (1981) have provided circumstantial evidence that N-nitroso compounds, including nitrosamines and nitrosamides which are used as food additives, might contribute to the production of type I diabetes, not in the consumer but in the progeny. Studies continue, to investigate and to identify other non-viral environmental agents that might be concerned in the pathogenesis of type I diabetes in genetically susceptible individuals.

Unifying hypotheses for the aetiology of Type I diabetes mellitus
The facts so far known are as follows:

1. There are inherited and genetically determined factors conferring susceptibility to type I diabetes that are significantly associated (or are in linkage disequilibrium) with certain HLA haplotypes
2. There appear to be at least two and probably three different HLA haplotypes that confer susceptibility
3. There is an association with viral infection and possibly other environmental factors
4. Antibodies to islet cell tissue are usually formed but not always sustained
5. In some patients there is an association with other organ-specific autoimmune diseases.

The facts that type IA and type IB diabetes are associated with different HLA haplotypes, that they have different islet cell antibody patterns and that type IB has an association with other autoimmune diseases and type IA does not, suggest that these two subgroups of insulin-dependent diabetes have different aetiologies. Any hypothesis used to explain the pathogenesis of type I diabetes first supposes the presence of immune response genes in linkage disequilibrium with certain HLA haplotypes, of differences in immune responsiveness in relation to different HLA haplotypes, or a combination of both these mechanisms. Individuals with these haplotypes are deemed 'susceptible'. In type IA diabetes the HLA haplotype conferring susceptibility is the S_2 axis and individuals with this specific immunogenetic constitution may be unusually susceptible to infection with various viruses (perhaps due to a deficient T-lymphocyte reaction) and may thus develop viral isletitis. The viral interaction with cell-membrane antigen leads to an immune response associated with pancreatic islet cell antibody formation, although this response is short-lived and circulating antibodies soon disappear. Such individuals may also develop islet cell damage as a result of other environmental triggers; some food additives might conceivably act in this way.

The aetiology of type IB diabetes is different. In this disorder there is a fundamental immunogenetic deficit (possibly mediated via B lymphocytes). In this disease environmental factors play a less important part and may not even be necessary. Type IB diabetes is associated with the S_1 axis and this hypothesis regards the disorder as a primary organ-specific autoimmune disease. However, although both type IB diabetes and other autoimmune endocrinopathies are associated with the presence of HLA-B8, Gorsuch et al (1980) have presented strong evidence that the B8-linked 'diabetogenic' and 'thyroid autoimmunity' genes are not identical.

Occasionally both the S_1 and the S_2 axes may occur in the same individual. Under these circumstances, susceptibility to diabetes is greatly increased and, presumably, either environmental (type IA) or autoimmune (type IB) factors or both play a part in pathogenesis — such patients are in double jeopardy. In addition, the presence of 'modifying' genes might well influence such aspects as age of onset, severity, or degree of insulinopenia. It is possible that the risk for microangiopathy may be affected not only by the immunogenetic constitution of the patient but also by such modifying genes, although this concept is, at present, purely theoretical.

THE TREATMENT OF DIABETES

Insulin therapy

Insulin is essential in the treatment of children and adolescents, and in all adults who are ketotic when first seen. It may sometimes be needed in type II diabetes as a temporary measure in those patients whose control has been severely disturbed by such factors as an intercurrent illness or a surgical operation. Over 20 different insulin types are currently available in the UK, differing in the time of onset and duration of their action, their source and their purity. Many of these insulins have little place in the present-day management of diabetes. The current plethora of insulins serves only to confuse doctors, nurses and patients, and physicians in North America look on in bewilderment as new types continue to become available in the UK.

In the UK, insulin is available in strengths of 40 and 80 U/ml; soluble (BP) is also available in a strength of 20 U/ml. Until recently, each type and each strength of insulin used in this country had a standard colour code. As the number of insulin types has proliferated and with the introduction of highly purified pork and beef insulins, the system of colour coding is disappearing. The standard insulin syringe used in the UK (BS 1619) is calibrated for insulin of strength 20 U/ml. It is not surprising therefore, that serious dosage errors can and do occur with the present strengths of insulin, even among medical and nursing staff (Bloom et al 1981). Insulin of strength 100 U/ml (U100) has already been adopted by the United States, Canada, Australia and New Zealand. Authoritative bodies have proposed the introduction of U100 insulin in this country, and this change will probably come about in the spring of 1983. New insulin syringes, appropriately calibrated, will be introduced at the same time.

Highly purified insulins

Soluble insulin (BP) is of bovine origin and of acid pH, and contains a proportion of altered insulin, insulin polymers, proinsulin and peptides derived from insulin and proinsulin. Bloom and his colleagues (1979) have termed soluble and other traditional insulin types 'dirty insulins' (Editorial, Lancet, 1979). Highly purified insulins, both of beef and of pork origin, have been freely available for some years; it is doubtful whether the traditional insulins now have a place in the treatment of type I diabetes, certainly in patients being started on insulin for the first time. Highly purified short-acting insulins include Actrapid® (Novo) and Velosulin® (Nordisk). Beef insulin is also available in a highly purified form— Neusulin® (Wellcome). The highly purified intermediate-acting insulins commonly used are Insulatard® (porcine isophane; Nordisk), Monotard® (porcine IZS Lente; Novo) and Neulente® (bovine IZS Lente; Wellcome). The other available insulins, with the exception of Ultratard® (long-acting IZS of beef origin; Wellcome), which is used in the regimen described by Holman & Turner (1977) and Phillips et al (1979), appear to be superfluous.

Lipodystrophy is a well-recognised and distressing complication of the use of the traditional insulin types. Whereas fat hypertrophy is still seen with highly purified insulins, lipoatrophy is extremely rare, although a small number of cases have been reported (Jones et al 1981). Reeves et al (1980) have suggested that insulin-induced lipoatrophy might have an immune pathogenesis. There is little doubt that, if injections are properly given, fibrosis and induration at the injection sites are seen very much less often when highly purified insulins are used. Reactions at the injection sites are also much less common and, when they do occur, they usually reflect allergy to the protamine component of isophane or the preservative used rather than to the insulin itself.

Human insulin

A human insulin may be prepared from human pancreas, by total chemical synthesis, by amino-acid substitution (semi-synthesis) of porcine insulin and by recombinant DNA technology using *Escherichia coli.* Preliminary studies of the immunogenicity, safety and efficacy of biosynthetic (Keen et al 1980; Baker et al 1981) and of semi-synthetic insulin (Owens et al 1981a, b) have been conducted and others are in progress. They have shown that these insulins are safe and effective. Keen et al (1980) found that the dose–response relationship of genetically synthesised human insulin might differ from that of porcine insulin, although Owens et al (1981a) found that the potency, onset and duration of effect of semi-synthetic human (SSHI) and of porcine insulin were identical. These workers have also demonstrated the efficacy of SSHI when given intramuscularly and intravenously (Owens et al 1981b). Commercial preparations of human insulin, both biosynthetic and semi-synthetic are now available. Whether they will have any striking advantages over highly purified beef and pork insulins in terms of antigenicity, long-term side effects and biochemical control remains to be seen.

Regimens of insulin therapy

The subcutaneous injection of short-acting insulin given morning and evening in combination with an intermediate-acting insulin is the most satisfactory treatment for most type I patients. As well as providing more flexibility in management and superiority of biochemical control, there is evidence that divided insulin administration delays the progression of microvascular complications (Job et al 1976, Eschwege et al 1979). The advantages and versatility of such regimens are particularly seen in patients who have been intensively educated to undertake home monitoring of their diabetes (see below). Twice-daily insulin should always be used in all patients whose control is brittle or unstable, in pregnant patients, in those who are to undergo surgery and when the total daily insulin requirements exceed about 30 U. The twice-daily regimen should also be used when control deteriorates in type II patients because of intercurrent infection or other illness, or when poor control develops under similar circumstances in patients previously stable on a small, once-daily insulin dose. In children and adolescents the use of an appropriately designed twice-daily dosage regimen is urged, although some children who retain significant residual endogenous insulin secretion and whose exogenous insulin requirements are very small might be managed adequately with a single daily insulin injection, using Monotard® plus Actrapid® (Werther et al 1980). However, none of these regimens can perfectly reproduce normal, 'physiological' control.

The short-acting insulin normally used in these divided-dose regimens is either

Actrapid® or Velosulin®, although highly purified short-acting beef insulin may be equally acceptable. Highly purified pork isophane (Insulatard®) is a very suitable intermediate-acting insulin to use in combination with one of the short-acting insulins, although some physicians prefer to use Monotard® as the intermediate component. Monotard® has the advantage of being an IZS rather than a protamine-modified insulin, and also has a longer duration of action than isophane. However, Monotard® has an earlier onset and this must be remembered when patients are stabilised or their insulin dose adjusted using the Actrapid®/Monotard® combination. Semitard® (short-acting porcine IZS; Novo) should not be used to supplement Actrapid® or Velosulin;® its duration of action is too short to achieve good control, particularly overnight.

Single-dose regimens

In the older, milder type I patient whose daily insulin requirements are less than 30 U, and in children with considerable residual endogenous insulin secretion, a single morning injection may prove adequate in achieving acceptable control. Neulente® or Monotard® are the best types to use — the duration of action of isophane is not usually long enough to ensure fasting normoglycaemia. It is often necessary to provide additional short- and rapid-acting insulin effect and this may be achieved by supplementing the dose of intermediate-acting insulin with an appropriate quantity of Actrapid®.

Alternative regimens

Injections of short-acting insulin before breakfast, lunch and dinner, with a dose of intermediate-acting insulin given in addition before dinner or before the late evening snack, is suggested by some workers. Holman & Turner (1977) have pointed out that since a predominant abnormality in diabetes (independent of postprandial hyperglycaemia) is a raised fasting blood glucose concentration, a logical initial therapeutic aim should be to lower the fasting glucose concentration to normal. They feel that this can be achieved in type II diabetics with a constant basal insulin supplement provided by an injection, each morning, of the long-acting insulin Ultratard®. Phillips et al (1979) felt that this therapeutic principle could also be used to treat type I patients. Once basal normoglycaemia has been achieved, short-acting insulin can be added to cover meals in these patients, whose insulin requirements are higher than those of type II patients. These authors suggest the use of morning doses of Ultratard® and Actrapid®, with a further injection of Actrapid® before the main evening meal.

Techniques of insulin administration

Attempts have been made, without success, to produce a formulation of insulin that can be given orally. Pontiroli et al (1982) have shown that insulin given intranasally lowers blood glucose, but the therapeutic implications of this observation are not clear. However, the conventional way of giving insulin is still by subcutaneous injection. Jet injection of insulin has been tried, but although there is less immediate pain when an injector gun is used, this advantage is offset by delayed pain and more bleeding (Worth et al 1980). These authors also found that the effect of insulin when given by jet injection was shorter-lasting than when the same dose was given by syringe and did not demonstrate any superiority of jet injection over conventional injection.

It is now accepted that disposable syringes and needles have many advantages over the traditional glass or glass and metal syringes and stainless steel needles (Greenough et al 1979). Disposable syringes are lighter, more robust and more easily carried. Disposable syringes can also be used for more than one injection (Greenough et al 1979, Oli et al 1982). Greenough and his colleagues advised their patients simply to replace the syringe and its attached needle in the packet after each injection and to store it in the fridge until next used. If the needle became blunt after 3 or 4 days it was replaced by another disposable one. With this technique, patients were able to use the same disposable syringe for up to 2 months, with no clinical or bacteriological evidence of infection. Hodge et al (1980) obtained similar results and, in fact, infection at injection sites is remarkably rare (Editorial, British Medical Journal 1981a). Used in this way, disposable syringes are less expensive than glass syringes. Disposable syringes calibrated for U100 insulin are already available, and it is a matter for regret that repeated appeals for plastic syringes to be made available on prescription free of charge to diabetic patients have been persistently rejected.

Insulin delivery systems

Many mechanical devices are now available for insulin delivery in diabetics. The closed-loop device ('artificial pancreas') comprises a glucose sensor, a computer and a pump and controls the infusion of insulin by a feedback mechanism based on plasma glucose. This system responds not only to *degree* of change but to the *rate* of change of plasma glucose (see below). By eliminating the glucose sensor, such devices can be miniaturised and battery-operated, but feedback control is lost and all insulin doses must be preprogrammed—an open-loop system. Such techniques have been used to infuse insulin intravenously, intramuscularly, subcutaneously and intraperitoneally. Using a small battery-driven syringe pump to infuse insulin subcutaneously, Pickup et al (1978) have treated a number of type I patients. Insulin was delivered through a fine nylon cannula implanted subcutaneously and the basal infusion rate of 0.9–3.2 U/h was electronically stepped-up eightfold before meals; the basal infusion rate was adjusted individually for each patient. Continuous subcutaneous insulin infusion (CSII) is now widely used and is an effective way of maintaining normoglycaemia (Pickup et al 1979a, b). Pickup et al (1981) found that patient motivation was more important to a favourable response than was occupation or intelligence. Most patients felt that their control was better with CSII than with conventional treatment and several felt subjectively better. Features such as the greater flexibility of diet and insulin delivery rates were appreciated, although a number of patients in this series were critical of the size of the device used, and this may be the major constraint to long-term use.

However, not all groups have found long-term CSII to be completely satisfactory (Barbosa et al 1981). Human error, needle slippage, leaking and kinking in the cannula, skin intolerance or pump and battery failure occurred in about 50% of patients in this group, and patient acceptance was by no means universal. Pickup et al (1981) have emphasised the importance of appreciating possible psychological reactions and difficulties with interpersonal relationships when CSII is introduced.

The CSII system has been used during pregnancy, to maintain diabetic control during and after operations under general anaesthesia, in brittle or unstable diabetes, in acute metabolic emergencies and to maintain control when intercurrent illness or trauma is present. The system has also been used in attempts to achieve the best possible metabolic control with the aim of delaying or reversing the progression of microangiopathy. It is still too soon to decide whether long-term CSII will be effective in this regard (Watkins 1980), but preliminary results are reasonably promising (Steno Study Group 1982). Pickup et al (1979b) and Tamborlane et al (1979) have shown that CSII provides strict control not only of blood glucose concentrations but also of major intermediary metabolites and of lipid and amino acid metabolism.

More recently, continuous intravenous infusion of insulin delivered by a totally implanted pump has been used (Buchwald et al 1981) and was found to be effective and acceptable. However, long-term continuous intravenous infusion of insulin clearly carries additional hazards.

Closed-loop delivery systems

In non-diabetics, insulin secretion is regulated from minute to minute by changes in blood glucose concentration. The 'artificial pancreas' is designed to create a normal relationship between insulin delivery and blood glucose concentration. In this system, venous blood is withdrawn continuously through the inner lumen of a double-lumen cannula sited in a forearm vein. Blood is diluted and prevented from clotting by heparin and edetic acid in saline (0.154 mol/l) pumped down the outer lumen of the cannula. Continuous measurement of blood glucose concentration is performed with a glucose electrode–glucose oxidase method. Results are obtained 90 s after sampling and are passed to a computer controlling an infusion system with options to infuse saline, saline and insulin or saline and dextrose through a second cannula. The response of the infusion system to the patient's blood glucose concentration or rate of change of blood glucose concentration is determined by two sets of preprogrammed algorithms and the response can be further modified by keyboard instructions about the desired blood glucose concentration in the patient. Glucose-controlled insulin-infusion systems restore to normal the relationship between blood glucose concentrations and insulin delivery and are effective in maintaining normoglycaemia in brittle diabetes (Albisser & Leibel 1977), in diurnal studies (Buckle et al 1977) and in labour (Nattrass et al 1978) in type I diabetics. The method has also been used to cover massive surgery (e.g. open-heart operations). In newly diagnosed insulin-dependent diabetics it has been claimed that a few days' treatment with the artificial pancreas will often induce a temporary remission ('honeymoon period') and that further temporary remissions may sometimes be brought about by subsequent treatment. The treatment of 'insulin-resistant' patients by this method will often produce a dramatic reduction in daily insulin requirements, at least for a time. However, enthusiasm for the artificial pancreas must be tempered by recognition of present limitations. The accurate and rapid measurement of blood glucose concentration and the degree of sophistication of the computer algorithms in determining infusion responses, at present depend entirely on maintaining a constant blood flow through the double-lumen cannula and this can often be a problem. An accurate, miniaturised glucose sensor which can be implanted beneath the skin has yet to be developed, although developments to date are quite promising (Goetz

1974). Ultimately, of course, not only the glucose sensor but also the power source, the computer, the insulin and glucose pumps and refillable glucose and insulin reservoirs will need to be reduced in size, while maintaining accuracy and reliability, to the extent that the whole system, if not actually implantable, will at least be easily portable. Furthermore, some system of measuring continuous glucose concentration which does not depend on the permanent removal of blood from the body is obviously necessary. Many problems have yet to be overcome, but with the silicon chip and with radioactive power sources, the time may come when such portable systems are feasible. However, it must be remembered that so far all such systems infuse insulin into the systemic rather than the portal circulation; whether the difference is important is not known. In addition, it is not known whether the absence of an 'A cell' in the artificial pancreas is likely to be significant.

Pancreatic and islet cell transplantation. So far, the results of whole pancreatic transplantation in man have been dismal. The alternative approach, of transplanting only endocrine tissue, has received much attention (Editorial, Lancet 1975). Islet transplantation in animals does work (Goetz 1974, Anderson 1979). Unfortunately, the islets are not immunologically privileged and clear evidence of rejection has been observed. Nevertheless, implantation of islets into the portal vein or intrasplenically has produced encouraging results. The problems of islet cell transplantation in man are formidable and need not be spelled out. Even in animal studies, progress has been slow and fraught with difficulties.

Problems of control in type I diabetics

Few insulin-treated patients attending a diabetic clinic could be described as well controlled, if by this we mean the maintenance of blood glucose levels as close as possible to those in the non-diabetic. Detailed monitoring shows that most of these patients have both considerable within-day and between-day variation in blood glucose concentrations. However, in spite of what is sometimes considerable blood glucose instability, most of these patients lead relatively normal lives and are seldom troubled by their diabetes.

Although divided-dosage insulin regimens give considerable flexibility, and despite the fact that home monitoring associated with intensive education and reinforcement has given many diabetic patients the opportunity to control their own diabetes rather than to allow it to control them, conscientious diabetic care can be very demanding. Furthermore, regimens based on twice-daily injections of short- and intermediate-acting insulins balanced by an appropriate carbohydrate intake, even with adjustments made on the basis of activity and special circumstances, are an extremely crude way of controlling blood glucose compared with the precision of blood glucose homeostasis pertaining in the non-diabetic individual. Nevertheless, sustained 'good' and asymptomatic biochemical control is possible in the diabetic and if this is not achieved, or if frequent episodes of instability punctuate a diabetic patient's progress, efforts should be made to find a cause.

Counter-regulatory hormone secretion is largely responsible for precipitating ketoacidaemia in otherwise stable patients during acute physical illness: increased secretion of, or increased sensitivity to, these hormones may be the reason why some patients develop ketoacidaemia within a few hours, a process that usually takes many hours or even several days in more stable patients. Emotional factors have long been recognised as a common cause of instability, particularly in children, who may use ketoacidosis as a refuge from unpleasant situations. Deliberate manipulation and fecklessness can enable a diabetic child or adolescent to compel attention. In adults, instability may coincide with some emotional or psychological stress such as loss of a job, bereavement, marital dysharmony or pressure of work. Carelessness or manipulation may also be seen in adults, enabling the patient to escape from situations or responsibilities that he is unable or unwilling to face. A surprisingly large number of patients may make regular errors in dosage, spill their insulin or even forget injections, but what may simply seem at first sight to be lack of care is often, in fact, lack of education or failure of communication. A common example of this is the patient who reduces or omits his insulin when he is anorectic or has a vomiting illness.

Overtreatment with insulin is surprisingly common and both doctor and patient may be responsible for this situation. Once again, failure of education and of communication are major causes. As a result of continued dietary indiscretions or carbohydrate binges (sometimes due to the overenthusiastic treatment of frequent hypoglycaemic attacks or to 'prophylactic' ingestion of carbohydrate to guard against the possible occurrence of such attacks, particularly at night) a patient's weight rises and his daily insulin dosage may be increased to enormously high levels in an attempt to maintain reasonable glycaemia. Presumably, in this situation there is 'down-regulation' of insulin receptors, and such insulin resistance may be corrected by a spell on the artificial pancreas or a period of low-dose insulin infusion (Dandona et al 1978). It is assumed that these treatments, which maintain normoglycaemia with more 'physiological' quantities of insulin, restore insulin receptor affinity to normal. However, with increasing obesity (an almost inevitable occurrence in these circumstances) comes an increasing degree of 'true' insulin resistance attributable to a reduction in insulin receptor population associated with the obese state. This is reversible, although not without difficulty, and the underlying reason for dietary non-compliance must be sought and, if possible, corrected. Overtreatment with insulin should always be considered if a patient's insulin requirements exceed 1 U/kg body weight per day. Excessive insulin dosage, often iatrogenic, plays a part in the Somogyi effect (Somogyi 1959) of rebound hyperglycaemia, which is further discussed below.

Regrettably, unsatisfactory insulin regimens are still a common cause of instability. Such regimens are usually those where twice-daily injections of short-acting insulin alone are used, or when Actrapid® (or Velosulin®) is combined with Semitard®. These regimens are a frequent cause of recurrent hypoglycaemia, often with a subsequent hyperglycaemic rebound. The action of intermediate and long-acting depot insulins such as Neulente®, protamine zinc and Monotard® may be erratic, and their use as a single daily dose in the totally insulin-deficient patient is inappropriate. If the total daily insulin requirement exceeds about 0.5 U/kg the use of twice-daily insulin is mandatory.

Other factors and situations which are liable to affect diabetic control or to be associated with it are discussed in a little more detail below.

Factors affecting the action of injected insulin

It has been appreciated for some years that *the time that elapses* between a subcutaneous injection of insulin being given and the subsequent meal, is critical.

Very different effects are observed if the injection is given as late as 5 min or as early as 30 min before a meal (Kinmonth & Baum 1980). These workers found that subsequent blood glucose concentrations were persistently lower with the early injection regimen than with the late, and pointed out the importance of the timing of insulin injections in the control of postprandial hyperglycaemia.

The *composition of the diet* is equally important in determining blood glucose response after a meal: although they may contain the same quantity of carbohydrate, a drink of apple juice will produce a more rapid and greater rise in blood glucose than will eating a raw apple. Similarly, a high-fibre diet will blunt the postprandial blood glucose peak (see below).

The *rate of absorption* of insulin from the injection site must be borne in mind (Editorial, Lancet 1980a), as it differs according to the anatomical site used for the injection and is also modified by the volume of the injection, the strength of insulin used and the type of insulin. In some cases insulin may be degraded by subcutaneous tissue, possibly because of the effect of a proteolytic enzyme, leading at times to apparent extreme insulin resistance (Dandona et al 1978).

Absorption of subcutaneously injected insulin is accelerated by *exercise* and also by *sauna bathing* (Koivisto 1980). *Smoking* may reduce insulin absorption from subcutaneous tissue (Klemp et al 1982). *Environmental temperature and the state of hydration* and of *vascular perfusion* are also factors that may modify the rate of absorption of insulin, as is the *depth of injection.*

The many variables affecting a patient's response to an injection of insulin are well recognised as important and common causes of unpredictable or unstable control.

Brittle diabetes

This term is often used to describe insulin-treated patients whose control fluctuates rapidly and unpredictably between extremes of hyperglycaemia and hypoglycaemia. It is said that the condition is typically associated with absent endogenous insulin secretion, an exaggerated counter-regulatory hormone response to physical and emotional stress (and, possibly, to hypoglycaemia) and a low circulating titre of insulin antibodies which are, none the less, avid binders of insulin. However, Gale & Tattersall (1979a) have pointed out that the term is frequently misused and often becomes an excuse or even a term of abuse when attempts to improve control have failed and the physician has become exasperated with his patient and the patient disenchanted with his physician. Tattersall (1977) and Gale & Tattersall (1979a) feel that it is more useful for the physician to reserve the term 'brittle diabetes' for a small but conspicuous minority of patients whose lives are 'constantly disrupted by episodes of hypo- or hyperglycaemia, *whatever* the underlying cause.' This is a sensible and practical definition and the term can therefore usefully be extended to include not only those patients whose diabetes is severely unstable as a result of humoral, metabolic or other factors but also those who are unstable because of one or more of the factors discussed in the preceding section.

Patients in this category are readily identifiable and make up a high proportion of emergency admissions. In time their physical, psychological and social problems become inextricably intertwined and unstable diabetes may become a way of life (Gale & Tattersall 1979a). Such patients are often depressed and frustrated, and these reactions often lead to carelessness. While it seems likely that some diabetics are inherently 'brittle', a vicious circle of increasing instability may develop due to the personality factors mentioned earlier, augmented by lack of sympathy on the part of the physician, as well as poor communication and lack of education. Self-monitoring leads to higher motivation and better control in most patients (Sönksen et al 1978; Walford et al 1978) and there is no substitute for continuity of care, a sympathetic and personal approach, effective communication and intensive and persistent education. Any obvious underlying causes such as a badly designed insulin regimen must be corrected, and with adequate training and access to techniques such as home glucose monitoring, most patients are perfectly capable of controlling their own diabetes, although they still need skilled advice and support. However, a minority of patients who are brittle in childhood and adolescence remain brittle well into adult life and demand much time and care. As Gale & Tattersall (1979a) wisely point out, 'brittle people make brittle diabetics.' Continuous intravenous insulin infusion has been used to manage brittle diabetes that seems unresponsive to conventional insulin treatment (Bayliss 1981). However, it must be appreciated that CSII and CIVII greatly increase the opportunities for manipulation and attention-seeking if such patients' lability is due primarily to psychological and personal factors and a feeling of rejection. The helplessness that the physician frequently feels when attempting to manage such patients will often be transmitted to the patients themselves.

The Somogyi effect

Somogyi (1959) suggested that overtreatment with insulin might itself be a cause of unstable diabetes and postulated that hypoglycaemia (which might be asymptomatic) triggered the release of counter-regulatory hormones leading to hyperglycaemia and insulin resistance. Gradual reduction in insulin dosage led to greatly improved control. Unrecognised nocturnal hypoglycaemia frequently leads to fasting hyperglycaemia, and Asplin et al (1980) have suggested that raised cortisol : creatinine ratios in overnight urine samples may indicate an otherwise unrecognised episode of nocturnal hypoglycaemia. However, although the Somogyi effect is well recognised, Gale & Tattersall (1979b) and Gale et al (1980) have pointed out that Somogyi's suggestion that rebound hyperglycaemia is caused by excessive secretion of counter-regulatory hormones has never been confirmed. These workers studied a group of unstable patients during and after episodes of nocturnal hypoglycaemia and found no difference in cortisol, growth hormone and glucagon levels between patients who showed post-hypoglycaemic hyperglycaemia and those with prolonged hypoglycaemia. On the other hand, they did find a very strong inverse correlation between blood glucose and free insulin, suggesting that hyperglycaemia, when present, was attributable to relative insulin deficiency in the latter part of the night. They concluded that early changes in blood glucose after untreated hypoglycaemia seem to be due to changes in free insulin rather than to a response to antagonistic hormones.

The risk of nocturnal hypoglycaemia, both clinical and subclinical, is high in insulin-treated patients and must be recognised (Editorial, Lancet 1980b). Such patients must be further subdivided into those who show 'rebound' hyperglycaemia and those whose blood glucose concentrations remain low. In the former patients, a reduction should be made in the evening dose of short-acting insulin and an increase in the evening dose of intermediate-acting insulin may need to be considered. The time at which nocturnal hypoglycaemia occurs (if this can be identified) will guide the physician in this regard. In the latter cases (those with persistently low blood glucose concentrations) an all-round reduction in the evening dose of insulin is necessary.

THE ASSESSMENT OF DIABETIC CONTROL

Home blood glucose monitoring

In addition to purely clinical criteria, 'control' in diabetes is still often judged simply by intermittent urine tests and occasional blood glucose estimations. These may be adequate in the type II patient but can be notoriously unreliable in the type I diabetic. Random blood glucose estimations can be particularly misleading because they can fluctuate so much in a day; they can never serve as a rational basis for the logical adjustment of insulin dosage. Carefully performed urine tests, regularly carried out and intelligently interpreted, can be more helpful, but one patient summed up the problem of the renal threshold for glucose by pointing out that adjusting insulin dose according to urine tests was like driving a car on roads with a 30 mph speed limit with a speedometer that began to work only at 70 mph (Sönksen et al 1978). The delayed and indirect relationship between urine and blood glucose means that even tests of double-voided urine provide only a crude means of evaluation. Furthermore, even those patients who are most conscientious in performing urine tests and recording the results have seldom been told how to alter their insulin dosage in response to these results — indeed, some patients are ordered *never* to change their insulin dose! Diurnal blood glucose series carried out at frequent intervals in outpatients can be much more helpful, particularly during pregnancy, but can still fluctuate considerably even in a stable patient. The factors that may upset diabetic control have been referred to in a previous section: exercise, intercurrent infection and emotional factors can lead to marked blood glucose fluctuation in a patient on a fixed dose of insulin.

The aim of management is to allow diabetic patients to live as normal a life as possible, taking into account the variations in activity level, size, timing of meals and other factors that must inevitably occur and which will affect diabetic control. Monitoring of control is therefore inextricably linked with the need to change insulin dosage in a logical way, and this in turn leads to the need for intensive education and continued advice, support and reinforcement. These are essential prerequisites of home monitoring, however performed.

Home blood glucose monitoring, where the patient adjusts his insulin dosage on the basis of the blood glucose results that he has obtained himself, is a realistic and practicable method both of assessing control and of obtaining the best possible biochemical stability. Various methods have been described, either using a reflectance meter (Sönksen et al 1978, Walford et al 1978, Tattersall 1979) or by direct visual reading of reagent strips (Howe-Davies et al 1978, Ferguson & Prosser 1980, Walford et al 1980). A number of reflectance meters are available in the UK; their performance characteristics have been described (Webb et al 1980). The Eyetone® (Ames) and Reflomat® (Boehringer) machines are mains-operated and expensive; the former displays the result on a needle scale and the latter on a calibrated dial. Battery machines that are easily portable and much less expensive include the Glucochek® (Medistron, Ltd), the Hypocount® (Hypoguard, Ltd) and the

Glucometer® (Ames). All of these machines have a digital read-out and the Hypocount® was the meter preferred by patients in the study by Webb and his colleagues (1980).

There are at present two principal blood glucose reagent strip systems available — Dextrostix® (Ames) and Reflotest® (Boehringer Mannheim). The Dextrostix® system comprises a single strip. The Reflotest® system, however, includes BM-Glycemie and BM-Hypoglycemie strips for meter-read blood glucose in the normal-to-high ranges and the low ranges respectively. More recently, the BM-Glycemie 20–800 strip has been introduced for visually read blood glucose estimation over both high and low ranges. This strip has two separate test pads whose indicators permit differentiation of eight pairs of colours corresponding to blood glucose concentrations from 1.1 to 44.4 mmol/l.

Of the reflectance meters referred to above, all except the Reflomat® use the Dextrostix® system. However, a new Hypocount® machine (Hypocount® II B) has recently been introduced which also uses the BM strip system.

All the available blood glucose test strips can be read visually against a colour scale; all except the BM 20–800 can also be read in a reflectance meter. A comparative study of test strips has been carried out (Worth et al 1981). These workers found that, when read visually, the BM 20–800 strip was more accurate than the Dextrostix® strip. Comparison of meter reading showed that the Reflotest® system was more accurate and precise than those using Dextrostix®. This was because the Reflotest® system was read closer to the end-point of colour development and because there was less subsequent colour fade than with Dextrostix®. The BM strips developed colours that were stable for at least two days after completion of the test if strips were stored in desiccant containers. Colour faded rapidly when Dextrostix® were stored in this way. The technique involved when Dextrostix® are used is more difficult to follow than with the other systems and therefore more prone to error, when nurses and patients carry out the tests. Accuracy of timing is particularly critical with Dextrostix®.

Current opinion favours the Reflotest BM® systems both for machine use and for visual reading. If a reflectance meter is to be used, the Reflomat® is recommended for hospital use and the Hypocount® II B for outpatients. However, the BM 20–800 strip can be used accurately and easily by most patients (Ferguson & Prosser 1980, Walford et al 1980, Worth et al 1981) and is recommended as the method of choice for home blood glucose monitoring. Graham et al (1980) have shown that defects of colour vision have no significant effect on patients' ability to use visual methods of estimating blood glucose: the main use of reflectance meters therefore seems to be for the initial stages of home monitoring, when some patients wish to check the accuracy of their visually read results in order to gain confidence with the method, and find the Hypocount® II B machine useful in this respect. This machine is also of great assistance to those diabetics with some degree of visual failure who are unable to read strips directly but who can read the digital display on this portable machine.

Home blood glucose monitoring, usually utilising the BM 20–800 strip, is now a fundamental addition to the conventional management of type I diabetic patients, but it must be recognised that no system can be effective unless the patient is very carefully instructed in its use and advised how to alter his insulin dosage in response to the results he obtains. Intensive education is vital and cannot be ignored — technology alone is not enough. There is evidence that home monitoring improves motivation (Sönksen et al 1978, Walford et al 1978) but it must be accepted that some patients cannot get to grips with the technique, either because they find it too complicated or inconvenient, they have difficulty in converting their results into action or they lack the confidence to make frequent and sometimes substantial changes in their insulin dosage. Self-monitoring is of particular value during pregnancy (Peacock et al 1979), but these patients are so highly motivated that excellent control is not difficult to achieve in most cases, whatever method of monitoring is used (Stubbs et al 1980). Home monitoring has also been used in type II patients (Paisey et al 1980). These authors suggest that control in such patients might be monitored satisfactorily by regular measurement of fasting or mid-morning blood glucose concentrations.

In some quarters, acceptance of home blood glucose monitoring has been more cautious (Editorial, Lancet 1980c) and it must again be emphasised that the ability of a patient to measure his blood glucose means nothing unless he responds in some way to the results he obtains. Those patients whose control is most in need of improvement, particularly children and adolescents who are manipulative and feckless, will also be those most likely to reject the offer of monitoring methods. In such children, holiday camps such as those run by the British Diabetic Association can make a dramatic contribution to the resolution of such behaviour disturbances and are strongly recommended (Editorial, Lancet 1980d). Nevertheless, most diabetologists would agree that the instruction of newly diagnosed patients in home-monitoring techniques is now as important as instruction in injection technique. The earlier that self-monitoring is introduced in the course of the disease, the more likely the patient is to accept it as part of his overall management and to make the best use of it.

Glycosylated haemoglobin

Apart from the estimation of 24 h urinary glucose excretion there was not, until a few years ago, any method available that could be used to assess effectively the accuracy of long-term blood glucose regulation. A possible method of doing this now seems to exist (Editorial, New England Journal of Medicine 1976, Editorial, British Medical Journal 1978, Boden et al 1980). Haemoglobin A_{Ic} (HbA_{Ic}) is one of three negatively charged minor haemoglobin compounds that are eluted on cation exchange resin chromatography before the main HbA peak. The beta-chain N terminus of HbA_{Ic} has a hexose attached (glycosylated haemoglobin) and has been shown to be increased in diabetes. The glycosylation of HbA to HbA_{Ic} is a post-translational modification of HbA occurring by a slow non-enzymatic process in the circulating red cell. The presence of haemoglobin and of glucose in high concentrations and the relative irreversibility (but see also below) of their ketoamine linkage (that present in HbA_{Ic}) result in the continuous formation and accumulation of glycosylated Hb within the red cells. All three HbA_I fractions are glycosylated and are now usually measured together in the assays currently used; the estimation of HbA_I is simpler and more rapid than measurement of its subfraction HbA_{Ic}.

It is now known that the process of glycosylation affects other proteins, including albumin. Indeed, because of its short half-life, it has been suggested that measurement of glycosylated albumin might provide an accurate indication of short-term diabetic control (Dolhofer & Wieland 1980).

Many studies have established what seems to be a correlation between HbA_1 and the blood glucose concentration. The value of measurements of HbA_1 is that they appear to reflect overall blood glucose concentrations independently of day-to-day fluctuations. Because HbA_1 reflects blood glucose control retrospectively, it may provide valuable information in circumstances such as the evaluation of control during the first trimester of pregnancy. Nevertheless, while the concept of glycosylated haemoglobin as an indicator of long-term diabetic control is now popular, the problems encountered with its estimation and its metabolism have hindered the interpretation of results. The amount of HbA_1 in the blood depends to some extent on red cell turnover, because its formation takes place during the whole life of the red cell. Values are reduced if the rate of red cell turnover is increased, as in haemolytic anaemia. Large quantities of HbA_1 are found in patients with iron-deficiency anaemia (Brooks et al 1980b) and, in uraemic patients, both high (De Boer et al 1980) and low (Dandona et al 1979) values have been recorded.

Many difficulties have been experienced with laboratory methods for the determination of HbA_1 — different methods give different results and, in those based on column chromatography, the temperature of the column is of critical importance. Prolonged storage of specimens, even when refrigerated, also leads to changes in HbA_1. It is probably stable for about 3 days when whole blood is stored at 4°C, but we have little reliable information about any changes that may occur when blood samples are left standing at room temperature (Editorial, British Medical Journal 1980).

In clinical practice, Gonen and his colleagues (1977) found that the level of HbA_1 in diabetic patients correlated closely with their physicians' ratings of their degree of control and their fasting blood glucose levels. Elkeles et al (1978) found that there was a significant correlation between HbA_1 and blood glucose measured at the same time and mean blood glucose measured over the preceding year. Fraser et al (1979) suggested that glycosylated Hb concentration reflected the average blood glucose concentration over the previous 1 to 2 months. However, the same average figure may be obtained both from a series of results that fluctuate very little and from a series that fluctuates markedly between very high and very low levels. A 'normal' HbA_1 concentration may not mean that the blood glucose concentration is uniformly stable. There are further problems in interpreting HbA_1 results in clinical practice. Brooks et al (1980a) measured HbA_1 in type I diabetics before, during and after a 7-day period of monitored poor control. There was considerable individual variation in the pattern and degree of change in HbA_1 concentration induced by poor control and the time when it occurred. Scobie et al (1981) measured blood glucose and HbA_1 concentrations during an oral glucose tolerance test and for 120 days afterwards in 20 normal subjects. Their results showed that a minor degree of hyperglycaemia led to a significant increase in glycosylated haemoglobin concentrations which appeared 10 days after the test and which remained raised for at least 30 days afterwards; levels did not return to normal until 60 days after the test. Marquat et al (1978) had observed similar results after an oral glucose load. These findings, and the discrepancies observed in unstable diabetics, can be explained by the fact that it is now known that an unstable component of HbA_1 exists, perhaps representing the Schiff base, which is formed as the initial step in the formation of glycosylated haemoglobin. Short-term hyperglycaemia can therefore cause relatively rapid changes in HbA_1 (fast glycosylation) and this reaction is reversible (Welch 1979, Svendsen et al 1980). The errors resulting from the presence of unstable HbA_1 may be large; the normal range of HbA_1 is about 4–8% of total HbA but this fraction may be increased in vitro by 3% or more because of fast glycosylation. In routine outpatient studies, however, the unstable fraction rarely accounts for more than 1.5% (Goldstein et al 1980). If measurement of HbA_1 is to be of value in the assessment of long-term diabetic control, account must be taken of the unstable component, which should preferably be removed before analysis. Svendsen et al (1980) recommend incubation of red cells in a low-glucose medium at 37° for several hours to eliminate the unstable fraction; alternatively, dialysis can be used. However, Welch (1979) found that washing diabetic red cells in glucose-free saline for 17 h did not result in any appreciable drop in HbA_1, and he felt that the phenomenon of fast glycosylation did not reduce in any way the potential value of such estimations in the assessment of diabetic control. As he points out, the aim of control is permanent rather than transient normoglycaemia, and the fact that the initial stage of glycosylation may be partly reversible is not, therefore, relevant. New cells entering the circulation and experiencing a lower blood glucose concentration will encounter a reduced glycosylation of their haemoglobin and this will be reflected in a lower blood HbA_1. Only if hyperglycaemia is more permanent, more pronounced or, possibly, more frequent will the result be the formation of true (stable) HbA_1.

Nevertheless, these observations on rapid glycosylation and unstable HbA_1 inevitably must cast doubt on the reliability of many of the earlier published reports. It is now known that close attention must be given to the storage of samples, elimination (if possible) of the unstable fraction and quality control of the laboratory methods. Under these circumstances, measurement of HbA_1 should still provide the unique retrospective assessment of long-term diabetic control which its advocates have claimed. In the diabetic clinic, a single estimation of HbA_1 provides limited information, although a series of values over months or years might prove very useful. This is particularly the case when diabetic control is monitored by this method during pregnancy.

Despite the present uncertainties, a normal HbA_1 concentration is likely to indicate good blood glucose control, particularly if this can be confirmed by diurnal blood glucose series and if nocturnal hypoglycaemia can be excluded (Gale & Tattersall 1979b, Gale et al 1979, Editorial, Lancet 1980b). Persistent elevation of HbA_1 demands detailed appraisal and action — the estimation is valuable if we use it properly and critically; uncritical acceptance of every result obtained is potentially dangerous.

FIBRE-RICH DIETS IN DIABETES MELLITUS

For several years there has been much interest in the possibility of improving diabetic control by the use of fibre-rich diets, the aim being to decrease postprandial hyperglycaemia by delaying gastric emptying and by slowing the rate of absorption of glucose from the small intestinal lumen (Editorial, Lancet 1981). Jenkins et al (1976) found that the addition of guar and pectin to a control meal markedly decreased the rise in blood glucose between 30 and 90 min after the meal and also resulted in significantly lower insulin concentrations between 30 and 120 min in a group of type II diabetics. Other reports have shown that the use of high-fibre or high-carbohydrate/high-fibre diets reduced fasting and postprandial blood glucose levels and allowed withdrawal of insulin when the daily dose of insulin was less than 20 units, although no beneficial effect was found in patients whose daily dose was 30 units or more (Anderson & Ward 1978, Miranda & Horwitz 1978).

Fibre supplementation has also been shown to improve some aspects of blood glucose control in type I diabetic patients (Monnier et al 1981). This study showed blunting of the postprandial blood glucose rises in patients who had been on high-fibre diets for 10–15 days, although this effect was seen only after lunch and dinner in labile diabetics and only after lunch in stable patients. Apart from lowering the postprandial blood glucose response, a high-carbohydrate leguminous-fibre diet has been shown to improve other aspects of diabetic control. Such a diet was found to reduce significantly total cholesterol in both type I and type II patients, and the HDL/LDL cholesterol ratio increased significantly in the type II patients (Simpson et al 1981). Jenkins et al (1979) demonstrated a reduction in 3-hydroxybutyrate excretion in diabetics taking guar.

Although the beneficial effects of a high-fibre diet on postprandial blood glucose have been confirmed on numerous occasions over the last few years, the fact remains that such changes are relatively small and, in all probability, might be obtained equally well if the patients were to eat less of anything and to pay more attention to the timing and content of their meals. Nor are high-fibre diets particularly pleasant or easy to follow. Postprandial blood glucose concentrations are influenced only when the fibre content is fivefold that of the normal British diet (Simpson et al 1981). The most effective forms of fibre are those such as guar and tragacanth, which are the most viscous. The greatest effect has been seen with guar, but this was abolished when hydrolysed non-viscous guar was substituted (Jenkins et al 1978). Viscous fibre preparations are difficult to incorporate into ordinary foods: it seems that the fibre must be intimately mixed with the main carbohydrate portion of the meal. When merely sprinkled over a 'normal' meal the effect is much less striking (Williams et al 1980). Guar and pectin crispbreads and biscuits are particularly unpalatable. Unfortunately, it is difficult to devise a naturally high-fibre diet without including an unacceptably large quantity of vegetables, especially beans. Breakfast in a diet used in the Oxford study (Simpson et al 1981) included 140 g of haricot beans and the evening meal 50 g each of red kidney beans and butter beans. A combination of leguminous seeds and guar may allow smaller quantities of each to be used (Jenkins et al 1980) but, overall, if is doubtful whether such a diet is much more acceptable than one based on either guar or on leguminous seeds alone. Patients taking such diets often complain of increased stool bulk, increased frequency of bowel action, easy satiety and excessive flatus.

For many years, the diets recommended for diabetics have varied regularly between low-carbohydrate/high-fat and high-carbohydrate/low-fat. Although low-fat diets have obvious appeal, and while there is no clear evidence that high-carbohydrate diets are inferior to low-carbohydrate, there is still disagreement about the desirable proportion of carbohydrate that should be used (Reaven 1980). Though the reduction in postprandial hyperglycaemia in diabetics taking a fibre-rich diet is undeniable, the benefits gained seem to be small when the monotony and unpalatability of such diets is considered. Certainly, it is wise to advise a diet which has a high natural-fibre content for both type I and type II patients, but in the long term, therapeutic advantages of a supplemented high-fibre diet are far from clear. It is not always easy for a diabetic patient to have ready access to expert dietetic advice and, even when such advice is given, it is sometimes overcomplicated, unimaginative and inconsistent (Thomas et al 1974). Furthermore, dietary compliance in diabetes is notoriously poor. It would probably be better to concentrate on the simpler and more fundamental aspects of dietary management, both in type I and in type II patients, than to advocate the widespread and uncritical use of high-fibre diets, either supplemented or of natural origin.

ORAL HYPOGLYCAEMIC AGENTS

Sulphonylureas

In 1970 the University Group Diabetes Program (UGDP) reported that patients with mild diabetes treated with a fixed dose of tolbutamide and diet fared no better than those on diet alone as regards life expectancy, and indeed the death rate from cardiovascular disease was significantly higher in the tolbutamide-treated group than in the diet alone (placebo) group or in the two groups of patients treated with insulin (fixed and variable dose). Patients treated with phenformin had a mortality rate similar to that seen in the tolbutamide group. This study provoked considerable criticism both from clinicians and statisticians. The results conflicted with those of Keen et al (1968) in a broadly comparable study: these workers had concluded that in mild and moderately severe diabetes tolbutamide provided a significant degree of primary protection against cardiovascular events. The argument continues perhaps because it has often been forgotten that the American investigators were careful to point out that their conclusions related only to the effects of tolbutamide and phenformin, prescribed in fixed dosage, in a population of overweight, middle-aged, asymptomatic maturity-onset diabetics. The results should not be extrapolated to include all other oral hypoglycaemic agents (OHA). Nevertheless, some later studies (Boyle et al, 1972, Hadden et al 1972) have yielded data which add some support to the UGDP conclusions. These studies indicated that patients treated with OHA had a frequency of myocardial infarction twice as great as those treated by diet alone, although these workers make the important point that patients who are not clearly insulin-dependent, yet who cannot be controlled by diet alone, may select themselves as a group with an inherently greater risk of ischaemic heart disease.

The publication of the UGDP study has generated much heat but has not greatly altered practice in the United Kingdom except in a few important regards — it was shown that there is no obvious benefit in the long term in treating mild overt diabetics routinely with OHA — a proper diet is the only treatment necessary in the majority and should certainly be the initial treatment for all patients. Furthermore, the study has emphasised the fact that these are potent and potentially dangerous drugs that should be prescribed only for patients likely to benefit from them, and with full knowledge of their possible unwanted effects. Sulphonylureas should be reserved for those type II diabetic patients who fail to respond to diet alone or who have marked hyperglycaemia and prominent symptoms at presentation, requiring a rapid clinical response. Sulphonylureas are of most value in type II patients who are of average weight or are only slightly overweight; however, they are not contraindicated even when significant obesity is present, although they should not be regarded as the treatment of first choice in this situation.

The use of sulphonylureas

The second generation sulphonylurea, glibenclamide, a potent hypoglycaemic agent with an intermediate duration of action, has been available for several years and is now a popular choice. The drug has a half-life substantially shorter than that of chlorpropamide. The maximum effective dose is about 20 mg daily, and if daily dosage requirements exceed 10 mg the dose is best divided and given in the morning and in the evening. An evening dose of glibenclamide in these circumstances is more likely to ensure a satisfactory fasting glucose level and to avoid mid-morning hypoglycaemia than is a higher dose given once daily. The very long half-life of chlorpropamide is a clear disadvantage, especially in older patients who may not maintain an adequate carbohydrate intake. Hypoglycaemia with chlorpropamide is often profound and tends to be prolonged and recurrent despite apparently adequate therapy.

Hypoglycaemia may occur with any of the sulphonylureas, and not infrequently this is a result of drug interaction. Oral anticoagulants, clofibrate, isoniazid, phenylbutazone, probenecid, β-blockers, salicylates, sulphaphenazole and other drugs all potentiate the hypoglycaemic action of sulphonylureas. Hypoglycaemia is a particular hazard when a previously stable patient voluntarily or involuntarily reduces his food intake or when any degree of renal failure is present. In this situation hypoglycaemic metabolites of the parent compound accumulate. The dosage of sulphonylureas must always be adjusted to clinical response, and Tomkins & Bloom (1972) have found that as many as one-third of patients established on sulphonylureas are able to discontinue their drugs and maintain satisfactory control on diet alone. Although patients who fail to respond to one sulphonylurea may sometimes respond to another, the practice of 'ringing the changes' between a wide range of different preparations is to be discouraged.

New sulphonylureas

A number of new second-generation sulphonylureas have been introduced over the last few years. These include glipizide, glibornuride, gliclazide and gliquidone. Glipizide has a rather short half-life and, except in the lowest dosages, is best given twice daily. It appears to offer no advantage whatsoever over chlorpropamide and glibenclamide. Glibornuride has a longer half-life, similar to that of glibenclamide, and is commonly effective in once-daily dosage. The metabolites of glibornuride are either devoid of hypoglycaemic activity or are much less active than the parent compound. Although the half-life of glibornuride is prolonged in patients with impaired renal function and dosage must be reduced, glibornuride seems to be a safer drug in this situation than other sulphonylureas and therefore seems to be of some value in older patients. Gliclazide has a half-life intermediate between those of glibenclamide and chlorpropamide. It can therefore be given once daily to good effect. It is metabolised in the liver: less than 5% of the dose is excreted unchanged in the urine. It would appear that its metabolites have only low hypoglycaemic activity: the drug can therefore safely be given to patients with mild impairment of renal function. This drug has been shown to reduce platelet adhesiveness and aggregation and to increase fibrinolytic activity. It is uncertain whether these effects are specific to gliclazide or are shared by other sulphonylureas; the clinical significance of these effects is not known. Gliquidone has a very short half-life and should be given two or three times daily. Metabolic degradation of gliquidone occurs in the liver and the metabolites are excreted via the bile into the faeces. Only 5% is excreted via the kidneys, largely as inactive metabolites. The drug is therefore safe in patients with renal impairment, although it seems to be a less potent hypoglycaemic agent than glibenclamide.

Mode of action of sulphonylureas

For many years after the introduction of the first sulphonylurea (tolbutamide) it was assumed that these drugs exerted their long-term hypoglycaemic effect solely by stimulating pancreatic insulin release. There can be no doubt that an acute action of sulphonylureas both in vitro and in vivo is to stimulate insulin release from the β cell. It has been confirmed that with chlorpropamide therapy the early phase of insulin secretion usually improves (Hecht et al 1973) and that in newly treated diabetics there is a transient increase in insulin output (Barnes et al 1974). Mutch & Stowers (1980) have claimed that chlorpropamide might reverse mild diabetes in children, presumably as a result of its insulinogenic effect. However, most type I patients established on insulin obtain little benefit from the addition of a sulphonylurea to their treatment (Ward et al 1981) and although patients with diabetes of recent onset with considerable residual beta-cell secretion might be aided, such patients already have fairly good diabetic control. It is also certain that some β-cell function must be present for these drugs to exert their hypoglycaemic action. Nevertheless, although continued use of the drug may maintain normoglycaemia, the increased output of insulin is short-lived and variable and does not correspond well with blood glucose levels. It appears that the main hypoglycaemic action of the sulphonylureas on long-term therapy is extrapancreatic (Hecht et al 1973, Jackson et al 1973, Barnes et al 1974). This effect may be due to a reduced hepatic output of glucose or to increased effectiveness of endogenous insulin. Reduced hepatic glucose output seems to be the main reason for sustained hypoglycaemia in patients treated with sulphonylureas and this action might be reversed by intramuscular glucagon.

Biguanides

Unwanted effects of the biguanides

Biguanides are seldom used in the USA and phenformin has been banned in some European countries because of the risk of lactic acidaemia. It is recommended that phenformin should *not* be used and that metformin should be prescribed only in carefully selected patients who should be reviewed regularly. Metformin undoubtedly has a hypoglycaemic effect in type II patients with adequate endogenous insulin secretion and, when used in combination with a sulphonylurea, the effect is synergistic. It does not cause biochemical hypoglycaemia when given alone. Metformin has a number of unwanted effects, including indigestion, general malaise and diarrhoea, which limit its value. The most dangerous unwanted effect of the biguanide group of drugs is lactic acidaemia (type B2; Alberti & Nattrass

1977). This condition has long been recognised as a significant and serious hazard of phenformin therapy and the risk is much increased in the presence of impaired renal or hepatic function and in hypoxic states. There has been no report in the United Kingdom of lactic acidaemia associated with the use of metformin. A small number of reports that this complication has occurred in patients treated with metformin have appeared on the Continent but, in virtually every case, serious associated disease which might have been expected to increase the likelihood of lactic acidaemia was also present. Nevertheless, it is suggested that metformin should be avoided in the following situations:

1. Impaired renal function (e.g. plasma creatinine of 133 μmol/litre or more, checked quarterly)
2. Impaired hepatic function
3. Patients prone to alcohol abuse
4. Serious cardiovascular disease (coronary insufficiency, cardiac failure, myocardial infarction)
5. Conditions which lead to or are associated with tissue hypoxia (gangrene, circulatory shock, acute blood loss, pulmonary embolism, chronic respiratory disease).

In high-dosage metformin therapy, malabsorption of vitamin B_{12} has been reported (Tomkin et al 1971).

DIABETIC COMPLICATIONS

Diabetic ketoacidaemia

The management of diabetic ketoacidaemia has altered little since the last edition of this book was published in 1978, although low-dose insulin infusion is now much more widely used in treatment and the rate of administration of insulin advised is lower than in the earlier days of this regimen. Nevertheless, in a recent survey (Tunbridge 1981), ketoacidaemia was shown to be the major cause of death in 15% of diabetics dying under the age of 50 years and the importance of this topic is therefore such that its management is again discussed in detail.

The importance of glucagon in the pathogenesis of diabetic ketoacidaemia (DKA) is now recognised. The condition should be regarded as a state of glucagon excess as well as of insulin deficiency (Alberti et al 1975), and hyperglucagonaemia is an important factor in determining the degree of hyperglycaemia and hyperketonaemia in the early stages of insulin deprivation. However, although somatostatin almost completely suppresses plasma pancreatic glucagon as well as plasma growth hormone, and while somatostatin may suppress hyperketonaemia in diabetic patients if administered as soon as insulin is withdrawn, somatostatin does not reverse the metabolic state if it is given only when DKA is well established (Lundbaek et al 1976). The role of residual insulin secretion in protecting against ketoacidaemia in type I diabetics has been emphasised (Madsbad et al 1979): even minimal residual secretion is important for metabolic well-being in diabetes and may prevent the development of severe ketoacidosis when insulin delivery is inadequate.

Treatment of DKA

When treatment of DKA is considered, some traditional and often cherished concepts have for some time been questioned; in some instances safer and more appropriate, convenient and simple therapeutic regimens have been recommended. The treatment of DKA will be considered under several headings.

General and supportive. If vomiting is a feature, as it usually is, a nasogastric tube should be passed and gastric aspiration commenced and it may be necessary to catheterise the unconscious patient. In a hypotensive patient in a critical state, transfusion of whole blood should be considered and, in the older patient, a central venous pressure line should be inserted as very large quantities of fluid will need to be given.

Insulin. The traditional treatment of DKA involved the use of frequent boluses of large quantities of soluble insulin, given intravenously or intramuscularly or more commonly by both routes simultaneously. Such therapy often produced a very rapid, precipitous and uncontrolled fall in the blood glucose concentration with a substantial risk of hypoglycaemia and osmotic disequilibrium, and also provoked a rapid shift of potassium into the cells, with associated hypokalaemia unless large potassium supplements were given. The dose of insulin used was far in excess of that which was physiologically appropriate, and the whole situation was fraught with anxiety, uncertainty and lack of control.

Alberti et al (1973) showed that frequent small intramuscular doses of soluble insulin were in most cases just as effective in restoring normoglycaemia as the bolus method. These workers used an initial dose of 10–20 units intramuscularly and thereafter continued with 5–10 units every hour by the same route. Plasma glucose fell at a regular rate (although the rate of fall was slower when infection was present), physiological levels of insulin were reproduced more closely and it appeared that sudden shifts in potassium and phosphate were minimised. However, the regimen is not always effective in hypotensive and severely dehydrated patients with advanced DKA. An alternative method of administering soluble insulin is by the intravenous route and, as the half-life of intravenous insulin is very short (about 4 min), a continuous intravenous infusion using low doses (4–8 units/h initially, reducing to 1–4 units/h thereafter) is the method of choice. This method produces a sustained (although not always linear) fall in blood glucose and is extremely effective; nevertheless, the possibility of larger insulin requirements in a few severely ketoacidaemic, comatose patients should be recognised and anticipated.

Soler and his collegues (1975) have suggested that small doses of insulin, although effective in most cases, may not be clearly superior to conventional treatment with large doses, although some of their conclusions have been challenged by Alberti (1976) and Page et al (1976b). As Page and his colleagues point out, it is easy to alter the infusion rate, and the technique is flexible and may be used in pregnant patients during labour. Junior hospital staff find it much easier to manage than the traditional, empirical regimen. In clinical practice there is no doubt that the use of either the repeated low-dose intramuscular regimen or the low-dose intravenous infusion has greatly simplified management of the great majority of patients with DKA and has removed much of the guesswork, although neither regimen excludes the need for frequent biochemical monitoring. Whereas lack of adjustable constant-rate infusion pumps and shortage of staff might make the intramuscular method the safer one to use in some centres, the low-dose intravenous infusion method seems in general to be preferable and is more adaptable to the patient's progress. It has been suggested that monocomponent insulin might be preferable to soluble insulin when low-dose intramuscular or intravenous infusion regimens are used. Repeated estimation of the blood glucose concentration (as well as of plasma electrolytes) is always necessary and the rate of insulin infusion should be adjusted to reach a blood glucose concentration of 10–14 mmol/l. There is no merit (and there is potential hazard) in lowering the blood glucose too rapidly.

Fluid. Isotonic saline is the intravenous fluid of choice. The first litre is given in 30 min and the second litre in 1 h, continuing at this rate; however, in patients with heart failure or known myocardial damage the rate should be slowed and central venous pressure monitored. If hypernatraemia is present, 0.45% saline (77 mmol/litre) should be substituted for isotonic saline and subsequent replacement guided by plasma sodium estimations. When the blood glucose concentration reaches about 10–14 mmol/litre, the saline is discontinued and administration of 4% glucose in 0.18% saline or 5% glucose in water is begun. At this stage the rate of insulin infusion is adjusted to maintain a satisfactory blood glucose concentration (perhaps 8–10 mmol/litre) and infusions of insulin and glucose are continued simultaneously until the patient is able to return to twice-daily insulin and a normal diet. Because of the very short half-life of intravenous insulin, the insulin infusion is continued until immediately before the first subcutaneous dose is given.

Potassium. Balance studies have shown a deficit of total body potassium of approximately 500 mmol in DKA. Despite this, it has often been stated that potassium should be withheld until some hours after insulin is first given or until there is a 'significant' fall in blood glucose. It is now generally accepted that, except in patients with known renal failure and those with hyperkalaemia when they first present, intravenous potassium should be given early, as the level is bound to fall once treatment is underway. The rate at which potassium should be given varies from patient to patient. A mean rate of 30 mmol potassium/litre of intravenous fluid was required to keep the serum potassium normal in the study by Soler et al (1972), and a satisfactory rate of infusion would be 15–30 mmol/h, although this might need considerable adjustment, and frequent estimation of plasma potassium concentration is vital. Smaller quantities of potassium are needed using the low-dose insulin infusion routine than with the high-dose insulin bolus methods. Low doses of insulin primarily inhibit hepatic gluconeogenesis and glucose release, and stimulation of cellular glucose uptake is much less marked than when large doses of insulin are used. There is thus a fall in blood glucose without a marked increase in the rate of entry of potassium into the cells. The most dangerously ill patients may present with a low plasma potassium. Here potassium must be given in large quantities from the outset, and monitoring of the ECG is mandatory.

Phosphate. There is a significant loss of phosphate during the development of DKA, and there seem to be good theoretical reasons for adding phosphate to the replacement fluid, although Malins (1971) did not find it to have any clinical advantage. Nevertheless, there is a fall in red cell 2,3-diphosphoglycerate (2,3-DPG) in DKA and this can be reversed by intravenous administration of phosphate. Such administration might improve tissue oxygenation by restoring 2,3-DPG to normal more rapidly.

Bicarbonate. It is now recognised that in milder degrees of acidaemia it is unwise to give large quantities of bicarbonate. Too-rapid correction of the blood pH can be harmful and can cause rapid movement of potassium into the cells. In addition, rapid correction of pH will shift the oxygen dissociation curve further to the left which, in association with low red cell 2,3-DPG levels, will result in poorer tissue oxygenation. Nevertheless, bicarbonate affords symptomatic relief to the severely acidotic patient and may reduce the risk of cardiac arrhythmias. Hockaday & Alberti (1972) have recommended that, if the blood pH is below 7.0, 125 mmol $NaHCO_3$ should be given, and if the pH is 7.0–7.1, 50 mmol $NaHCO_3$ should be given, repeating the dose 30 min later. The pH is measured again 1–2h after the bicarbonate and further treatment is given accordingly. Correction of acidaemia will lead to an increased shift of potassium into the cells and each infusion should be covered with 15–20 mmol of potassium. However, it must be remembered that potassium chloride *must not be added* to sodium bicarbonate infusions. The sodium bicarbonate infusion used should preferably be the isotonic (300 mmol/litre; 2.5%) solution. Sodium lactate should never be used.

CHRONIC COMPLICATIONS OF DIABETES MELLITUS

Autonomic neuropathy

Autonomic neuropathy is not at all uncommon in long-standing diabetics and often coincides with the presence of peripheral neuropathy, retinopathy and nephropathy. The complication is responsible for a wide range of troublesome and distressing symptoms, including dependent oedema of the lower limbs, disturbances of sweating, neurogenic bladder symptoms, gastric stasis and vomiting, bowel disturbances (notably nocturnal diarrhoea), impotence and postural hypotension.

Measurement of beat-to-beat heart rate (Page & Watkins 1977) and of the cardiovascular response to sustained hand-grip (Ewing et al 1974) have been used as accurate tests for autonomic neuropathy. Sundkvist et al (1979) have described a simple test of autonomic nervous function based on changes in the R–R interval on the ECG during maximal inspiration and expiration. They defined an E:I ratio of the mean of the longest R–R interval during maximal expiration to the mean of the shortest interval during maximal inspiration. An E:I ratio of 1.10 or less (which corresponds to a difference in heart rate between deep inspiration and expiration of 10% or less) appears to indicate autonomic dysfunction. Impaired secretion of pancreatic polypeptide in response to hypoglycaemia may also serve as an early sign of autonomic neuropathy (Krarup et al 1979).

However, the manifestations of autonomic neuropathy are not only unpleasant and inconvenient but may be life-threatening. Ewing et al (1976) studied 37 patients with symptoms and clinical features of autonomic neuropathy. Over a 33-month period, 10 of the 20 patients with abnormal Valsalva or hand-grip tests died — six of renal failure and the others of various causes; there was one 'sudden death'. These authors concluded that abnormal cardiovascular responses indicating autonomic neuropathy are associated with a high mortality. Page & Watkins (1978) described 12 episodes of cardiorespiratory arrest in eight young diabetics with severe autonomic neuropathy; three of these episodes were fatal and five occurred during or immediately after anaesthesia. They suggested that the arrests were caused by defective respiratory rather than cardiovascular reflexes and that such arrests appear to be a specific feature of diabetic autonomic neuropathy. Rees et al (1981) reported sleep apnoea in such patients. Thirty or more periods of apnoea lasting 10 seconds or longer during one night's sleep were demonstrated in three of the eight diabetic patients with autonomic neuropathy studied. These authors felt that such apnoeic episodes might be related to the high incidence of cardiac arrests reported in such patients. Ewing et al (1981) observed an increased resting heart rate in diabetics. They felt that in some patients this might be due to cardiac parasympathetic damage alone, and in others to combined parasympathetic and sympathetic damage. Their observations support the view that the vagus nerve is affected before the cardiac sympathetic nerves. It is therefore mandatory to screen all long-standing diabetic patients, particularly those in whom a surgical operation under general anaesthesia is planned, for autonomic neuropathy, using one of the methods described above. Beat-to-beat variation of the ECG is the simplest and is sufficiently accurate.

Impotence in diabetes mellitus

Although there is general agreement that impotence is commoner in diabetic than in non-diabetic men, there is less agreement about its exact incidence. It is often claimed that as many as 50% of diabetic men have some degree of impotence, although this high figure has recently been challenged (Hosking et al 1979, Lester et al 1980). Hosking and his colleagues studied nocturnal erections in 30 diabetic patients who complained of impotence and in 11 healthy volunteers. The maximal increase in penile circumference was measured by a penile strain gauge and recorded on a portable tape recorder; an external oculogram was recorded simultaneously to identify periods of REM sleep. Only six of the diabetic patients showed a maximal increase in penile circumference of less than 15 mm, whereas all but one of the healthy subjects showed maximum increases above this value. Of the six diabetics, five complained of total impotence and had other features of autonomic neuropathy that suggested an organic basis for their problem. The other patient complained of partial impotence which was probably caused by psychological factors. These findings suggest that the prevalence of *organic* impotence among diabetics has been greatly overestimated. In a small study, Lester and her colleagues found that the prevalence of impotence in diabetic men attending a hospital outpatient clinic was little different from that in non-diabetic men of the same age attending other outpatient clinics. The use of the penile strain gauge is a valuable technique for the investigation of impotence in diabetics, and can be expected to give useful therapeutic and diagnostic information that will guide management.

Diabetic nephropathy

Proteinuria is present in about 4% of patients with diabetes of less than one year's duration (although this is not usually associated with demonstrable basement membrane thickening (BMT) in the glomerular capillaries), increasing to a frequency of 16% or more in patients who have been known to have the disease for more than 10 years. In a significant number of the latter patients, proteinuria is due to lesions such as pyelonephritis, nephrosclerosis or hypertension. However, it has been estimated that at least 10% of patients who have had diabetes for more than 20 years will show histological glomerular lesions, and changes of diabetic glomerulosclerosis are observed in 40% of all diabetics at autopsy.

Diabetic glomerulosclerosis usually begins as a functional change marked by increased protein filtration through the glomeruli. Initially, this increased protein excretion will not usually be detected by the routine methods normally used. This slight proteinuria is present from the very onset of diabetes and probably reflects a generalised increase in capillary permeability. Over the next few years, particularly if diabetes is not well controlled, the basement membranes of the glomerular capillaries thicken and some of the glomeruli become occluded. Renal filtration and function decreases, ultimately leading to renal failure. The severe proteinuria that precedes and accompanies renal failure is always associated with the presence of marked BMT. Nephropathy is almost invariably associated with some degree of retinopathy and, commonly, neuropathy. As with retinopathy, it has been suggested that cigarette smoking may be a significant factor in the pathogenesis of nephropathy (Christiansen & Nerup 1978). McVerry et al (1980) gave mice repeated injections of plasma proteins glucosylated in vitro. Five of the seven mice treated in this way showed glomerular basement membrane thickening on electron microscopical examination, whereas no changes were observed in mice given multiple injections of non-glucosylated plasma proteins and in untreated mice. These experimental results suggest a link between plasma protein glucosylation and diabetic nephropathy, and it is now generally accepted that nephropathy, like the other lesions attributable to microangiopathy, has a close relationship with poor diabetic control.

The *clinical course* of renal complications may be insidious. At first, protein loss is slight and intermittent, but later it becomes massive and is unselective. A nephrotic syndrome may develop, but hypertension is a comparatively late feature. Heavy proteinuria is an ominous finding, and once significant impairment of renal function is observed, deterioration is progressive. Although such progression varies considerably from one patient to another, its rate is constant in individuals. Jones et al (1979a) have shown that for each patient there is a linear relationship between the interval in months which elapses from the time that the serum creatinine exceeds 200 μmol/l and the inverse (and also the log) of the serum creatinine concentration. Thus the time at which end-stage renal failure will develop can be predicted. More recently it has been shown that in type I diabetics with proteinuria, plasma concentrations of β_2-microglobulin correlate more closely than plasma creatinine concentrations or creatinine clearance with glomerular function, as measured by clearance of ^{51}Cr-labelled EDTA (Viberti et al 1981). In this study the plasma β_2-microglobulin concentration was raised in all patients with diminished glomerular filtration rate. These authors suggest that measurement of β_2-microglobulin concentrations is a simple and accurate (although expensive) method of detecting minor degrees of renal impairment in diabetics, and of monitoring the progress of the disease and the effects of treatment.

Treatment

No formal treatment has been shown to alter the progress of diabetic nephropathy, although in all cases it is important to treat coexisting urinary infection and hypertension. Sustained improvement in diabetic control may slow the rate of progression of nephropathy (Steno Study Group 1982), and this must remain a prime aim. The probability is that continuous subcutaneous insulin infusion (CSII) will achieve the desired level of control more readily and consistently than will traditional multiple subcutaneous insulin injections. Long-term haemodialysis is not well tolerated by diabetics and serious complications may occur (Jones et al 1979b). Continuous ambulatory peritoneal dialysis (CAPD) has been used as effective treatment for patients with renal failure caused by diabetes (Rubin et al 1977). Balducci and his colleagues (1981) have combined CAPD with intraperitoneal instillation of insulin, which seems effectively to control the diabetes and to avoid the need for subcutaneous insulin.

However, in suitable patients, well-timed live-related renal transplantation offers the best chance of survival with a good quality of life. Cadaver transplantation is less successful. The Minneapolis group recorded a 2-year cumulative patient survival for diabetics of 65% for a cadaver transplant and of over 80% for an HLA-identical live-related transplant from a sibling (Najarian et al 1977). A Joint Scandinavian Report (1978) showed a mean 2-year survival of around 67% — again, the results were better in live-donor transplants. This group found that survival was significantly reduced in patients with heart disease and impaired vision attributable to diabetic retinopathy, and in those with a long history of diabetes. Survival was not influenced by age, sex, neuropathy or pretransplantation dialysis. Diabetic retinopathy progressed slowly after successful transplantation but progression of large-vessel disease was common, leading to amputation(s) in 18 of the 146 insulin-dependent patients studied. Nevertheless, the quality of life of those who had successful transplantation was improved, and the main contraindication to renal transplantation would seem to be the presence of clinically significant large-vessel disease. Jones and his colleagues (1979a, b) suggested a programme of treatment for diabetic renal failure. Treatment should start early when the serum creatinine reaches 400–500 μmol/l and where possible a live-related transplant should be performed when the serum creatinine reaches 700–800 μmol/l. If this is not possible, the choice between similarly timed cadaver transplantation and maintenance dialysis must be made. Many would recommend the use of CSII in patients who are potential transplant candidates once the serum creatinine has exceeded 200 μmol/l, and Slama et al (1978) have suggested that the use of a biostator ('artificial pancreas') makes management during and immediately after transplantation much easier. Glomerulosclerosis may develop in transplanted kidneys, so biochemical control of the diabetes cannot be relaxed.

COMPLICATIONS OF DIABETES MELLITUS — PROGNOSIS AND PREVENTION

In middle age the death rate among diabetics is two to six times higher than that of the general population, and this increased mortality is largely accounted for by cardiovascular and renal disease. The overall mortality is such that 56% of a cohort of young diabetics were dead 40 years after diagnosis of their disease compared with only 10% of a control population. Rather less than a third of the deaths were due to uraemia and about a quarter were the result of a cardiovascular event (Deckert et al 1978a). In addition, diabetes remains the most common cause of blindness in Britain among people below the age of retirement. However, there is another side to this depressing picture. In practice, follow-up studies have shown that at least one-third of long-surviving diabetics are free of retinopathy and over 80% are free from incapacitating complications (Oakley et al 1974, Deckert et al 1978b). Long-standing diabetes is therefore compatible with good health (Editorial, British Medical Journal 1981b). Furthermore, all of these figures refer to diabetic patients who were diagnosed in the 1940s or 1950s — diabetic management was much less rigorous and more permissive then than in recent years. Two-thirds of long survivors are women.

The angiopathic complications of diabetes occur irrespective of the genetic nature of the diabetic trait; even 'MODY' type diabetes is not entirely benign (Fajans et al 1978). Vascular complications increase in frequency with increasing duration of diabetes. Few obese patients are found among long survivors, and leanness may be related to low insulin dosage, normal triglyceride concentrations and increased insulin sensitivity — these factors have been associated with long survival. Whether some of the other abnormalities that have been reported as associations of vascular complications precede or are a consequence of them is not known. Diabetic nephropathy is more common among cigarette smokers (Christiansen & Nerup 1978), and retinopathy is associated with abnormal blood viscosity, increased antithrombin III and factor VII, immune complexes and high titres of insulin antibodies, as well as smoking. Hypertension is rare in patients with long-standing diabetes (Oakley et al 1974, Deckert et al 1978b), but when present it accelerates the rate of decline in renal function in patients with nephropathy. Martin & Warne (1975) studied 51 type I diabetics over a period of 7 years. In patients with clinical vascular disease, hypertension and fasting hypertriglyceridaemia were bad prognostic signs. Acute insensitivity to intravenous insulin was correlated with the presence of initial vascular disease and was significantly related both to death and to clinical deterioration in either large-vessel or small-vessel disease.

It has long been debated whether good biochemical control might delay or lessen the severity of the manifestations of small-vessel disease (Cahill et al 1976). The problem is that the great majority of type I diabetic patients are, by any criteria, not well controlled for much of the time. A major difficulty in the past has been our inability to assess accurately the degree of hyperglycaemia on a long-term basis. In this regard, home monitoring and the use of serial estimations of glycosylated haemoglobin may well prove to be helpful. However, there are now many reports which indicate that 'good' control does pay dividends (Pirart 1978, Tchobroutsky 1978, Eschwege et al 1979). In particular, the superiority of divided-dose insulin regimens over single daily injections has been demonstrated (Job et al 1976). Until we understand better the aetiology of small-vessel disease and its relationship to the observable metabolic defects in diabetes, early diagnosis and the best possible biochemical control must be fundamental aims.

It is quite possible that those patients who are most difficult to stabilise have a particularly 'severe' form of the disease and are therefore more at risk of developing vascular complications. Cause and effect are still not clearly separable. Nevertheless, the conviction that diabetic control influences microangiopathy is sufficient to justify attempts to improve it by new methods of treatment (Watkins 1980). Such techniques, which involve continuous insulin infusion, have proved successful in the short term and seem to avoid serious hypoglycaemia (Pickup et al 1979a, b). Their continued development during the next few years will show whether or not they prove as successful in preventing, delaying or reversing the vascular complications of diabetes. Preliminary reports give grounds for cautious optimism. An interim report from Denmark (Steno Study Group 1982) has studied the effects of 6 months of strict metabolic control upon eye and kidney function in 32 type I diabetics randomised either to unchanged conventional treatment (UCT) or to continuous subcutaneous insulin infusion (CSII). Although the UCT group showed significant deterioration in all indices of retinal function, patients treated with CSII showed a distinct improvement. Glomerular filtration rate fell by 9% in the CSII group and rose 2% in the UCT patients. However, urinary albumin excretion fell by 12% with CSII and rose by 56% with UCT. This report supports the view that long-term control which achieves near-normal blood glucose levels may arrest or even reverse some of the features associated with diabetic microangiopathy.

DIABETES AND PREGNANCY

The definitions and diagnosis of impaired glucose tolerance during pregnancy and of gestational diabetes have already been referred to. The use of twice-daily insulin during pregnancy has been emphasised and home monitoring and the value of serial estimations of glycosylated haemoglobin in assessing control have been discussed.

It is now well established that maternal hyperglycaemia is the primary factor jeopardising the outcome of the diabetic pregnancy, and recent studies of HbA_1 during the course of pregnancy in the diabetic patient have provided further support for this conclusion. Diabetic control during pregnancy should be precise to the point of obsession and the value of continuous antenatal supervision by a single specialised team is generally accepted. Throughout the greater part of pregnancy, control is achieved by weekly or fortnightly visits to adjust insulin dosage and dietary needs (the diet will usually need to be supplemented to allow for increased urinary glucose loss). Blood glucose estimations provide an accurate basis for control; an increasing number of patients carry out regular home monitoring, usually using BM 20–800 reagent strips, but sometimes with the aid of a battery-operated reflectance meter. The ease with which capillary blood samples are obtained may be greatly increased by the use of 'Autolet®' (Owen Mumford, Ltd) or 'Autoclix®' (Boehringer Mannheim) devices. Blood glucose concentrations should be maintined at less than 7–8 mmol/l; after 32 weeks the aim is to maintain levels below 5.5–6 mmol/l. Potter et al (1980) have described the use of continuous subcutaneous insulin infusion in diabetics during the third trimester of pregnancy; this method may be useful in limiting possible diurnal fluctuations of blood glucose. However, motivation is usually so high during pregnancy that with frequent and close supervision allied to continued education and advice, good control should not be difficult to achieve in the great majority of patients using conventional twice-daily subcutaneous injections. Troublesome hypoglycaemia is seldom a problem. Accurate control of blood glucose results in a smaller baby, greatly improves fetal outcome and almost certainly reduces the incidence of polyhydramnios and of pre-eclampsia.

The optimum time for delivery is at about the 38th week, although special reasons such as renal or cardiovascular disease, polyhydramnios, antepartum haemorrhage and pre-eclampsia might modify this policy. Some would advise allowing the pregnancy to proceed to the 39th week, but even with apparently tight control, occasional late intrauterine death might occur and the baby may still be larger than average, so the risk of a difficult delivery remains. The choice of the mode of delivery is less important than the time at which it is undertaken. The decision whether to induce labour or to advise elective Caesarean section will take into account obstetric and fetal factors, the personality of the patient, the severity and stability of the diabetes, the presence or absence of other complicating factors and the patient's past obstetric history.

During labour, the keynotes of management are meticulous supervision and constant biochemical monitoring. The method adopted to maintain control during labour depends on the facilities available, but a sine qua non is that a physician should be available constantly to advise and direct management and to participate in discussion should a change of plan be considered. A number of different regimens are available (Anderson 1980); local practice, facilities and experience will determine which is used. Immediately after delivery, insulin requirements fall markedly, reaching pre-pregnancy levels or even lower. A useful rule of thumb is to cut insulin doses immediately after delivery either to the pre-pregnancy level or to 50% (at most) of the dosages that achieved stability immediately before labour began, whichever is the lower. Breast-feeding is not contraindicated in diabetes but, if this is undertaken, additional dietary carbohydrate will usually be needed. Patients with gestational diabetes and impaired glucose tolerance must be reviewed and if necessary followed up after delivery.

With careful supervision, fetal loss should not exceed 5–6% in insulin-dependent patients and in many large centres is even lower. However, a disturbingly high incidence of congenital malformation is observed in infants born to diabetic patients. Soler et al (1976) reported an incidence of 8.1% in 701 infants born to diabetic mothers — a rate about four times higher than that in the normal population. Provided that gestational diabetes and impaired glucose tolerance are diagnosed as early as possible and are appropriately treated (insulin must not be withheld if diet fails to maintain blood glucose concentrations below about 6–6.5 mmol/l), fetal loss and congenital abnormalities should not exceed those rates observed in the non-diabetic patient. However, if these disorders are not detected or are not effectively treated, the risk of fetal loss increases.

It is now universally accepted that control during the first 8–10 weeks is particularly critical. More and more centres are therefore running pre-pregnancy clinics so that diabetics can be adequately educated in techniques of home monitoring, their control can be optimised before conception and pregnancy is diagnosed as early as possible. Effective screening techniques for the detection of gestational diabetes and impaired glucose tolerance have been described by Lind & McDougall (1981). The more carefully these disorders are sought, the more frequently they will be diagnosed.

REFERENCES

Alberti K G M M 1976 Comparison of different insulin regimens in diabetic ketoacidosis. Lancet 1: 83

Alberti K G M M, Nattrass M 1977 Lactic acidosis. Lancet 2: 25–29

Alberti K G M M, Hockaday T D R, Turner R C 1973 Small doses of intramuscular insulin in the treatment of diabetic 'coma'. Lancet 2: 515–521

Alberti K G M M, Christensen N J Iversen J, Ørskov H 1975 Role of glucagon and other hormones in development of diabetic ketoacidosis. Lancet 1: 1307–1311

Albisser A M, Leibel B S 1977 The artificial pancreas. Clinics in Endocrinology and Metabolism 6: 457–474

Anderson J 1980 Diabetes mellitus. In: Hall R, Anderson J, Smart G A, Besser G M (eds) Fundamentals of clinical endocrinology, 3rd edn. Pitman Medical, London, p 483–582

Anderson J 1981 Disorders of metabolism I. In: Davies D M (ed) Textbook of adverse drug reactions, 2nd edn. Oxford University Press, Oxford, p 314–329

Anderson J W, Ward K 1978 Long-term effects of high carbohydrate, high fibre diets on glucose and lipid metabolism: a preliminary report on patients with diabetes. Diabetes Care 1: 77–82

Andersson A 1979 Islet implantation normalises hyperglycaemia caused by streptozotocin-induced insulitis. Lancet 1: 581–584

Asplin C M, Hockaday T D R, Smith R F, Moore R A 1980 Detection of unrecognised nocturnal hypoglycaemia in insulin-treated diabetics. British Medical Journal 2: 357–360

Baker R A, Schmidtke J R, Ross J W, Smith W C 1981 Preliminary studies on the immunogenicity and amount of *Escherichia coli* polypeptides in biosynthetic human insulin produced by recombinant DNA technology. Lancet 2: 1139–1142

Balducci A, Slama G, Rottembourg J, Baumelou A, Delage A 1981 Intraperitoneal insulin in uraemic diabetics undergoing continuous ambulatory peritoneal dialysis. British Medical Journal 283: 1021–1023

Barbosa J 1977 HLA and diabetes mellitus. Lancet 1: 906–907

Barbosa J, Menth L, Sutherland D, Eaton J, Najarian J 1981 Long-term, ambulatory subcutaneous infusion vs multiple daily injections in brittle diabetics. Diabetes Care 3: 351–358

Barnes A J, Garbien K J T, Crowley M F, Bloom A 1974 Effect of short-and long-term chlorpropamide treatment on insulin release and blood-glucose. Lancet 2: 69–72

Bayliss J 1981 Brittle diabetes: long-term control with a portable, continuous, intravenous insulin infusion system. British Medical Journal 283: 1207–1209

Bloom A, Hayes T M, Gamble D R 1975 Register of newly diagnosed diabetic children. British Medical Journal 3: 580–583

Bloom A, Keen H, Watkins P J 1981 A change to 100-unit insulin dosage will reduce errors. British Medical Journal 283: 33–34

Bloom S R, Adrian T E, Barnes A J, Polak J M 1979 Autoimmunity in diabetics induced by hormonal contaminants of insulin. Lancet 1: 14–17

Boden G, Master R W, Gordon S S, Shuman C R, Owen O E 1980 Monitoring metabolic control in diabetic outpatients with glycosylated haemoglobin. Annals of Internal Medicine 92: 357–360

Bottazzo G F, Doniach D 1976 Pancreatic autoimmunity and HLA antigens. Lancet 2: 800

Bottazzo G F, Dean B M, Gorsuch A N, Cudworth A G, Doniach D 1980 Complement-fixing islet-cell antibodies in type-I diabetes: possible monitors of active beta-cell damage. Lancet 1: 668–672

Boyle D, Bhatia S K, Hadden D R, Montogomery D A D, Weaver J A 1972 Ischaemic heart disease in diabetics. A prospective study. Lancet 1: 338–339

British Diabetic Association Medical Advisory Committee 1978 Draft memorandum regarding diagnostic criteria for diabetes mellitus.

Brooks A P, Nairn I M, Baird J D 1980a Changes in glycosylated haemoglobin after poor control in insulin-dependent diabetics. British Medical Journal 2: 707–710

Brooks A P, Metcalfe J, Day J L, Edwards M S 1980b Iron deficiency and glycosylated haemoglobin A_1. Lancet 2: 141

Buchwald H, Barbosa J, Varco R L, Rohde T D, Rupp W M, Schwartz R A et al 1981 Treatment of a type II diabetic by a totally implantable insulin infusion device. Lancet 1: 1233–1235

Buckle A L J, Nattrass M, Cluett B E, Stubbs W A, Walton R J, Alberti, K G M M et al 1977 Blood metabolite concentrations in diabetics: effect of normalization of blood glucose using a glucose controlled insulin infusion system (GCIIS). Diabetologia 13: 385

Cahill G F Jr, Etzwiler D D, Freinkel N 1976 'Control' and diabetes. New England Journal of Medicine 294: 1004–1005

Christiansen J S, Nerup J 1978 Smoking and diabetic nephropathy. Lancet 1: 605

Cudworth A G 1976 The aetiology of diabetes. British Journal of Hospital Medicine 16: 207–216

Cudworth A G Woodrow J C 1976 Genetic susceptibility in diabetes mellitus: analysis of the HLA association. British Medical Journal 2: 846–848

Cudworth A G, Gamble D R, White G B B, Lendrum R, Woodrow J C, Bloom A 1977 Aetiology of juvenile-onset diabetes. Lancet 1: 385-388

Dandona P, Freedman D, Moorhead J F 1979 Glycosylated haemoglobin in chronic renal failure. British Medical Journal 1: 1183–1184

Dandona P, Foster M, Healey F, Greenbury E, Beckett A G 1978 Low-dose insulin infusions in diabetic patients with high insulin requirements. Lancet 2: 283–285
De Boer M-J, Miedema K, Casparie A F 1980 Glycosylated haemoglobin in renal failure. Diabetologia 18: 437–440
Deckert T, Poulsen J E, Larsen M 1978a Prognosis of diabetics with diabetes onset before the age of 31. I. Survival, causes of death and complications. Diabetologia 14: 363–370
Deckert T, Poulsen J E, Larsen M 1978b Prognosis of diabetics with diabetes onset before the age of 31. II. Factors affecting the prognosis. Diabetologia 14: 371–377
Dolhofer R, Wieland O H 1980 Increased glycosylation of serum albumin in diabetes mellitus. Diabetes 29: 417–422
Editorial 1976 Glycosylated hemoglobin and diabetic control. New England Journal of Medicine 295: 443–444
Editorial 1978 Glycosylated haemoglobin and diabetic control. British Medical Journal 1: 1373–1374
Editorial 1980 Haemoglobin A_1 and diabetes: a reappraisal. British Medical Journal 281: 1304–1305
Editorial 1981a Insulin injections and infection. British Medical Journal 282: 340
Editorial 1981b Prolonged disease-free survival in diabetics. British Medical Journal 282: 1339–1340
Editorial 1975 Islet-cell transplantation. Lancet 2: 909–910
Editorial 1979 Highly purified insulins. Lancet 1: 363–364
Editorial 1980a Subcutaneous injections and absorption of insulin. Lancet 1: 1005–1006
Editorial 1980b Diabetic control at night. Lancet 2: 297–298
Editorial 1980c Home blood-glucose monitoring: revolution, revelation or rip-off? Lancet 2: 187–188
Editorial 1980d Behaviour disorders in diabetic children. Lancet 2: 188–189
Editorial 1981 High-fibre diets and diabetes. Lancet 1: 423–424
Editorial 1982 Genetics of insulin-dependent diabetes. Lancet 1: 263.
Elkeles R S, Wu J, Hambley J 1978 Haemoglobin A_1, blood glucose, and high-density lipoprotein cholesterol in insulin-requiring diabetics. Lancet 2: 547–549
Eschwege E, Job D, Guyot-Argenton C, Aubry J P, Tchobroutsky G 1979. Delayed progression of diabetic retinopathy by divided insulin administration: a further follow-up. Diabetologia 16: 13–15
Ewing D J, Campbell I W, Clarke B F 1976 Mortality in diabetic autonomic neuropathy. Lancet 1: 601–603
Ewing D J, Campbell I W, Clarke B F 1981 Heart rate changes in diabetes mellitus. Lancet 1: 183–186
Ewing D J, Irving J B, Kerr F, Wildsmith J A W, Clarke B F 1974 Cardiovascular responses to sustained handgrip in normal subjects and in patients with diabetes mellitus: a test of autonomic function. Clinical Science and Molecular Medicine 46: 295–306
Fajans S S, Cloutier M C, Crowther R L 1978 Clinical and etiologic heterogeneity of idiopathic diabetes mellitus. Diabetes 27: 1112–1125
Ferguson S D, Prosser R 1980 Are reflectance meters necessary for home blood glucose monitoring? British Medical Journal 281: 912
Fitzgerald M G, Keen H 1964 Diagnostic classification of diabetes. Lancet 1: 1325–1326
Flier J S, Kahn R, Roth J 1979 Receptors, antireceptor antibodies and mechanisms of insulin resistance. New England Journal of Medicine 300: 413–419
Fraser D M, Smith A F, Gray R S, Borsey D Q, Sinclair M E, Clarke B F et al 1979 Glycosylated haemoglobin concentrations in newly diagnosed diabetics before and during treatment. British Medical Journal 1: 979–981
Gale E A M, Tattersall R B 1979a Brittle diabetes. British Journal of Hospital Medicine 22: 589–597
Gale E A M, Tattersall R B 1979b Unrecognised nocturnal hypoglycaemia in insulin-treated diabetics. Lancet 1: 1049–1052
Gale E A M, Kurtz A B, Tattersall R B 1980 In search of the Somogyi effect. Lancet 2: 279–282
Gale E A M, Walford S, Tattersall R B 1979 Nocturnal hypoglycaemia and haemoglobin A_1. Lancet 2: 1240–1241
Gamble D R 1980 Relation of antecedent illness to development of diabetes in children. British Medical Journal 281: 99–101
Goetz F C 1974 Conference on beta cell function, transplantation, and implantable glucose sensors: a summary. Metabolism 23: 875–884
Goldstein D E, Peth S B, England J D, Hess R L, Da Costa J 1980 Effects of acute changes in blood glucose on HbA_{1c}. Diabetes 29: 623–628
Gonen B, Rubenstein A H, Rochman H, Tanega S P, Horwitz D L 1977 Haemoglobin A_1: an indicator of the metabolic control of diabetic patients. Lancet 2: 734–737
Gorsuch A N, Dean B M, Bottazzo G F, Lister J, Cudworth A G 1980 Evidence that type I diabetes and thyrogastric autoimmunity have different genetic determinants. British Medical Journal 280: 145–147

Graham K, Kesson C M, Kennedy H B, Ireland J T 1980 Relevance of colour vision and diabetic retinopathy to self-monitoring of blood glucose. British Medical Journal 281: 971–973

Greenough A, Cockcroft P M, Bloom A 1979 Disposable syringes for insulin injection. British Medical Journal 1: 1467–1468

Hadden D R, Montgomery D A D, Weaver J A 1972 Myocardial infarction in maturity-onset diabetics. A retrospective study. Lancet 1: 335–338

Hecht A, Gershberg H, Hulse M 1973 Effect of chlorpropamide treatment on insulin secretion in diabetics: its relationship to the hypoglycaemic effect. Metabolism 22: 723–733

Helgason T, Jonasson M R 1981 Evidence for a food additive as a cause of ketosis-prone diabetes. Lancet 2: 716–720

Hockaday T D R, Alberti K G M M 1972 Diabetic coma. Clinics in Endocrinology and Metabolism 1: 751–788

Hodge R H Jr, Krongaard L, Sande M A, Kaiser D L 1980 Multiple use of disposable insulin syringe-needle units. Journal of the American Medical Association 244: 266–267

Hodge S E, Anderson C E, Neiswanger K, Field L L, Spence M A, Sparkes R S et al 1981 Close genetic linkage between diabetes mellitus and Kidd blood group. Lancet 2: 893–895

Holman R R, Turner R C 1977 Diabetes: the quest for basal normoglycaemia. Lancet 1: 469–474

Hosking D J, Bennet T, Hampton J R, Evans D F, Clark A J, Robertson G 1979 Diabetic impotence: studies of nocturnal erection during REM sleep. British Medical Journal 2: 1394–1396

Howe-Davies S, Holman R R, Phillips M, Turner R C 1978 Home blood sampling for plasma glucose assay in control of diabetes. British Medical Journal 2: 596–598

Irvine W J, Gray R S, McCallum C J 1976 Pancreatic islet-cell antibody as a marker for asymptomatic and latent diabetes and prediabetes. Lancet 2: 1097–1102

Irvine W J, McCallum C J, Gray R S, Campbell C J, Duncan L J P, Farquhar J W et al 1977 Pancreatic islet-cell antibodies in diabetes mellitus correlated with the duration and type of diabetes, coexistent autoimmune disease, and HLA type. Diabetes 26: 138–147

Jackson W P U, Van Mieghem W, Keller P 1973 Observations on the mechanism of action of the sulfonylureas under clinical conditions. Metabolism 22: 1155–1162

Jarrett R J, Keen H 1976 Hyperglycaemia and diabetes mellitus. Lancet 2: 1009–1012

Jenkins D J A, Goff D W, Leeds A R, Alberti K G M M, Wolever T M S, Gassull M A et al 1976 Unabsorbable carbohydrates and diabetes: decreased postprandial hyperglycaemia. Lancet 2: 172–174

Jenkins D J A, Hockday T D R, Wolever T M S, Nineham R, Goff D V, Haisman P et al 1979. Dietary fibre and ketone bodies: reduced urinary 3-hydroxybutyrate excretion in diabetics on guar. British Medical Journal 2: 1555

Jenkins D J A, Wolever T M S, Leeds A R, Gassull M A, Haisman P, Dilawari J et al 1978 Dietary fibre, fibre analogues, and glucose tolerance: importance of viscosity. British Medical Journal 1: 1392–1394

Jenkins D J A, Wolever T M S, Taylor R H, Barker H M, Fielden H, Jenkins A L 1980 Effect of guar crispbread with cereal products and leguminous seeds on blood glucose concentrations of diabetics. British Medical Journal 281: 1248–1250

Job D, Eschwege E, Guyot-Argenton C, Aubry J P, Tchobroutsky G 1976 Effect of multiple daily insulin injections on the course of diabetic retinopathy. Diabetes 25: 463–469

Joint Scandinavian Report 1978 Renal transplantation in insulin-dependent diabetics. Lancet 2: 915–917

Jones G R, Statham B, Owens D R, Jones M K, Hayes T M 1981 Lipoatrophy and monocomponent porcine insulin. British Medical Journal 282: 190

Jones R H, Hayakawa H, Mackay J D, Parsons V, Watkins P J 1979a Progression of diabetic nephropathy. Lancet 1: 1105–1106

Jones R H, Rudge C J, Watkins P J, Bewick M, Parsons V 1979b Renal transplantation in insulin-requiring diabetics. Lancet 1: 153

Keen H, Jarrett R J, Chlouverakis C, Boyns D R 1968 The effect of treatment of moderate hyperglycaemia on the incidence of arterial disease. Postgraduate Medical Journal 44: 960–965

Keen H, Glynne A, Pickup J C, Viberti G C, Bilous R W, Jarrett R J et al 1980 Human insulin produced by recombinant DNA technology: safety and hypoglycaemic potency in healthy men. Lancet 2: 398–401

Kinmonth A L, Baum J D 1980 Timing of pre-breakfast insulin injection and postprandial metabolic control in diabetic children. British Medical Journal 280: 604–606

Klemp P, Staberg B, Madsbad S, Kølendorf K 1982 Smoking reduces insulin absorption from subcutaneous tissue. British Medical Journal 284: 237

Koivisto V A 1980 Sauna-induced acceleration in insulin absorption from subcutaneous injection site. British Medical Journal 280: 1411–1413

Krarup T, Schwart T W, Hilsted J, Madsbad S, Verlaege O, Sestoft L 1979 Impaired response of pancreatic polypeptide to hypoglycaemia: an early sign of autonomic neuropathy in diabetics. British Medical Journal 2: 1544–1546

Lendrum R, Walker G, Cudworth A G, Theophanides C, Pyke D A, Bloom A et al 1976 Islet-cell antibodies in diabetes mellitus. Lancet 2: 1273–1276

Lernmark A, Freedman Z R, Hofmann C, Rubenstein A H, Steiner D F, Jackson R L et al (1978) Islet-cell surface antibodies in juvenile diabetes mellitus. New England Journal of Medicine 299: 375–380

Lester E, Grant A J, Woodroffe F J 1980 Impotence in diabetic and non-diabetic hospital outpatients. British Medical Journal 281: 354–355

Lind T, McDougall A N 1981 Antenatal screening for diabetes mellitus by random blood glucose sampling. British Journal of Obstetrics and Gynaecology 88: 346–351

Lundbaek K, Christensen S E, Hansen A P, Iversen J, Orskov H, Seyer-Hansen K et al 1976 Failure of somatostatin to correct manifest diabetic ketoacidosis. Lancet 1: 215–218

MacCuish A C, Jordan J, Campbell C J, Duncan L J P, Irvine W J 1975 Cell-mediated immunity in diabetes mellitus: lymphocyte transformation by insulin and insulin fragments in insulin-treated and newly-diagnosed diabetes. Diabetes 24: 36–43

McVerry B A, Fisher C, Hopp A, Huehns E R 1980 Production of pseudodiabetic renal glomerular changes in mice after repeated injections of glucosylated proteins. Lancet 1: 738–740

Madsbad S, Alberti K G M M, Binder C, Burrin J M, Faber O K, Krarup T, Regeur L 1979 Role of residual insulin secretion in protecting against ketoacidosis in insulin-dependent diabetes. British Medical Journal 2: 1257–1259

Malins J M 1971 The management of diabetic coma. Journal of the Royal College of Physicians of London 6: 75–82

Marquat F X, Poynard J P, Borel J P, Leutenegger M 1978 Evolution of haemoglobin A_{Ic} after oral glucose. Lancet 2: 431–432

Martin F I R, Warne G L 1975 Factors influencing the prognosis of vascular disease in insulin-deficient diabetes of long duration: a seven-year follow up. Metabolism 24: 1–9

Menser M A, Forrest J M, Bransby R D 1978 Rubella infection and diabetes mellitus. Lancet 1: 57–60

Miranda P M, Horwitz D L 1978 High fibre diets in the treatment of diabetes mellitus. Annals of Internal Medicine 88: 482–486

Monnier L H, Blotman M J, Colette C, Monnier M P, Mirouze J 1981 Effects of dietary fibre supplementation in stable and labile insulin-dependent diabetics. Diabetologia 20: 12–17

Morris P J, Vaughan H, Irvine W J, McCallum F J, Gray R S, Campbell C J et al 1976 HLA and pancreatic islet-cell antibodies in diabetes. Lancet 2: 652–653

Mutch W J, Stowers J M 1980 Reversible mild diabetes in children after treatment with chlorpropamide. Lancet 1: 1158–1161

Najarian J S, Sutherland D E R, Simmons R L, Howard R J, Kjellstrand C M, Mauer S M et al 1977 Kidney transplantation for the uremic diabetic patient. Surgery, Gynaecology and Obstetrics 144: 682–690

Nattrass M, Alberti K G M M, Dennis K J, Gillibrand P N, Letchworth A T, Buckle A L J 1978 A glucose-controlled insulin infusion system for diabetic women during labour. British Medical Journal 2: 599–601

Nelson P G, Pyke D A, Cudworth A G, Woodrow J C, Batchelor J R 1975 Histocompatibility antigens in diabetic identical twins. Lancet 2: 193–194

Nerup J, Ortved Anderson O, Bendixen G, Egeberg J, Poulsen J E 1971 Antipancreatic cellular hypersensitivity in diabetes mellitus. Diabetes 20: 424–427

Nerup J, Platz P, Anderson O O, Christy M, Lyngsøe J, Poulsen J E et al 1974 HLA antigens and diabetes mellitus. Lancet 2: 864–866

Oakley W G, Pyke D A, Tattersall R B, Watkins P J 1974 Long-term diabetes. A clinical study of 92 patients after 40 years. Quarterly Journal of Medicine 43: 145–156

Oli J M, Gugnani H C, Ojiegbe G C 1982 Multiple use of ordinary disposable syringes for insulin injections. British Medical Journal 284: 236

Owens D R, Jones M K, Hayes T M, Heding L G, Alberti K G M M, Home P D et al 1981a Human insulin: study of safety and efficacy in man. British Medical Journal 282: 1264–1266

Owens D R, Jones M K, Hayes T M, Heding L G, Alberti K G M M, Home P D et al 1981b Comparative study of subcutaneous, intramuscular, and intravenous administration of human insulin. Lancet 2: 118–122

Page M McB, Watkins P J 1977 The heart in diabetes: autonomic neuropathy and cardiomyopathy. Clinics in Endocrinology and Metabolism 6: 377–388

Page M McB, Watkins P J 1978 Cardiorespiratory arrest and diabetic autonomic neuropathy. Lancet 1: 14–16

Page M M, Asmal A C, Edwards C R W 1976a Recessive inheritance of diabetes: the syndrome of diabetes insipidus, diabetes mellitus, optic atrophy and deafness. Quarterly Journal of Medicine 45: 505–520

Page M M, Pyke D A, Watkins P J 1976b Comparison of different insulin regimens in diabetic ketoacidosis. Lancet 1: 83–84

Paisey R B, Bradshaw P, Hartog M 1980 Home blood glucose concentrations in maturity onset diabetes. British Medical Journal 280: 596–598

Peacock I, Hunter J C, Walford S, Allison S P, Davison J, Clark P et al 1979 Self-monitoring of blood glucose in diabetic pregnancy. British Medical Journal 2: 1333–1336

Phillips M, Simpson R W, Holman R R, Turner R C 1979 A simple and rational twice daily insulin regime. Quarterly Journal of Medicine 48: 493–506

Pickup J C, Keen H, Parsons J A, Alberti K G M M 1978 Continuous subcutaneous insulin infusion: an approach to achieving normoglycaemia. British Medical Journal 1: 204–207

Pickup J C, Keen H, Viberti G C, Bilous R W 1981 Patient reactions to long-term outpatient treatment with continuous subcutaneous insulin infusion. British Medical Journal 282: 766–768

Pickup J C, Keen H, Parsons J A, Alberti K G M M, Rowe A S 1979a Continuous subcutaneous insulin infusion: improved blood-glucose and intermediary metabolite control in diabetics. Lancet 1: 1255–1258

Pickup J C, White M C, Keen H, Parsons J A, Alberti K G M M 1979b Long-term continuous subcutaneous insulin infusion in diabetics at home. Lancet 2: 870–873

Pirart J 1978 Diabetes mellitus and its degenerative complications: a prospective study of 4400 patients observed between 1947 and 1973. Diabetes Care 1: 168–188

Pontiroli A E, Alberetto M, Secchi A, Dossi G, Bosi I, Pozza G 1982 Insulin given intranasally induces hypoglycaemia in normal and diabetic subjects. British Medical Journal 284: 303–306

Potter J M, Reckless J P D, Cullen D R 1980 Subcutaneous continuous insulin infusion and control of blood glucose concentration in diabetics in third trimester of pregnancy. British Medical Journal 280: 1099–1101

Raum D, Alper C A, Stein R, Gabbay K H 1979 Genetic marker for insulin-dependent diabetes mellitus. Lancet 1: 1208–1210

Reaven G M 1980 How high the carbohydrate? Diabetologia 19: 409–413

Rees P J, Prior J G, Cochrane G M, Clark T J H 1981 Sleep apnoea in diabetic patients with autonomic neuropathy. Journal of the Royal Society of Medicine 74: 192–195

Reeves W G, Allen B R, Tattersall R B 1980 Insulin-induced lipoatrophy: evidence for an immune pathogenesis. British Medical Journal 280: 1500–1503

Rittner C, Bertrams J 1981 On the significance of C2, C4 and factor B polymorphisms in disease. Human Genetics 57: 235–247

Rubin J, Orepoulos D G, Blair R D G, Chisholm L D J, Meema H E, De Veber G A 1977 Chronic peritoneal dialysis in the management of diabetics with terminal renal failure. Nephron 19: 265–270

Sartor G, Schersten B, Carlström S, Melander A, Norden A, Persson G 1980 Ten-year follow-up of subjects with impaired glucose tolerance. Prevention of diabetes by tolbutamide and diet regulation. Diabetes 29: 41–49

Scobie I N, Onyanga-Omara F, Singaraveloo M, Forrest A R W, MacCuish A C, Manderson W G 1981 Changes in glycosylated haemoglobin after oral glucose load. British Medical Journal 283: 877–878

Simpson H C R, Simpson R W, Lusley S, Carter R D, Geekie M, Hockaday T D R et al 1981 A high carbohydrate leguminous fibre diet improves all aspects of diabetic control. Lancet 1: 1–5

Slama G, Klein J C, Meroccani A, Frantz P 1978 Artificial pancreas for renal transplantation in a diabetic. Lancet 1: 665

Soler N G, Bennett M A, Dixon K, FitzGerald M G, Malins J M 1972 Potassium balance during treatment of diabetic ketoacidosis. Lancet 2: 666–667

Soler N G, Walsh C H, Malins J M 1976 Congenital malformations in infants of diabetic mothers. Quarterly Journal of Medicine 45: 303–315

Soler N G, Wright A D, FitzGerald M G, Malins J M 1975 Comparative study of different insulin regimens in management of diabetic ketoacidosis. Lancet 2: 1221–1224

Somogyi M 1959 Exacerbation of diabetes by excess insulin action. American Journal of Medicine 26: 169–191

Sönksen P H, Judd S L, Lowy C 1978 Home monitoring of blood glucose. Lancet 1: 730–732

Steno Study Group 1982 Effect of 6 months of strict metabolic control on eye and kidney function in insulin-dependent diabetics with background retinopathy. Lancet 1: 121–124

Stubbs S M, Brudenell J M, Pyke D A, Watkins P J, Stubbs W A, Alberti K G M M 1980 Management of the pregnant diabetic: home or hospital, with or without glucose meters? Lancet 1: 1122–1124

Sundkvist G, Almér L-O, Lilja B 1979 Respiratory influence on heart rate in diabetes mellitus. British Medical Journal 1: 924–925

Svendsen P A, Christiansen J S, Segaard U, Welinder B S, Nerup J 1980 Rapid changes in chromatographically determined haemoglobin A_{Ic} induced by short-term changes in glucose concentrations. Diabetologia 19: 130–136

Tamborlane W V, Sherwin R S, Genel M, Felig P 1979 Restoration of normal lipid and aminoacid metabolism in diabetic patients treated with a portable insulin-infusion pump. Lancet 1: 1258–1261

Tattersall R B 1977 Brittle diabetes. Clinics in Endocrinology and Metabolism 6: 403–419

Tattersall R B 1979 Home blood glucose monitoring. Diabetologia 16: 71–74

Tattersall R B, Fajans S S 1975 A difference between the inheritance of classical juvenile-onset and maturity-onset type diabetes of young people. Diabetes 24: 44–53

Tchobroutsky G 1978 Relation of diabetic control to development of microvascular complications. Diabetologia 15: 143–152

Thomas B, Truswell A S, Brown A 1974 Diabetic diet sheets used in Great Britain. I. Aspects of presentation and content. Nutrition 28: 297–312

Thomsen M, Nerup J, Platz P, Christy M, Ortved Anderson O, Ryder L P et al 1975 MLC typing in juvenile diabetes mellitus and idiopathic Addison's disease. Transplantation Reviews 22: 125–147

Tomkins A M, Bloom A 1972 Assessment of the need for continued oral therapy in diabetics. British Medical Journal 1: 649–651

Tomkin G H, Hadden D R, Weaver J A, Montgomery, D A D 1971 Vitamin-B_{12} status of patients on long-term metformin therapy. British Medical Journal 2: 685–687

Tunbridge W M G 1981 Factors contributing to deaths of diabetics under 50 years of age. Lancet 2: 569–572

University Group Diabetes Program 1970 A study of the effects of hypoglycemic agents on vascular complications in patients with adult-onset diabetes. Diabetes 19 (suppl. 2): 787-830

Viberti G C, Keen H, Mackintosh D 1981 Beta$_2$-microglobulinaemia: a sensitive index of diminishing renal function in diabetics. British Medical Journal 282: 95–98

Walford S, Gale E A M, Allison S P, and Tattersall R B 1978 Self-monitoring of blood-glucose. Lancet 1: 732–735

Walford S, Clarke P, Paisey R, Hartog M, Allison S P 1980 Home blood-glucose measurements without reflectance meter. Lancet 1: 653–654

Walsh C H, Cooper B T, Wright A D, Malins J M, Cooke W T 1978 Diabetes mellitus and coeliac disease: a clinical study. Quarterly Journal of Medicine 47: 89–100

Ward E A, Ward G M, Turner R C 1981 Effect of sulphonylurea on insulin secretion and glucose control in insulin-treated diabetics. British Medical Journal 283: 278

Watkins P J 1980 Insulin infusion systems, diabetic control, and microvascular complications. British Medical Journal 280: 350–352

Webb D J, Lovesay J M, Ellis A, Knight A H 1980 Blood glucose monitors: a laboratory and patient assessment. British Medical Journal 280: 362–364

Welch S G 1979 Fast glycosylation of haemoglobin. Lancet 1: 728

Werther G A, Jenkins P A, Turner R C, Baum J D 1980 Twenty-four-hour metabolic profiles in diabetic children receiving insulin injections once or twice daily. British Medical Journal 281: 414–418

WHO Expert Committee on Diabetes Mellitus. Second report 1980 Who Tech Rep Ser No. 646

Williams D R R, James W P T, Evans I E 1980 Dietary fibre supplementation of 'normal' breakfast administered to diabetics. Diabetologia 18: 379–383

Worth R, Anderson J, Taylor R, Alberti K G M M 1980 Jet injection of insulin: comparison with conventional injection by syringe and needle. British Medical Journal 281: 713–714

Worth R, Harrison K, Anderson J, Johnston D G, Alberti K G M M 1981 A comparative study of blood glucose test strips. Diabetes Care 3: 407–411

Yoon J W, Austin M, Onodera T, Notkins A L 1979 Virus-induced diabetes mellitus. Isolation of a virus from the pancreas of a child with diabetic ketoacidosis. New England Journal of Medicine 300: 1173–1179

3

Clinical immunology

P. L. Amlot and M. H. Lessof

MONOCLONAL ANTIBODIES

The monoclonal immunoglobulins which occur naturally in man are, in general, the products of malignant plasma cells from patients with myeloma. Through their use, much has been learned about immunoglobulin structure, properties, sequence and synthesis. However, only rarely have these molecules been shown to have antibody activity — that is, the ability to bind to antigen. In August 1975, Köhler & Milstein reported their discovery that normal B lymphocytes could be fused with myeloma cell lines and that such hybridomas secreted monoclonal antibodies coded for by the normal B lymphocytes. The impact of this discovery is so wide-ranging that it is worth expanding on its implications.

Normally, when man or mouse is immunised with an antigen the antibody response is polyclonal. In other words the product is a heterogeneous mix of antibody molecules (of differing classes, affinity and recognising different parts of the antigen molecule). This polyclonal range of antibodies represents the net output of a range of plasma cells, each producing a monoclonal antibody specific for the antigen. The precursor of each plasma cell is a B lymphocyte bearing on its surface the variable, antigen-binding region of the immunoglobulin molecule which it will subsequently mass-produce when it differentiates into a plasma cell. However, normal plasma cells have little potential to divide and have a finite life span, so continual production cannot be guaranteed. The ingenuity shown by Köhler and Milstein has now provided the basis for interminable division as well as immunoglobulin synthesis. This has been achieved by fusing a myeloma cell line with the genetic material coding for a specific immunoglobulin sequence contained in a normal B lymphocyte.

Most work on hybridisation and production of monoclonal antibodies has been done using mice and rats in which suitable myeloma cell lines are available. Mice are immunised on two occasions with an antigen of interest to the investigator in order to expand the number of antigen-sensitive B lymphocytes. At the optimum time (3–4 days) after the second immunisation, the mouse's spleen is removed and the spleen cells fused with a mouse myeloma cell line, using polyethylene glycol to achieve this fusion. Here another ingenious technological step was added to prevent overgrowth by the myeloma cell line. The myeloma cells used have been selected to lack a purine salvage pathway and they die in selective HAT medium — except for those cells which have fused with normal lymphocytes and have so been provided with the necessary enzyme pathway. The surviving cells are thus either hybridoma cells or unfused lymphocytes. The latter die naturally over the next few weeks, but the remaining steps require a great deal of work. The hybridoma supernates have to be screened to find which cells are producing the relevant specific antibody. Finally, individual clones are separated in order to produce a truly monoclonal antibody of relevance for the investigator. The hybridomas can then be grown in vitro and the culture supernatants harvested, or more profitably, they can be injected intraperitoneally to produce an ascitic fluid which is rich in monoclonal antibody. For a review see Guarneota & Parkhouse (1981).

These monoclonal antibodies have enormous advantages over conventional polyclonal antisera. First, their potency is far greater than that of normal antisera, not only because they have a single specificity but also because little or no non-specific immunoglobulin is produced by the type of myeloma cell lines now commonly used. Secondly, a stock of such hybridomas can be relied upon to produce monoclonal antibodies when needed without any further purification steps and is of such purity that it can be used immediately, for example, in radioimmunoassay procedures or to identify antigens in tissues. Thirdly, a clearly defined monoclonal antibody has the potential to become a standard for a particular antigenic determinant — as reliable as pure chemical reagents — and will not suffer some of the vagaries that bedevil conventional antisera. Fourthly, and most exciting for immunologists, the technique allows clean antisera to be raised against weak antigenic determinants. A good example is in the field of cellular membrane antigens. Raising antisera to T cells has always been difficult and controversial, requiring extensive absorption, even for the production of weak antisera. Now, however, there are several commercially available, good monoclonal antisera, not only to human T cells but also to human T cell subsets. A fuller discussion of this application will follow this section.

There are a number of disadvantages to monoclonal antibodies. As predicted, they do not produce good precipitating antisera unless two or more monoclonal antibodies to different antigenic sites on the same molecule are mixed. Furthermore, not all monoclonal antibodies, even when they are of the IgM class, necessarily fix complement. Therefore, monoclonal antibodies have to be selected if they are to be used in a complement-fixing assay. Lastly, care has to be taken not to grow hybridomas in culture for long periods because they may deviate into non-producers of immunoglobin.

Using mouse and rat systems it will be possible to produce a complete range of diagnostic antisera with a precision and accuracy hitherto unknown. Once established, their final economy, both in time and animals, will make them sufficiently cheap to allow their use in industrial processes. Definition of cell-membrane antigens by monoclonal antibodies will allow even better standardisation of HLA systems, as well as differentiation of antigens in other cellular systems. It will be possible to use reagents of this kind to analyse the antigenic variation which occurs in infective agents. By means of affinity chromatography, such antibodies can also be used to select and purify individual antigens from a more crude mixture. These pure antigens can then be used in diagnostic tests or in the preparation of vaccines for such diseases as malaria. Lastly, by producing hybridomas using human B lymphocytes and human myeloma cells (Olsson & Kaplan 1980) considerable therapeutic possibilities are opened up. It should now be possible to give patients specific antibody which does not contain protein of non-human origin and is therefore free from the injurious effects of anaphylaxis and serum sickness. Antisera to Rhesus antigen, hepatitis virus antigens, rabies and a wide range of venoms and toxins may thus become available for prophylactic and therapeutic use.

In one area, the use of monoclonal antibodies has so far given disappointing results — that is, in the treatment of cancer by the administration of antibody which is directed specifically against cancer cells. One part of the problem has arisen from a failure to produce antibodies which react with tumour cells alone. Those antibodies which cross-react with other types of cell may well have an affinity for normal differentiation antigens rather than for a specific tumour component and their selectivity is therefore rather suspect. Attempts to destroy tumour cells in this way are, in any case, fraught with difficulty. Antibody which binds to cell-surface antigen but fails to cause the destruction of the cell could have an 'enhancing' effect of the type seen with transplanted animal tumours, in which the body's own immune response to the tumour is altered by the presence of antibody on the cell surface and the rate of tumour growth is increased. Even if this danger is avoided and the viability of the tumour cell is impaired in some way by the antibody, it is possible — as with the use of cytotoxic drugs — that the resistance of the tumour will be altered as the more susceptible cells are destroyed. Alternatively, the cell-surface antigen might itself be eliminated in the presence of antibody.

One of the nearest approaches to the successful use of a specific anti-tumour antibody in man has depended on the development of monoclonal antibodies which react with subsets of T lymphocytes. Using an antibody to Leu-1 (see below), produced by a mouse hybridoma, attempts were first made to treat a patient with a T-cell leukaemia. It was then found that the tumour cells developed an antigenic change (as had been predicted) and a 'loss of control' followed. In addition, there was an immediate release of free antigen following the administration of antibody which, on theoretical grounds, might have provided a competing substrate for the binding of anti-T-cell antibody. The investigators concerned (Miller & Levy 1981) then treated a patient with cutaneous T-cell lymphoma and noted that the antigenic modulation which was detectable in the circulating T lymphocytes after the administration of antibody disappeared after a time. The patient was given twice-weekly injections for a period of 10 weeks: a striking but incomplete clinical response was noted in skin, lymph nodes and blood. A similar response was subsequently noted in a second patient. As the remaining diseased cells were antigen-positive, a failure to eradicate all the tumour cells could not have been the result of immunological selection (which would have allowed only antigen-negative cells to survive). This method of treatment thus remains an imperfect one, and alternative approaches have been suggested such as the coupling of a cytotoxic drug to a tumour-specific antibody, which might then be expected to deliver a chemotherapeutic effect at the site where it is most needed.

One of the observations of interest in this experimental treatment of T-cell lymphoma was that no immunological response to mouse globulin could be demonstrated. It remains to be seen whether this was the result of the disease itself or of the use of anti-T-cell antibody. An alternative possibility proposed by the authors is that the route of administration and the aggregate-free form of the globulin used may have favoured the induction of tolerance to the foreign protein.

LYMPHOCYTE FUNCTION AND DYSFUNCTION

Subsets of human T lymphocytes

Some of the most impressive results of monoclonal technology have involved the detection of weak antigenic determinants on the membranes of cells, with the help of a range of antisera which are usually code numbered and will be referred to by their number in the following text. Using such antisera, the presence of specific molecules on the surface of T lymphocytes can be linked to their helper or suppressor function. When inbred strains of mice are cross-immunised, antisera can be produced which identify T-helper lymphocytes (LyI +ve) or T-suppressor lymphocytes (Ly1, 2, 3 +ve). In man this has been more difficult and until recently the most widespread marker used for human T cells has been the sheep red cell (E) rosette. Painstaking collaborative work between Schlossman and co-workers and the Ortho company has, however, led to the production of antisera (OKT8) which identify human T-cell membrane markers associated with suppressor or cytotoxic function on the one hand and antisera (OKT4) which identify helper or inducer function on the other (Reinherz & Schlossman 1980). Corresponding monoclonal antisera have been produced by Becton and Dickinson, identifying suppressors (Leu 2a) and helper (Leu 3a) T cells.

As the available antisera are better defined, it is hoped that the molecules they detect can be analysed and their structure related to function. It is now possible to detect the membrane changes which occur as the human thymocyte matures during its transit through the thymus (Reinherz et al 1980a, Janossy et al 1981). The sheep red blood cell (E) rosette has been an approximate marker for human T cells for a decade and there is now a monoclonal antibody (OKT 11) which identifies the same erythrocyte receptors. A specific thymocyte marker is detected by OKT 10 and is lost as the T cell matures. Undifferentiated cortical thymocytes are identified by another monoclonal antibody (OKT 6), but within the medulla of the thymus there is further differentiation into either helper (T4) or suppressor (T5) cells. Medullary thymocytes gain HLA molecules on their surface and appear to remain unchanged thereafter, both in function and in their surface markings (Fig. 3.1). These changes coincide with an ability to react in the mixed lymphocyte response.

The mature T cells which are present in the peripheral lymphoid tissue, spleen and blood have lost the thymocyte marker (identified by OKT 10) but in other respects react like medullary thymocytes. In these mature T cells it is very rare to find overlap between helper and suppressor markers. The functional properties of these two sets of T cells are set out in Table 3.1.

In these and other ways, lymphocytes which appear to be identical under light microscopy can be separated into subpopulations. E-rosetting cells have also been separated into two populations on the basis of receptors for the Fc portion of IgG or IgM. These have become known as T_γ and T_μ cells respectively. The T_γ cells have been equated with suppressor function and have been shown to react with a monoclonal antibody (OKM) which is largely, but not entirely, specific for monocytes (Reinherz et al 1980b). T_μ cells have mainly been associated with helper function, although it should be noted that, in culture conditions, the presence of γ and μ receptors change with time, especially after stimulation by antigens or mitogens.

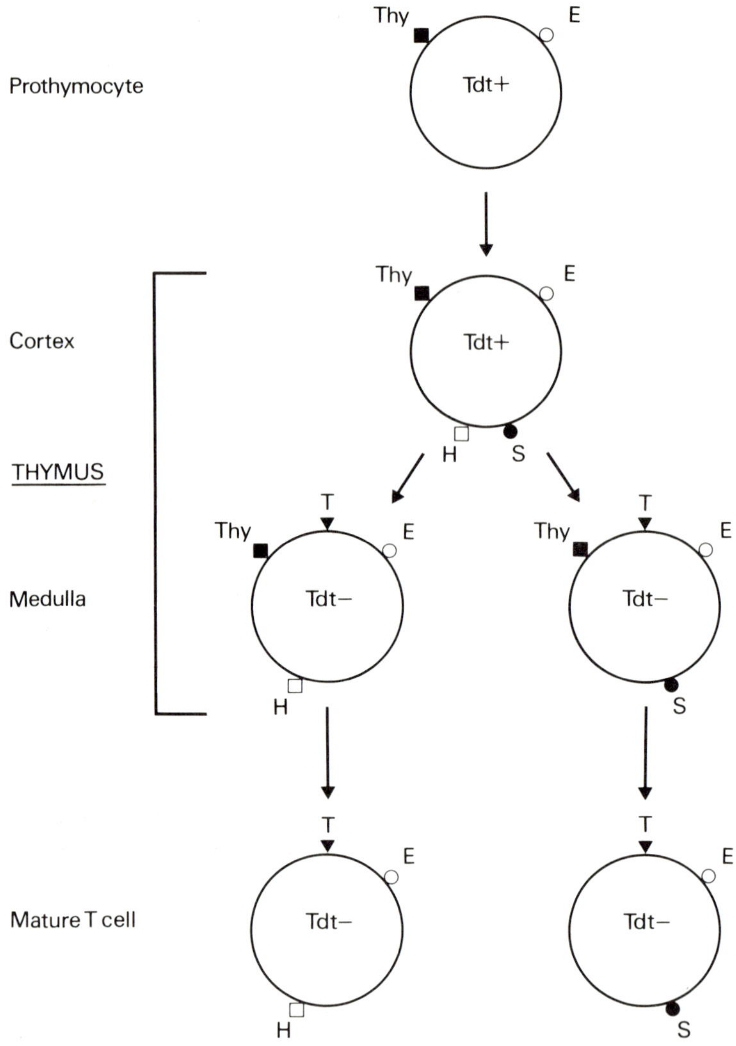

Fig. 3.1 Membrane phenotypes of maturing T cells. Tdt = terminal deoxynucleotidyl transferase; Thy = thymocyte marker (OKT 10); E = sheep red blood cell marker (OKT 11); H = helper marker (OKT 4 or BD Leu 3a); S = suppressor marker (OKT 8 or BD Leu 2a); T = pan mature T-cell marker (OKT 1 or 3).

The type of cell on which a surface marker appears may also vary in different circumstances. Ia is a molecule normally expressed on B cells and monocytes, but it also appears on T cells which have become activated (Reinherz et al 1981). In bacterial infections Ia appears on helper T cells, while in viral infections it appears on cytotoxic T cells. It is thus possible that T-cell help for antibody production is stimulated by bacterial infection, while viral infection is more likely to generate cytotoxic effector cells which react with viral antigens on cell surfaces. In keeping with this is the observation that, in infectious mononucleosis, the circulating abnormal mononuclear cells carry the phenotype of a cytotoxic T cell.

Table 3.1 Characteristics of helper (T_H) and suppressor (T_S) lymphocytes in peripheral blood and tissues

Characteristics	Type of lymphocyte T_H	T_S
Effect upon T- and B-cell responses:		
Helper or inducer	+	–
Suppressor or cytotoxic	–*	+
Proliferation with soluble antigen	+	–
Proliferation with lectins (concanavalin, phytohaemagglutinin)	+	±
Ability to produce activators (mitogenic, colony-forming, osteoclast-activating)	+	–

*Induces production of T_S cells but no direct action

The ever-expanding heterogeneity of T cells is slowly providing a clearer understanding of how the immune response is controlled, and this may in time make it possible to achieve a more exact manipulation of the immune system in disease states. Attempts of this kind have already been made. Thus OKT 3 was injected into a patient in Boston who was rejecting a kidney transplant. The rejection episode was successfully reversed.

Enzyme defects, lymphocytes, and immune deficiency

With the discovery of the association between deficiences of purine metabolic enzymes and certain inherited forms of immunodeficiency in man, some precise biochemical defects have been identified which have a specific toxic effect on lymphocytes (reviewed by Pollara et al 1979). These conditions are too rare to be of direct importance to the majority of clinicians. Their interest lies, however, in the light which they shed on mechanisms which may also apply to some of the common causes of secondary immune deficiency, including malnutrition, infection, burns, renal failure, cancer, cytotoxic and antibiotic drugs — and old age.

There is good evidence that adenosine deaminase (ADA) deficiency leads to one form of the combined immunodeficiency syndrome, with decreased numbers of T and B cells. It now appears that children who are deficient in purine nucleoside phosphorylase (PNP) have a more selective deficiency of T cells; in addition, an association has been reported recently between a deficiency of 5′-nucleotidase and various forms of agammaglobulinaemia (Johnson et al 1977, Edwards et al 1978). As these enzymes are widespread in the body, their selectively toxic effect on lymphatic tissue is puzzling. However, it is possible that these enzyme deficiencies have their main expression in lymphocytes or lymphocyte subpopulations because of the intracellular accumulation of toxic substances in these cells. According to this 'trapping' hypothesis, deoxyadenosine, which is excreted by many tissues, is selectively taken up in lymphocytes because of the high concentration of the enzyme purine deoxyribonucleoside kinase in those cells. In the absence of ADA the deoxyadenosine which is trapped within thymus-derived lymphocytes then accumulates to toxic levels. In PNP deficiency, a similar trapping mechanism increases the concentration of deoxyguanosine, which is taken up in lymphocytes through the action of the same enzyme.

Children with PNP deficiency usually have a defect which is confined to T cells. This defect may even be confined to a T-cell subpopulation, for it is now known that suppressor T-cell activity, affecting IgM production by human cells in vitro, can be abrogated by deoxyguanosine in concentrations 1000 times lower than those required to inhibit the activity of T-helper cells or the differentiation of precursor B lymphocytes (Dosch et al 1980). The mechanisms are complex and may depend on the sequential effect of two or more enzymes. Furthermore, the ability of suppressor cells to cause defective cellular immunity may depend on their release of prostaglandins (Goodwin et al 1977), particularly PGE_1 and PGE_2. Even in the present limited state of our knowledge it is clear that defects of more than one enzyme pathway may be capable of producing specific disorders of the immune system. The clinical consequences of PNP deficiency and defective T-cell function are a susceptibility to infections, especially viral, and a tendency to develop autoimmune phenomena including a Coombs-positive haemolytic anaemia, a positive antinuclear factor, and the presence of LE cells in the blood.

The clinical effects of gross congenital enzyme defects are thus sufficiently well known to provide some indication of the clinical syndromes which might be expected to occur with either major or minor deficiences of PNP. With this in mind, screening programmes are now under way for detecting incomplete deficiencies of the purine metabolic enzymes in a variety of clinical conditions. Theoretically, as with other congenital enzyme deficiency syndromes, these disorders should be correctable: as advances are made in genetic engineering there is the hope that, once identified, the deficient enzyme can be manufactured in cell culture conditions, using hybridised DNA. Alternatively, the defect might be correctable by the transplantation of fetal liver or other stem cells.

IMMUNOLOGY AND CARDIOVASCULAR DISEASE

Post-infectious cardiomyopathy

It is possible that viruses trigger some episodes of cardiomyopathy or myocardial fibrosis. However, viruses are so commonly recovered from human cardiac tissue that it is difficult to know when their presence is incidental or a cause of disease. In some cases of congestive cardiomyopathy the patient's illness begins with fever (Cambridge et al 1979) and in these patients high neutralisation titres of antibody against Coxsackie B viruses are commonly found. However, there is a paradox, for it has not proved to be possible to isolate virus in many fatal cases of poliomyelitis or influenza, despite the presence of obvious cardiac damage. This suggests that the presence of virus is not sufficient to account for the damage seen. This has led to the 'infectious-immune theory' of Kawai (1971) which postulates that, when viral antigen is fixed in the heart, a hypersensitivity or autoallergic response may follow and lead to damage of the myocardium, heart valves, pericardium and pleura. In support of this theory, Kawai noted many similarities between idiopathic cardiomyopathy and the heart disease of rheumatic fever, Chagas' disease and toxoplasmosis, all of which are known to follow infection.

These conclusions are somewhat speculative. In the case of neonatal endocardial fibroelastosis (EFE) the evidence is stronger (reviewed by Lessof & Olsen 1981). Noren and his colleagues found a delayed skin hypersensitivity to mumps in almost all cases of endocardial fibroelastosis. In the absence of circulating antibody, this finding was thought to indicate a primitive, fetal type of immunological response to intrauterine mumps infection, and the same type of 'split immunological recognition' has been demonstrated in the offspring of rhesus monkeys after an infection with mumps virus during pregnancy (St Geme et al 1972). Furthermore, an interstitial, possibly viral, myocarditis has been demonstrated histologically in 41 out of 64 children with EFE (Hutchins & Vie 1972). In those children who had survived the longest, there was less evidence of active myocarditis but the features of fibroelastosis were more prominent. Factor (1978) studied one case in great detail and, apart from a widespread chronic inflammatory reaction in the heart, found virus-like particles in many myocardial and endothelial cells.

Inevitably, a comparison has also been drawn with round heart disease, a spontaneous myocarditis of turkeys, in which a similar progression can be traced from neonatal myocarditis through to endocardial fibroelastosis (Noren et al 1971). In this disease of turkeys, particles resembling avian leucosis virus are present in the myocardial cells, and collagen accumulation can be demonstrated beneath the endocardium within a day or two of hatching. Within a month, these changes progress to produce marked endocardial fibroelastotic changes, often with mitral valve and papillary muscle involvement.

These various findings are highly suggestive, although it should be noted that evidence of a cellular reaction is not always present in the human disease. Factor (1978) has suggested that microvascular obliteration could be an important common factor, which can complicate viral infection in utero and lead to a variety of cardiac manifestations at different stages of fetal development.

Immunological aspects of atherosclerosis

The established changes of atherosclerosis represent an end stage in vascular damage. Several types of physical injury to the intima of arteries can provoke a common sequence of events. The adherence of platelets in the early stages is followed by proliferation of intimal cells, deposition of lipids, and the more advanced changes that accompany lipid imbibition and thrombus encrustation. It is clear that the rate at which these changes occur is also influenced by the level and composition of lipids in the blood.

Among the agents which can initiate vascular damage and lead to atherosclerosis — at least experimentally — are virus infections. It has been claimed that herpes virus infection contributes to atherosclerosis in chickens (Fabricant et al 1978); in both animals and man, Burch (1978) has suggested that Coxsackie B viruses are capable of initiating a similar process. In patients who had suffered a myocardial infarct, Nicholls & Thomas (1977) found a rise in the titre of Coxsackie B virus antibodies but not influenza A antibody, suggesting a significant role for Coxsackie virus infection. In order to explain these findings, it has been suggested that damage to the arterial wall may be mediated by an immune reaction against virus-infected cells, or that a virus infection is followed by the development of damage due to immune-complex formation.

Immune-complex damage

It has long been suspected that immune-complex-mediated vascular injury contributes to the development of atherosclerotic change. In classic serum sickness the arterial lesions are seen in the coronary arteries and at the bifurcation of major vessels. Although the histological appearances are those of arteritis, the distribution is the same as in atherosclerosis (Cochrane & Koffler 1973). When the pathological changes are studied sequentially, the development of endothelial damage appears to be followed by an infiltration of polymorphonuclear leucocytes. If the animal is depleted of these circulating leucocytes there is evidence that this reduces the severity of the lesions and prevents fibrinoid necrosis (reviewed by Poston 1981). Even before the stage of leucocyte involvement, a consistent and early finding has been the presence of circulating immune complexes. Complexes which are not removed by phagocytic cells thus appear to be concerned in the initiation of local vascular lesions, though whether this is by deposition at the site of previous injury in the walls of the vessels or by the attraction of leucocytes remains to be established.

There may also be a synergistic effect between serum sickness and the consequences of a raised serum lipid level, as in the rabbit experiments of Roberts (1960), in which cholesterol feeding was used as a means of increasing the circulating lipids. Immunological changes and the effects of lipids have also been shown to potentiate each other in primates. Howard and his colleagues (1971) induced serum sickness in baboons by giving a series of injections of bovine serum albumin and found that this caused only trivial lesions in the aorta; however, the combination of these injections with a lipid-rich diet resulted in the development of extensive plaques which, after 6 months' treatment, covered about half of the aorta. Once lesions had been caused by a combination of immune-complex injury and lipid feeding, they regressed more slowly than those caused by either factor alone (van Winkle & Levy 1970).

The extrapolation of these results to man depends on circumstantial evidence only. A number of groups, including Füst and his colleagues (1978), found immune complexes in the blood of myocardial infarction patients, but this could well be explained in terms of a reaction to the breakdown of necrotic or infarcted tissue. Their importance in man thus remains unresolved.

Atherosclerosis and transplantation

When transplant rejection occurs in experimental animals, there is evidence — as in serum sickness — that vascular damage and disease may depend on the combined effect of immunological damage and of changes in lipid metabolism. Laden et al (1973) grafted hearts between outbred rats and rabbits and produced intimal thickening in the coronary arteries. When, in addition, cholesterol was fed, this accumulated in the damaged arteries. In these circumstances Alonso et al (1977) showed that the transplanted aorta became severely atheromatous, with plaque covering much of its surface.

In man, the development of accelerated atherosclerosis after the transplantation of the heart and other organs has further stimulated an interest in these immunological and metabolic aspects. Chronic immune-complex deposition has been assumed to be the main cause (Cooper et al 1980), and it has also been postulated that there is a damaging effect due to lymphocytotoxic antibodies (Laden et al 1973).

However, the implantation of foreign tissue and the rejection process may not be the only factors. The administration of corticosteroids, which is a feature of the management of these patients, may itself be associated with an increase in the incidence of coronary disease or atherosclerosis, as has been shown in diseases such as systemic lupus (Bulkley & Roberts 1975) and rheumatoid arthritis (Kalbak 1972). As corticosteroids lead to a reduction in the fraction of cholesterol which is bound to high-density lipoprotein (Lessof et al, 1979), it is possible that an effect equivalent to that of a high-lipid diet is achieved. Anti-rejection therapy with corticosteroids might therefore combine with immune-complex deposition in its pathological effects.

ALLERGY

Food antigens and the intestinal tract

There is a paradox in the body's apparent acceptance of food antigens which are absorbed through the bowel, as contrasted with its brisk reaction to bacterial infection or to oral immunisation with viral or bacterial pathogens. The discriminating power of the gut is remarkable; when it fails, however, parasites or microorganisms may be allowed to enter the body without provoking a reaction. There is also the opposite danger when immunological reactions are unduly vigorous. In that case, food proteins, instead of being tolerated, may provoke an inappropriate immune response and lead to allergic or immune-complex-mediated reactions. What, perhaps, is most surprising is that adverse immune reactions to food are not an everyday occurrence.

Two per cent of the plasma cells in the normal gut mucosa contain immunoglobulin E (IgE). However, the major lymphoid tissue of the intestines is located within the Peyer's patches, and these contain B lymphocytes which are principally concerned with immunoglobulin A (IgA) production. It now appears that these lymphocytes are activated by 'microfold' or 'M' cells, which were first described by Owen & Jones (1974). These cells avidly take up antigenic material from the lumen of the bowel. It is thought that this material is then processed with the help of T lymphocytes and presented to the B cells within the Peyer's patch.

Apart from this mechanism for IgA antibody production, there exists a separate inhibitory mechanism which prevents inappropriate immune responses to ingested and absorbed dietary substances. In experimental animals, agents which are capable of causing sensitisation when injected intracutaneously can be prevented from doing so if they are first given by the oral route (Asherson et al 1977). Oral feeding can thus induce immune tolerance: however, if the liver is by-passed by anastomosing the portal vein to the inferior vena cava this tolerance no longer occurs (Triger et al 1973).

It is only when these mechanisms fail, that substances introduced by mouth can provoke an allergic response. The events which initiate this allergic response are still poorly understood, but it has been noted that specific food intolerance may follow a severe infection, usually a gastroenteritis. In neonates and small children, gastroenteritis can sufficiently damage the intestinal epithelium to cause a transient deficiency of disaccharidases, and also lead to a temporary increase in mucosal permeability which allows an increased absorption of whole milk proteins and the development of cow's-milk-protein sensitisation (Harrison et al 1976). In patients recovering from an infective gastroenteritis it has been shown (Iyngkaran et al 1979) that a recurrence of diarrhoea may be provoked by cow's milk and can be accompanied by a pattern of small-bowel mucosal damage after a cow's-milk challenge. In infants who develop a secondary sugar or milk intolerance while recovering from infective enteritis, consideration should therefore be given to the possible need to withdraw cow's-milk protein and lactose from the diet. As a point in differential diagnosis, naturally occurring lactose intolerance should also be given particular consideration in such cases, although its prevalence varies in different populations.

Clinical features of milk allergy

The most immediate symptoms of milk allergy include vomiting, diarrhoea, hypotension and bronchospasm. These features of anaphylactic shock may develop within minutes but later symptoms also occur, including abdominal pain, bloating and constipation. In some cases repeated challenges are necessary, over a period of days or weeks, before eczema, asthma, irritability or weight loss develop. Exceptionally, there may be more complex features, and the development of iron deficiency anaemia and intestinal bleeding, eosinophilia, steatorrhoea and hypoproteinaemia have all been documented in occasional cases.

Because of the problems associated with a long-term milk-exclusion diet, small-bowel biopsy has become the simplest method of providing the diagnostic confirmation which, when villous atrophy is present, is an indication for withdrawing milk and repeating the biopsy after clinical recovery has occurred. The cautious re-introduction of milk after six months or more may sometimes demonstrate the transient nature of the condition, but symptoms can recur and a further biopsy may be needed in doubtful cases. In addition, there is an association with gluten enteropathy in occasional cases; similar jejunal reactions to challenge have been described also in a child who was intolerant of soya flour and another who proved to be allergic to chicken.

Food reactions in adults

The re-awakening of interest in food allergy has been considerably stimulated by the study of small-bowel changes in infancy but, ironically, there is little to suggest that these particular changes are IgE-mediated. Their similarity to the villous atrophy seen in gluten enteropathy shows that similar appearances can arise in a disease in which the evidence for an IgE reaction is virtually absent. Although milk allergy is sometimes combined with other evidence of allergic disease such as asthma, eczema, a high serum IgE level and a positive radio-allergosorbent test to milk proteins, the evidence suggests a disorder which is complex and involves more than one type of immunological reaction. The same is true of food intolerance in adults, but mucosal atrophy is not a feature of adult cases and, unless there is evidence of changes in intestinal mucosal permeability (Jackson et al 1981), it may be difficult to demonstrate the presence of even a functional disorder of the bowel. Despite the frequent association with a more widespread allergic reaction, including asthma, eczema, urticaria, angioedema, rhinorrhoea or anaphylaxis in 93 out of 100 cases in a recent series confirmed by challenge methods (Lessof et al 1980), food intolerance due to non-allergic causes always needs to be considered in the differential diagnosis. Such non-allergic causes include disaccharidase deficiencies, cystic fibrosis, low-grade intestinal infections, gallstones, psychological illness, or the pharmacological effects of caffeine or of the amines contained in red wine or cheese. It has therefore been suggested that the diagnosis of food intolerance should be changed to that of food allergy only if there are clear anaphylactic symptoms or a strongly positive skin or radio-allergosorbent test (RAST).

When symptoms are delayed in onset, or occur after repeated administration of the appropriate food, the diagnosis is easily missed. Not surprisingly, IgE skin tests and RAST are likely to be negative in such cases, and a recent case of severe intractable thrombocytopenia which was reversed on a milk-free diet (Caffrey et al 1981) not only confirmed reports of similar cases in the older literature but has also shown the difficulty in proving either the diagnosis or the mechanism, even in patients with life-threatening disease. The situation may be even more complicated in the occasional case in which milk-induced exacerbation (and IgE changes) occur in a disease such as rheumatoid arthritis (Parke & Hughes 1981).

In terms of management, the offending foods, colouring agents or preservatives need to be identified and excluded from the diet. It seems possible that some of the gastrointestinal symptoms are mediated by prostaglandins and in some the symptoms may be prevented by salicylates or indomethacin (Buisseret et al 1979). It should, however, be noted that salicylates may themselves cause symptoms in other patients. Oral cromoglycate is of prophylactic value in some, but not all, patients with confirmed food allergy.

MacKie (1981) has noted that oral cromoglycate can also be of benefit in patients with atopic skin disease who have no evidence of food-induced reactions at all. The subject has been further reviewed by Lessof & Buisseret (1981).

NEW IMMUNOTHERAPEUTIC PROCEDURES

Cyclosporin A

Cyclosporin A (CSA) is a product isolated from a soil fungus *(Trichoderma polysporum)* and has a novel cyclic endecapeptide structure. Like many fungal products, it was originally screened for antibiotic activity, of which it has a narrow spectrum; it achieved prominence because of its potent immunosuppressive properties comparable with antilymphocyte globulin and azathioprine (Borel et al 1976). However, unlike cytotoxic immunosuppressants, it lacks antimitotic activity and thus does not cause myelosuppression. Even at very high dosage (50 mg/kg) it produces only a mild thrombocytopoenia and lymphopoenia. In addition, it does not affect inflammatory responses nor phagocytosis by granulocytes and monocytes (Gordon & Singer 1979). In clinical use, CSA is thus free from the major hazard of all potent immunosuppressants, namely bacterial infection.

Data on the mode of action of cyclosporin A are conflicting, largely as a result of the insolubility of the product in aqueous solutions. CSA is soluble in lipids and organic solvents; its bioavailability, both in vitro and in vivo, is still poorly understood. CSA has a selective effect on T-cell function, with B cells being relatively unaffected. It inhibits resting T cells from entering blast transformation and, whereas early experiments suggested that it led to clonal deletion of lymphocytes, it appears now that its inhibition is reversible once it has been thoroughly removed from either in vitro or in vivo conditions (Borel & Weisinger 1979). It probably interferes at an early stage (the first 6–8 h) in the stimulation of T-helper cells and subsequently establishes T-suppressor-cell control of immune responses. In animal experiments it inhibits T-dependent antibody production if given within 24 h of immunisation, and inhibits contact hypersensitivity, dinitrochlorobenzene sensitisation and recall delayed hypersensitivity, as well as Freund's adjuvant arthritis and experimental allergic encephalitis. Its potential for transplantation was realised when it was found that, even after short exposure to CSA ranging from 4 to 14 days, there was markedly prolonged survival of cardiac and renal allografts in a large number of animal species. With short courses of CSA treatment, acute rejection could be suppressed but chronic rejection appeared to require continuous administration. Furthermore, in bone marrow transplantation, graft-versus-host reactions could be suppressed and chimaeras produced after short courses of CSA, probably due to the induction of suppressor cells (Tutschka et al 1979). The only adverse effects noted in animal studies were reversible renal and hepatic toxicity at high dosage and, more seriously, the alarmingly frequent development of lymphomas (10%) in non-human primates (Bieber et al 1980).

So exciting were CSA's possibilities that it was rapidly introduced into human clinical studies. The first reported study was on its use in 30 renal, two pancreatic and two liver transplants (Calne et al 1979). Here, unfortunately, its toxic renal and hepatic effects were not initially realised and, in the setting of predominantly renal transplantation, were misinterpreted as indicating rejection. This led to over-suppression with added corticosteroids and azathioprine and consequently a disproportionate number of deaths from severe infection. A disturbing number of lymphomas (3 out of 34), as in the non-human primates, was seen in this study. One gastroduodenal lymphoma occurred in a patient treated with CSA only, one pulmonary lymphoma in a patient treated with CSA and steroids, and one jejunal lymphoma in a patient also receiving azathioprine. A subsequent study by the same group using CSA alone has not encountered any lymphoma development but the inordinately high incidence of lymphomas will still shadow its undoubted immunosuppressive success. CSA has transformed the clinical outlook for patients undergoing bone marrow transplantation. In a pioneering study of 23 patients, mostly suffering from acute myeloblastic leukaemia, who had achieved complete remission before transplantation, 15 survived in good health, and no lymphomas were reported (Powles et al 1980).

Side effects in humans have been a dose-dependent renal toxicity, hepatotoxicity, stimulation of body-hair growth and mild tremors. Patients treated with CSA are also liable to herpes zoster infections and reactivation of viruses such as cytomegalovirus. In relation to lymphomagenesis, it is noteworthy that CSA added to in vitro cultures of lymphoid cells is extremely efficient in promoting the establishment of lymphoblastoid cell lines infected with the Epstein-Barr virus. In 15 out of 92 patients treated with CSA there was a fourfold or greater rise in anti-EBV capsid antibody (Nagington 1981).

Undoubtedly, the startling incidence of lymphomas in patients treated with CSA may provide an insurmountable obstacle to its widespread clinical use. However, studies examining its short-term use at lower dosage and without the concurrent use of other immunosuppressants may negate these fears.

Plasma exchange

Plasmapheresis is a technique whereby noxious components of pathological plasma are removed to alleviate the symptoms they cause. Thus it has been used in the hyperviscosity syndrome which occurs in some cases of Waldenström's macroglobulinaemia and other myelomas. In plasmapheresis whole blood is removed from the patient. It is then separated by centrifugation into blood cells and plasma, and the cells returned to the patient. The volume removed is limited in extent by the hypovolaemia which ensues from the progressive removal of plasma. In plasma exchange this technique is taken a step further by replacing the pathological plasma with fresh frozen normal plasma (FFP), highly purified albumin solution (PPF) or, in some instances, crystalloids. This avoids hypovolaemia and allows much more extensive removal of the patient's own plasma. It was first used in the effective treatment of severe rhesus disease by plasma exchange either of the mother, of the fetus in utero or of the neonate (Clarke et al 1970).

Plasma exchange can be carried out as a continuous replacement procedure with an IBM or Aminco cell separator, or more frequently nowadays as a semicontinuous method using a Haemonetics® machine. It is a relatively safe procedure but requires good vascular access to be performed effectively. This means flow rates of 70–100 ml/min: rates below 40 ml/min result in clotting and continuous interruption. Difficulty can arise if patients start with anaemia of <8 g/dl. Side effects include hypokalaemia, hypocalcaemia and occasional vascular spasm with fast infusion rates. When FFP is used, febrile, urticarial and occasionally anaphylactic reactions can occur, as well as the danger of hepatitis (HBsAg).

Plasma exchange alone leads to a short-lived amelioration of symptoms which recur when abnormal proteins, usually autoantibodies, reach their previous levels. The rate at which proteins are synthesised makes it an impractical procedure when used alone; therefore, almost invariably, plasma exchange is combined with effective immunosuppression for lasting benefit.

There is an increasing list of immunological diseases in which autoantibodies have an important causative role, and in many of these plasma exchange can play a therapeutic part by bringing symptoms under control rapidly. A good example of this is seen in Goodpasture's syndrome. This rare disease is caused by the appearance of antiglomerular basement membrane (GBM) antibodies and, untreated, it has a fulminating and fatal course. A number of specialist centres has found that extensive plasma exchange combined with immunosuppression (corticosteroids and cyclophosphamide) is the most effective means of controlling lung haemorrhage and stabilising or reversing renal damage (Lockwood et al 1976, Walker et al 1977). Plasma exchange is extensive and should be continued until no further anti-GBM antibody can be detected in the patient's plasma. This usually means a minimum of 12 × 4-litre exchanges. The stimulus to antibody production ensuing from plasma exchange may potentiate the effect of immunosuppression, leading to clonal deletion of the abnormal antibody-producing cells. No improvement in renal function has been observed in patients already anuric at the start of treatment. However, it has been noted that the same immune damage to transplanted kidneys will follow if transplantation is performed before anti-GBM antibodies have been eliminated.

In contrast myasthenia gravis — a disease in which plasma exchange is temporarily beneficial — is bedevilled in the long term by a lack of effective immunosuppression.

In myasthenia gravis, disease unresponsive to conventional drugs may be improved temporarily by the removal of anti-acetylcholine receptor (AChR) antibodies (Pinching et al 1976). However, the disease rapidly relapses, because adequate means of immunosuppression have not been found. There are a number of other diseases in which autoantibodies are implicated in the pathogenesis and in which plasma exchange has been of reported benefit: these include bullous pemphigoid, idiopathic thrombocytopenic purpura, cold agglutinin disease, thyrotoxicosis due to LATS, and insulin-resistant diabetes. Furthermore, there have been anecdotal reports of improvement in certain immune complex diseases such as rapidly progressive glomerular nephritis and systemic lupus erythematosus.

A word of caution should be raised. Control trials have not been performed and the necessary controls (sham plasma exchange) may sometimes be ethically unjustifiable. In diseases like Goodpasture's syndrome the effective regime of plasma exchange, combined with immunosuppression, may already be established. However, in most other diseases the usefulness of plasma exchange should be tested by controlled trials to see if there is justification for the expense and time involved.

REFERENCES

Monoclonal antibodies

Guarneota G, Parkhouse R E 1981 Hybridisation of lymphocytes, techniques and applications. In: Weeral H W, Luderer A A (eds) Diagnostic immunology. Human Press Inc., New Jersey

Köhler G, Milstein C 1975 Continuous cultures of fused cells secreting antibody of predefined specificity. Nature 256: 495–497

Miller R A, Levy R 1981 Response of cutaneous T cell lymphoma to therapy with hybridoma monoclonal antibody. Lancet 2: 226–230

Olsson L, Kaplan H S 1980 Human-human hybridomas producing monoclonal antibodies of predefined antigenic specificity. Proceedings of the National Academy of Sciences of the United States of America 77: 5429–5431

Lymphocyte function and dysfunction

Dosch H M, Mansour A, Cohen A, Shore A, Gelfand W 1980 Inhibition of suppressor T-cell development following deoxyguanosine administration. Nature 285: 495–496

Edwards N L, Magillavry D B, Cassidy J T, Fox I H 1978 Lymphocyte ecto-5′-nucleotidase deficiency in agammaglobulinaemia. Science 201: 628–630

Goodwin J S, Bankhurst A D, Messner R P 1977 Suppression of human T-cell mitogenesis by prostaglandin. Journal of Experimental Medicine 146: 1719–1734

Janossy G, Tidman N, Papageorgiou E S, King D C, Goldstein G 1981 Distribution of human T cell subsets in the human bone marrow and thymus. Journal of Immunology 126: 1608–1613

Johnson S M, Asherson G L, Watts R W E, North M E, Allsop J, Webster A D B 1977 Lymphocyte purine 5′-nucleotidase deficiency in primary hypogammaglobulinaemia. Lancet 1: 168–170

Pollara B, Pickering R J, Meuwissen H J, Porter I H (eds) 1979 Inborn errors of specific immunity. Academic Press, New York

Reinherz E L, Schlossman S F 1980 The differentiation and function of human T lymphocytes. Cell 19: 821–827

Reinherz E L, Morimoto C, Penta A C, Schlossman S F 1981 Subpopulations of the T4+ inducer T cell subset in man. Journal of Immunology 126: 67–70

Reinherz E L, Kung P C, Goldstein G, Levey R H, Schlossman S F 1980a Discrete stages of human intrathymic differentiation. Proceedings of the National Academy of Sciences of the United States of America 77: 1588–1592

Reinherz E L, Moretta L, Roper M, Beard J M, Mingari M C, Cooper M D et al 1980b Human T lymphocyte subpopulations defined by FC receptors and monoclonal antibodies. Journal of Experimental Medicine 151: 969–974

Immunology and cardiovascular disease

Alonso D R, Starek P K, Minick C R 1977 Studies on the pathogenesis of atheroarteriosclerosis induced in rabbit cardiac allografts by the synergy of graft rejection and hypercholesterolaemia. American Journal of Pathology 87: 415–418
Bulkley B H, Roberts W C 1975 The heart in SLE and the changes induced in it by corticosteroid therapy. American Journal of Medicine 58: 243–264
Burch G E 1978 Atherosclerosis in infants and viral infection. American Heart Journal 96: 558–559
Cambridge G, MacArthur C G C, Waterson A P, Goodwin J F, Oakley C M 1979 Antibodies to coxsackie B viruses in congestive cardiomyopathy. British Heart Journal 41: 692–696
Cochrane C G, Koffler D 1973 Immune complex disease in experimental animals and man. Advanced Immunology 16: 185–253
Cooper D K C, Charles R G, Fraser R C, Beck W Barnard C N 1980 Long-term survival after orthotopic and heterotopic cardiac transplantation. British Medical Journal 281: 1093–1096
Factor S M 1978 Endocardial fibroelastosis: myocardial and vascular alterations associated with viral-like nuclear particles. American Heart Journal 96: 791–801
Fabricant C G, Fabricant J, Litrenta M M, Minick C R 1978 Virus-induced atherosclerosis. Journal of Experimental Medicine 148: 335–340
Füst G, Szondy E, Szekely J, Nanai I, Gerö S 1978 Studies on the occurrence of circulating complexes in vascular diseases. Atherosclerosis 29: 181–190
Howard A N, Patelski J, Bowyer D E, Gresham G A 1971 Atherosclerosis induced in hypocholesterolaemic baboons by immunological injury and the effects of i.v. polyunsaturated phosphatidyl choline. Atherosclerosis 14: 17–29
Hutchins G M, Vie S A 1972 The progression of interstitial myocarditis to idiopathic endocardial fibroelastosis. American Journal of Pathology 66: 483–496
Kalbak K 1972 Incidence of arteriosclerosis in patients with rheumatoid arthritis receiving long-term corticosteroid therapy. Annals of Rheumatic Diseases 31: 196–200
Kawai C 1971 Idiopathic cardiomyopathy. A study on the infectious-immune theory. Japanese Circulation Journal 35: 765–770
Laden A M, Sinclair R A, Ruskiewicz M 1973 Vascular changes in experimental cardiac allografts. Transplantation Proceedings 5: 737–739
Lessof M H, Olsen E G J 1981 Cardiac muscle disease. In: Lessof M H (ed) Immunology of cardiovascular disease. Marcel Dekker Inc., New York, ch 5, p 157–188
Lessof M H, Jefferys D N, Lehner T, Mattock M 1979 Corticosteroids and azathioprine: their use in Behçet's syndrome. In: Lehner T, Challacombe S (eds) Behçet's syndrome. Academic Press, London, p 267–275
Nicholls A C, Thomas M 1977 Coxsackie virus infection in acute myocardial infarction. Lancet 1: 883–884
Noren G R, Staley N A, Jenkins E F, Stevenson J E 1971 Myocarditis in round heart disease of turkeys. Virchows Archiv für pathologische Anatomie 352: 285–295
Poston R N 1981 Immunological aspects of atherosclerosis. In: Lessof M H (ed) Immunology of cardiovascular disease. Marcel Dekker Inc., New York, ch 12, p 361–386
Roberts J C 1960 Effect of serum sickness of cholesterol atherosclerosis in the rabbit. Circulation 22: 657
St Geme J W, Peralta H, van Pelt L F 1972 Intra-uterine infection of the rhesus monkey with mumps virus. Journal of Infectious Diseases 126: 249–256
van Winkle M, Levy L 1970 Further studies on the reversibility of serum sickness cholesterol-induced atherosclerosis. Journal of Experimental Medicine 132: 858–867

Allergy

Asherson G L, Zembala M, Perera M, Mayhew B, Thomas W R 1977 Production of immunity and unresponsiveness in the mouse by feeding contact sensitizing agents and the role of suppressor cells in the Peyer's patches, mesenteric lymph nodes and other lymphoid tissue. Cellular Immunology 33: 145–150
Buisseret P D, Youlten L J, Heinzelman D, Lessof M H 1979 Prostaglandin synthetase inhibitors and food intolerance. Monographs in Allergy 14: 197–202
Caffrey E A, Sladen G E, Isaacs P E T, Clark K G A 1981 Thrombocytopenia caused by cow's milk. Lancet 2: 316
Harrison M, Kilby A, Walker-Smith J A, France N E, Wood C B S 1976 Cow's milk protein intolerance: a possible association with gastroenteritis, lactose intolerance and IgA deficiency. British Medical Journal 1: 1501–1504
Iyngkaran N, Davis K, Robinson M J, Boey C G, Sumithran E, Yadav M et al 1979 Cow's milk protein-sensitive enteropathy. Archives of Disease in Childhood 54: 39–43

Jackson P G, Lessof M H, Baker R W R, Ferrett J, MacDonald D M 1981 Intestinal permeability in patients with eczema and food allergy. Lancet 1: 1285–1286
Lessof M H, Buisseret P D 1981 Gastrointestinal reactions. In: Lessof M H (ed) Immunological and clinical aspects of allergy. MTP Press Ltd, Lancaster, p 141–177
Lessof M H, Wraith D G, Merrett T G, Merrett J, Buisseret P D 1980 Food allergy and intolerance in 100 patients — local and systemic effects. Quarterly Journal of Medicine 49: 259–271
Mackie R M 1981 Intestinal permeability and atopic disease. Lancet 2: 155
Owen R L, Jones A L 1974 Epithelial cell specialisation within human Peyer's patches: an ultrastructural study of intestinal lymphoid follicles. Gastroenterology 66: 189–203
Parke A L, Hughes G R V 1981 Rheumatoid arthritis and food: a case study. British Medical 2: 2027–2029
Triger D R, Cynamon M H Wright R 1973 Studies on hepatic uptake of antigen. I. Comparison of inferior vena cava and portal vein routes of immunization. Immunology 25: 941–950

New immunotherapeutic procedures

Bieber C P, Reitz B A, Jamieson S W, Oyer P E, Stinson E B 1980 Malignant lymphoma in cyclosporin-treated allograft recipients. Lancet 1: 43
Borel J F Weisinger D 1979 Studies on the mechanism of action of cyclosporin A. British Journal of Pharmacology 66: 66P–67P
Borel J F, Feurer C, Gubler H U, Staehlin H 1976 Biological effects of cyclosporin A: a new anti-lymphocytic agent. Agents Actions 6: 468–475
Calne R V, Rolles K, White D J G, Thru S, Evans D B, McMaster P et al 1979 Cyclosporin A initially as the only immunosuppressant in 34 recipients of cadaveric organs: 32 kidneys, 2 pancreases and 2 livers. Lancet 2: 1033–1036
Clarke C A, Elson C J, Bradley J, Donohoe W T A, Lehane D, Hughes-Jones N C 1970 Intensive plasmapheresis as a therapeutic measure in rhesus immunised women. Lancet 1: 793–798
Gordon M Y, Singer J W 1979 Selective effects of cyclosporin A on colony-forming lymphoid and myeloid cells in man. Nature 279: 433–434
Lockwood C M, Rees A J, Pearson T A, Evans D J, Peters D K, Wilson C B 1976 Immunosuppression and plasma exchange in the treatment of Goodpasture's syndrome. Lancet 1: 711–715
Naginton J 1981 Cyclosporin A immunosuppression and Epstein-Barr antibody. Lancet 1: 196
Pinching A J, Peters D K, Newsom-Davis J 1976 Remission of myasthenia gravis following plasma exchange. Lancet 2: 1373–1376
Powles R L, Clink H M, Spence D, Morgenstern G, Watson J G, Selby P J et al 1980 Prevention of GVHD following allogeneic bone marrow transplantation using cyclosporin A. Lancet 1: 327–329
Tutschka P J, Beschorner W E, Alison A C, Burns W H, Santos A W 1979 Use of cyclosporin A in allogeneic bone marrow transplantation in the rat. Nature 280: 148–151
Walker R G, D'Apice A J F, Becker G J, Kincaid-Smith P, Cresswell P W J 1977 Plasmapheresis in Goodpasture's syndrome with renal failure. Medical Journal of Australia 1: 875–879

4

Cardiology

D. G. Julian

NUCLEAR CARDIOLOGY

Apparatus for nuclear imaging of the heart is now available in most major cardiac centres and in many district hospitals. Cardiac scintigraphy has established itself as an important research tool and has an increasing part in diagnosis, but its final place alongside such other techniques as echocardiography and exercise testing has yet to be established.

There are three major ways in which nuclear imaging may help in cardiac diagnosis: the demonstration of myocardial perfusion abnormalities, the detection of myocardial infarction, and the evaluation of left ventricular function.

Myocardial perfusion

Some radiopharmaceutical substances become concentrated in the myocardium in direct relationship to coronary blood flow, provided that the perfused cells have the ability to extract them. Although a number of radio-isotopes have been employed for this purpose in the past, thallium-201 is now in almost universal use. This isotope, which has a physical half-life of about 3 days, is usually injected intravenously in a dose of 1.5–2 mCi. It is important to recognise that the image of the heart that thallium provides gives information about the relative, but not absolute, perfusion of different parts of the heart, so that with overall hypoperfusion there will be no defect, but if some region of the heart is relatively poorly perfused compared with the rest, a 'cold spot' can be detected.

In the patient with angina pectoris, there is usually relatively uniform perfusion at rest and no abnormality may be detected. During stress, and particularly during exercise, blood flow increases markedly to the normal myocardium but remains restricted in the area supplied by a stenotic vessel (Ritchie et al 1979).

'Cold spots' may be present at rest if there has been a new or old myocardial infarction or in cases of 'rest angina', such as Prinzmetal's angina. In some cases, the cardiomyopathic heart has areas which do not take up thallium, presumably because of scarring, in spite of an unimpaired coronary blood flow.

In 'cold spot' imaging for the detection and assessment of angina pectoris, an exercise test is usually undertaken. A needle or cannula is inserted into a vein, and the patient then exercises maximally or submaximally on a bicycle ergometer or treadmill. An attempt should be made to maintain the peak exercise level, in spite of symptoms, for at least half a minute. Imaging should preferably start within 5 minutes of the injection. Other forms of stress have been utilised, such as isometric exercise, the use of dipyridamole (to produce differential increase in blood flow), and such drugs as dobutamine.

If stress-induced ischaemia is present, a thallium defect is detected shortly after exercise. It may take 3 or 4 hours for a normal scan to be restored; a further image should be recorded at that time. A normal thallium scan 3 hours after a 'cold spot' has been demonstrated is strongly suggestive of myocardial ischaemia.

Thallium scintigraphy has established itself as a quite sensitive and specific test for coronary artery disease, as detected on coronary angiography. However, it is found to be of most value in cases of single- or double-vessel coronary disease, and less so in triple-vessel disease when there is very widespread but relatively equal hypoperfusion. The chief disadvantages of thallium scintigraphy are the expense of the isotope, relatively poor reproducibility and the degree of skill and experience that is necessary for optimal interpretation.

Thallium scintigraphy perhaps has its major role in the diagnosis of angina pectoris when this is strongly suspected but when the exercise ECG is not confirmatory. It has also been found to be of particular value in determining whether coronary artery bypass grafting has relieved ischaemia.

Detection of myocardial infarction

Thallium-201 may be used for the detection of myocardial infarction when a 'cold spot' is shown in the region of the infarction; it has been reported to have a high sensitivity for acute infarction within the first 6 hours (Wackers et al 1975). However, the disadvantages include the expense of the isotope, the inability to visualise certain aspects of the heart, particularly the apex, posterior wall and basal parts of the ventricle, and, because of its long half-life, an inability to repeat the test in less than 3 days. Furthermore, thallium imaging cannot differentiate old from fresh infarction or ischaemia from infarction with confidence.

An alternative and, on the whole, a more helpful approach is to use 'hot spot' detection, using tracers that can be described as 'infarct-avid'. $^{99}Tc^{m}$ has proved the most suitable for this purpose; it is a relatively cheap radio-isotope, which may be used in a variety of forms such as the pyrophosphate, imidodiphosphate, and glucoheptonate. This and similar isotopes are taken up in the area of necrosed myocardial cells. The advantage of 'hot spot' imaging is that it is nearly always positive in transmural infarction, although it is much less sensitive in detecting subendocardial infarction (Willerson et al 1975a,b Walton et al 1978). Unfortunately, 'hot spots' can also be detected in some cases of unstable angina pectoris (although this may, in fact, be detecting infarction), some cases of left ventricular aneurysm and after cardioversion. A major drawback is that a 'hot spot' usually does not appear for some 12 to 36 h after the onset. 'Hot spot' scans are particularly helpful when a major infarction occurs in the presence of left bundle-branch block or old infarction when ECG features obscure the development of new changes. It has also been found useful in detecting infarction after coronary artery bypass surgery (Burdine et al 1979).

Radionuclide angiography

Of the techniques available for studying the heart by scintigraphy, radionuclide angiography, which involves labelling of red cells rather than of myocardium, is probably proving the most helpful. Two major methods are used — first-pass studies and equilibrium studies.

In first-pass studies, a bolus is injected into a vein and the initial passage of the isotope is detected. Satisfactory first-pass scans usually require a multicrystal camera which is large and not portable. However, they do permit rapid visualisation of the heart with good separation of right and left ventricles, and are useful for demonstrating shunts.

Equilibrium studies usually use technetium-labelled red cells to allow imaging of the blood pool. In vivo labelling is achieved by injecting stannous pyrophosphate, which becomes attached to red cells, and subsequently injecting $^{99}Tc^{m}$ which combines with it. The ventricles can then be visualised by a gamma camera over a period of several hours. By gating techniques, using the ECG, segments of the cardiac cycle from successive beats can be superimposed. In its simplest form, end-systolic and end-diastolic images can be obtained, but with multiple-gated acquisition (MUGA) it is possible to obtain 20 or more exposures during the cardiac cycle. Multiple-gated blood-pool scanning permits the radionuclide equivalent of a cineangiogram. It has the advantage of being non-invasive and, unlike left ventriculography, does not induce ectopic beats. On the other hand, resolution is less good, and overlying of adjacent chambers as well as background radiation can cause problems.

It is relatively easy to obtain a first-pass scan during or at the end of exercise, but because of the need of averaging techniques over several minutes, multiple-gated pool scanning is less suitable for such stress studies. Radionuclide angiography provides evidence of a number of characteristics of left ventricular function. The ejection fraction may be estimated at rest and on exertion and has been found to be similar to that obtained by invasive left ventriculography. Regional wall abnormalities can also be detected, as can ventricular aneurysms.

Unlike echocardiography, nuclear imaging has a relatively small part to play in the assessment of valvular heart disease, but may be of value in estimating left ventricular dimensions and, for example, their increase in cases of progressive aortic regurgitation. It may, therefore, prove to be of value in defining the appropriate time for aortic valve replacement.

Nuclear angiography has been particularly useful in assessing right ventricular function. This applies not only to myocardial infarction, but also to pulmonary arterial hypertension and chronic obstructive pulmonary disease.

As yet, nuclear imaging has little part to play in the evaluation of congenital heart disease, although it allows accurate measurement of left-to-right cardiac shunts.

ELECTROCARDIOGRAPHIC MONITORING

Long-term electrocardiographic monitoring (dynamic, Holter or 24-hour monitoring) has now become an established part of cardiological practice, being used in many district hospitals. It has been predominantly employed for the detection of arrhythmias and disorders of conduction in patients complaining of syncope or palpitation, but it is also capable of detecting the ST changes of myocardial ischaemia, provided that the appropriate apparatus is employed.

There are, in fact, a number of different ways in which electrocardiographic information can be obtained about paroxysmal arrhythmias or conduction disturbances. Most commonly, single-channel Holter recording is employed, using small portable tape-recorders and chest electrodes, and obtaining a record similar to V5 in most cases. In this country, the most commonly used apparatus is the Oxford Medilog® recorder which uses standard C120 tapes and is geared to allow a continuous 24-hour recording. When the tape has been recorded, it must be analysed on a system which allows rapid replay so that a 24-hour recording can be scanned in less than half an hour.

There are many potential pitfalls in 24-hour recording. The application of the electrodes is of primary importance; skin preparation and electrode application must be optimal. It is wise for anyone undertaking this kind of work to visit a centre of expertise in this field to see the procedures in action, so that technicians can be trained to attach the electrodes correctly. It is preferable to use a technique which allows the selection of the best lead for the individual patient. Artefacts and variable running of the tape can give rise to spurious arrhythmias and periods of apparent bradycardia or asystole. Analysis is facilitated by a variety of high-speed scanning systems, one of which is made by Oxford Instruments and another, the Pathfinder®, by Reynolds Medical Instruments. Two-channel recorders are in increasing use and have the advantage that they help in the recognition of P waves and in determining whether ectopic beats are truly similar to the prevailing sinus beats. Patients using the apparatus should keep a careful diary of their symptoms during the recording: in general, analysis of the tape is seldom of diagnostic value unless symptoms and rhythm disturbances can be correlated.

Other methods of detecting rhythm abnormalities in ambulatory patients include transmission by telephone and 'event-recorders'. The former technique is simple and requires only a relatively cheap transmitter and receiver, but the GPO must approve the system and the telephone lines must be reliable. This is of value only if the patient is aware of arrhythmias — it is of no use for syncope. An 'event-recorder', which is a tape-recorder activated by the patient or automatically by an arrhythmia, is of particular value if episodes are infrequent.

CALCIUM ANTAGONISTS

Calcium has a vital role both in the electrophysiological and in the mechanical function of the myocardium. Calcium also has important effects on contraction of smooth muscle elsewhere.

The fast initial depolarisation of myocardial cells starts with a rapid inrush of sodium ions. Closely following this, but at a slower pace, calcium ions enter the cell and are partly responsible for depolarisation and for the plateau phase of the action potential. In certain tissues, notably the atrioventricular node, the slow calcium current, rather than the fast sodium current, is responsible for depolarisation.

Calcium is essential for myocardial contraction because it acts by repressing tr[illegible]in which otherwise inhibits the interaction between actin and myosin. [illegible]er, intracellular calcium is not available during relaxation as it is bound to many structures including the nucleus, mitochondria, sarcolemma, the T system and, in particular, the sarcoplasmic reticulum. The small amount of calcium which enters the cell during depolarisation and the plateau phase is insufficient, in itself, to trigger contraction but appears to release a large quantity of calcium from the sarcoplasmic reticulum (the 'calcium-induced' calcium release). During relaxation, calcium returns to the sarcoplasmic reticulum, releasing troponin which now inhibits actin–myosin interactions. The rate at which the tension of the myocardium is increased is related to changes in the rate at which calcium is made available, and the total tension developed depends upon the quantity of calcium delivered to the myofilaments.

A number of calcium-antagonist drugs are available (Opie 1980b); the two in most common use are verapamil and nifedipine. Perhexilene and prenylamine, both of which have been found to have anti-anginal effects, are also calcium antagonists but have additional actions.

Although verapamil and nifedipine share calcium antagonism as their major pharmacological characteristic, they differ markedly in their therapeutic action.

Verapamil has a potent effect on the function of the atrioventricular node and can, in high concentration, cause atrioventricular block. It has been found to be particularly effective when used intravenously in the treatment of supraventricular tachycardias but is of little use in ventricular arrhythmias (Singh et al, 1978). Intravenous verapamil should not be given to patients who are under the influence of β-adrenergic blocking drugs. It is effective in treating coronary artery spasm of the Prinzmetal type, but also suppresses exercise-induced angina (Bala Subramanian et al 1980, Simoons et al 1980). In this situation it is effective when given on its own, and there are doubts about its safety when given in association with oral β-adrenergic blocking drugs. The dose is 5–10 mg given slowly by intravenous injection over 5–10 minutes. Quite apart from the risks of bradycardia and atrioventricular block, the drug has a negative inotropic effect and should be given with caution to patients with severely compromised ventricular function. It may be given by mouth in a dose of 40–120 mg four times a day but blood levels are variable, due to a first-pass effect. Its chief uses are in slowing the ventricular response to atrial fibrillation when digitalis alone has failed, and in the treatment of those patients for whom β-blocking drugs have either proved ineffective or are contraindicated because of obstructive airways disease. Apart from the bradycardiac and negative inotropic effects of verapamil, its main side effect is that of constipation.

Nifedipine differs from verapamil in having little effect on the atrioventricular node; it is therefore of little value in the treatment of supraventricular arrhythmias. It is a potent vasodilator of both coronary and peripheral arteries and is effective in the treatment of coronary arterial spasm (Antman et al 1980). It is also of value in exercise-induced angina, but its peripheral vasodilating effect often results in a tachycardia which may be undesirable. However, the combination of β-blockade and nifedipine appears to be safe and effective in controlling angina (Ekelund & Orö 1979, Lynch et al 1980). Nifedipine has also been found to be a useful antihypertensive drug, especially if combined with β-blockers or other antihypertensives (Guazzi et al 1980). The usual dose is 10–20 mg three times a day.

Nifedipine has a negative inotropic effect and can, occasionally, exacerbate cardiac failure. Other side effects are not uncommon and include oedema of the feet and ankles (in the absence of cardiac failure), hypotension and syncope, flushing and headache. In spite of these, the majority of patients tolerate the drug well.

INFECTIVE ENDOCARDITIS

Despite advances in antibiotic therapy and in knowledge of prophylaxis, infective endocarditis continues to be a dangerous and not infrequent condition. Some 20–35% of hospitalised patients die: many cases are first recognised at autopsy, so the overall mortality may, in fact, be in the region of 50% (Smith et al 1976). With the diminishing incidence of rheumatic heart disease, mitral valve endocarditis is becoming less frequent but with the ageing population the aortic value is more often involved. New forms of endocarditis secondary to prosthetic heart valves and drug abuse are being seen more often and approximately one-quarter of cases now involve what were apparently previously normal valves. Streptococcus (especially *Streptococcus viridans*) is the most common causative organism, but staphylococci have become more frequently implicated; enterococci and a wide variety of other organisms are responsible for the remaining cases.

Blood culture from three separate venepunctures will usually allow the identification of the infecting organism. However, special efforts must be made to identify anaerobes and fungi and in all suspected cases (particularly in patients with evidence of liver dysfunction) Rickettsia *(Coxiella burnetti)* must be sought by the appropriate tests.

Non-invasive techniques, especially two-dimensional echocardiography, have proved valuable in assessing progress. Thus, bacterial vegetations may be demonstrated, as may the prolapse of valve cusps, abscesses and pericardial effusions. The effects of the disease on ventricular function may also be observed.

Antibiotic therapy continues to be modified as new drugs become available. Oakley & Darrell (1980) have recently reviewed current recommendations. Two unresolved issues concern the choice of antibiotic for dental and other forms of prophylaxis, and the timing and role of cardiac surgery. The use of penicillin or other parenterally administered antibiotics before dental extraction has been widely recommended, but the logistic difficulties in administering a drug in this way, and the fact that dentists are not authorised to do so, has meant that relatively few patients at risk have received appropriate antibiotic prophylaxis. It is probable that a single dose of 3 g of amoxycillin given orally will provide equally effective protection and will permit more reliable administration.

Death from infective endocarditis is now most commonly attributable to cardiac failure or embolism rather than uncontrolled infection. Frequently, the surgeon is asked to operate on a patient with gross aortic regurgitation in an advanced state of failure. Early surgery is usually successful even in the presence of infection, although it is clearly preferable that the infection should be brought under control before a prosthetic value is inserted. Surgery is particularly likely to be needed in staphylococcal and fungal infections and, in the former, myocardial abscesses commonly occur and the aortic wall may be weakened by direct infection.

Because of the largely unpredictable risks to which victims of endocarditis are exposed, there is much to be said for all such patients being admitted to a cardiac centre so that the patient can be closely observed by cardiologists and surgeons, and operation undertaken without delay, if necessary.

THE REPLACEMENT OF CARDIAC VALVES

In spite of the decline of rheumatic valvular disease in Western Europe and North America, valve replacement continues to be a relatively common cardiac operation, particularly for calcific aortic stenosis in the middle-aged and elderly and for the replacement of previously inserted valvular prostheses which have failed to function properly.

In spite of a wide variety of new valve designs, some of the older types of valvular prosthesis continue to function as well as, if not better than, the newer models. Thus, Starr-Edwards silastic ball-valve prostheses have been functioning satisfactorily since 1966 (Starr et al 1977), and the Bjork-Shiley valve since 1969 (Pluth 1981). Many surgeons prefer one or other of these valves but acknowledge that problems may arise because of the need for anticoagulant therapy in most cases.

Relatively fresh homograft valves, sterilised in antibiotic, have given satisfactory results but have been used on a large scale in only a few centres. This probably reflects the difficulty of obtaining this form of bioprosthesis, as well as the undoubtedly superior skill required in its insertion.

A more popular form of bioprosthesis at present is the porcine tissue valve. Such a value has the advantage, at least in the aortic position, of not requiring long-term anticoagulant treatment. However, anticoagulant treatment may be necessary for elderly patients requiring an aortic bioprosthesis, and is certainly desirable in the mitral valve area, especially if atrial fibrillation is present or likely to develop. A further question relates to the long-term durability of these valves. Unfortunately, heterograft valves seem most likely to degenerate in the young, particularly in those under the age of 10 years. As Kirklin (1981) has observed: 'Most experienced cardiac surgeons would agree that the risks and imponderables associated with both mechanical devices and bioprostheses highlight the importance of preserving the patient's own valve by deferring operation — not for too long but until intervention is clearly indicated — and by repairing rather than replacing the patient's valve whenever possible'.

VASODILATOR THERAPY OF CARDIAC FAILURE

The concept of vasodilatation in the management of heart failure is a relatively new one, although most of the drugs now used for this purpose have been employed therapeutically with different concepts in mind in the past.

It is important to differentiate drugs which cause venodilatation (such as glyceryl trinitrate and isosorbide dinitrate) from those that are arteriolar dilators (e.g. hydrallazine). Other drugs (including prazosin and captopril) have roughly equivalent effects on arteries and veins.

Venodilating drugs increase the volume of the capacitance vessels and blood tends to pool in the venous compartment. This reduces, at least temporarily, the venous return to the heart. Whether or not this is beneficial depends on whether the left ventricle is overloaded in the sense of having too high a filling (or end-diastolic) pressure. It has been found that, in most cases of cardiac failure, the optimal filling pressure lies between 15 and 20 mmHg. If the pressure is higher than this, the ventricle is over-distended and the heart is working on the flat part or descending limb of the Starling curve. In this situation, a reduction in filling pressure will result in an improvement in left ventricular function, which may then be able to cope with the venous return and, consequently, there will be a rise in cardiac output. Ideally, before using a venodilator, the filling pressure should be measured either directly or, more conveniently, by recording pulmonary capillary wedge pressure by means of a Swan-Ganz balloon-tipped catheter. It is important not to administer a venodilating drug to patients with normal or low filling pressures, particularly in the presence of myocardial infarction, as a marked fall in cardiac output and blood pressure may occur.

The principle behind arteriolar dilatation is quite different. Such drugs reduce after-load, that is the resistance or impedance against which the heart muscle contracts. Since the blood pressure is dependent upon the product of the cardiac output and the systemic vascular resistance, it tends to fall in line with any fall in systemic vascular resistance, unless this is compensated by an increase in cardiac output. The normal heart usually responds to 'impedance reduction' by drugs such as hydralazine or prazosin by a fall in blood pressure. The heart that is failing in the face of an increased vascular resistance may well respond to a fall in this resistance by an increase in output with no significant change in blood pressure.

The drugs in most widespread use at present are isosorbide dinitrate (given orally or intravenously), nitroprusside (given intravenously), and hydralazine and prazosin (given orally).

In most patients with raised filling pressures (over 15 mmHg), isosorbide is likely to produce a fall in pulmonary capillary wedge and right atrial pressures, followed by a rise in stroke volume and cardiac output. There may be some slight decrease in arterial pressure but the heart rate usually does not change.

Nitroprusside acts as both arteriodilator and venodilator, but must be given intravenously (Cohn & Burke 1979). Very careful monitoring is necessary and treatment is best administered in an intensive care environment with pulmonary- and systemic-arterial monitoring. It should be started in a low dose, for example 0.25 μg/kg per min with close observation of the arterial pressure. Administration of nitroprusside should not be continued beyond 48 h, because of the risks of thiocyanate or cyanide poisoning. Other toxic effects include nausea, convulsions and cyanosis caused by methaemoglobinaemia.

Prazosin is also both an arteriodilator and venodilator (Awan et al 1977, Rubin et al 1979). Although hypotensive reactions are unusual in patients in cardiac failure, particularly in those confined to bed, treatment should start with a relatively small dose which should then be progressively increased. A dosage of 0.5 mg three times a day may be used initially but this can be gradually built up to 5 mg three or four times a day. Some reports have suggested that tachyphylaxis develops rapidly, but others have demonstrated a persisting effect over several months.

Arteriolar dilators are particularly effective in patients with a high systemic vascular resistance associated with a low cardiac output. In this situation, hydralazine may be particularly beneficial (Koch-Weser 1976, Fitchett et al 1979). The initial dose is 25–50 mg three or four times a day; it is probably wiser to avoid doses in excess of 200 or 300 mg daily, because of the risk of a lupus-like syndrome. Reflex tachycardia may also be a problem.

Captopril, the angiotensin-converting enzyme, also has venodilator and arteriodilator activities and is as effective as, or more effective than, other vasodilator drugs in treating heart failure (Turini et al 1979).

Experience with vasodilator therapy is still relatively limited and largely confined to its use in severe cases of cardiac failure that do not respond to other therapy. Currently, it is recommended mainly for patients who have failed to respond to conventional therapy, but it is probable that in the future, particularly in selected forms of cardiac failure, vasodilator drugs will be used concurrently with, or in place of, other forms of therapy such as digitalis or diuretics. For example, infusion of isosorbide dinitrate may be particularly effective in acute pulmonary oedema and, indeed, more so than intravenous frusemide which is commonly employed. However, it should be mentioned that both morphine and frusemide have some venodilator action which may contribute to their value in the management of acute pulmonary oedema.

Acute mitral regurgitation, which can follow rupture of papillary muscles or chordae tendineae, may benefit strikingly from arteriolar vasodilators. Nitroprusside and hydralazine, in particular, have been shown to be of value in this context as they lower aortic impedance and encourage forward output at the expense of mitral regurgitation. The lowering of systemic vascular resistance also reduces regurgitant volume in acute aortic regurgitation. However, vasodilators should be used cautiously in this situation as they may lower aortic diastolic pressure.

EPIDEMIOLOGY AND PREVENTION OF CORONARY HEART DISEASE

Mortality trends

Much publicity has been given to the fact that mortality from ischaemic heart disease in the United States has been declining progressively since about 1967 (Walker 1977). This decline now amounts to almost 25% and has affected white and coloured men and women. A similar fall in mortality has been observed in Australia, New Zealand, Canada and Norway. In Britain, after a period of rising mortality, there has been a plateau for some years, but in other countries, including Sweden, Denmark, Ireland and the countries of Eastern Europe, there still seems to be a progressive increase (Rose 1981).

These trends, particularly their variation between different countries, are not readily explained. Certainly, in the United States, Australia and New Zealand, there has been a greater attempt to influence public behaviour in lowering the lipid content of the diet and in anti-smoking campaigns and there has also been more widespread detection and treatment of hypertension. On the other hand, it was in these same countries that both coronary care and coronary artery surgery gained acceptance most rapidly. The fall in mortality is unlikely to be due to any one single factor, but is probably the consequence of a combination of prophylactic and therapeutic measures. Furthermore, there is the possibility of some changing, but as yet unrecognised, factor.

It is of interest that, in the United Kingdom, there was a progressive fall in deaths from coronary heart disease in doctors between 1954 and 1971, whereas in all males there was a slight increase during this period (Royal College of Physicians 1977). One undoubted difference in the behaviour of doctors compared with the rest of the community is the degree to which they gave up smoking over this period. It is much less certain that they changed their dietetic habits, were treated for hypertension, or received better medical care. However, it is also pertinent that mortality from ischaemic heart disease has been continuing to rise in the social classes III–V, but not in classes I and II.

Controlled intervention trials

There have been several trials which have attempted to control individual risk factors. In the Los Angeles study on Veterans and the Helsinki Mental Hospital study (Dayton et al 1969, Miettinen et al 1972), there was some evidence of a reduction in non-fatal infarction, and a less convincing reduction in coronary death in individuals who received a high fat diet with a very high proportion of polyunsaturated fats.

In the Hypertension Detection and Follow-up Program (Hypertension Detection and Follow-up Program Co-operative Group 1979) in the United States, patients were assigned either to 'stepped care' or to 'referred care'. In the 'stepped care' group, antihypertensive therapy was administered in special centres and treatment was increased in a step-wise fashion to ensure blood pressure control. Patients in the 'referred care' group were referred back to their usual medical attendant. Some evidence of a reduction in myocardial infarction was observed in the better-controlled patients.

In the Australian Therapeutic Trial in mildly hypertensive individuals, 3232 subjects with diastolic pressures between 95 and 109 mmHg were assigned to antihypertensive medication or placebo (Management Committee 1980). In men and women with diastolic pressures of 100 mmHg or more, in the treated group there was a reduction in cerebrovascular disease, but only a non-significant reduction in fatal ischaemic heart disease. A number of multi-factorial prevention trials are in progress (Beevers et al 1981), but as yet there are no satisfactory data on the results thereof.

Drug therapy in lowering lipids

A very large trial (under the auspices of WHO) involved the use of clofibrate in some 15000 men who were selected from volunteers in Edinburgh, Budapest and Prague (Committee of Principal Investigators 1978). Those in the top tertile of plasma cholesterol levels, who agreed to participate, were randomly allocated to clofibrate or placebo and compared with another group of men in the lowest tertile of cholesterol levels, who received only placebo. Cholesterol levels in those receiving clofibrate were reduced by 9% (less than the expected 15%). The treated group had a higher overall mortality (by 37%). This was partly accounted for by the effect of clofibrate on the biliary concentration and solubility of neutral steroids, with the result that 25 patients required cholecystectomy and three of these died. However, there was a greater mortality from a variety of causes including gastrointestinal cancer. It was claimed that there was a reduction in the incidence of non-fatal ischaemic heart disease, but paradoxically the actual mortality rate from acute ischaemic attacks was higher in the clofibrate-treated individuals.

The disappointing results of this large and long-term trial raise the question as to whether similar attempts to lower lipid levels will be equally ineffective and, indeed, will increase the risk of death from other causes. It is possible that even the substitution of polyunsaturated fats or the lowering of cholesterol itself may increase the risk of intestinal neoplasm.

CORONARY ARTERY BYPASS SURGERY

There have been no recent major technical advances in coronary artery bypass surgery, but its place in management is becoming more clearly defined and results are improving with better selection of patients and increasing experience. It has been established convincingly that this operation can improve symptoms and objective measurements of cardiac function during stress, in 80–90% of cases. The mortality of the procedure, in the absence of complicating factors, should not be greater than 2%; however, when left ventricular function is severely compromised, the mortality rises sharply. The procedure is most clearly indicated in relatively young people whose livelihood or major social activities are seriously limited. The success and low mortality have encouraged cardiac surgeons to accept for operation the elderly and those with poorer myocardial function. There is little evidence that myocardial performance at rest is improved by the procedure but if angina is a major symptom, poor left ventricular function is not an overriding contraindication.

Controversy continues as to the effects on prognosis. The European Coronary Artery Bypass Study (European Coronary Surgery Study Group 1980) concerned 768 men aged less than 65 years, with angina pectoris, with 50% or more reduction demonstrable in at least two coronary arteries, and with good left ventricular function. All patients have been followed up for a minimum of 5 years and many for up to 8 years. This study has provided good evidence that, in those with disease affecting all three coronary vessels, there is a significant improvement in prognosis up to 8 years after the operation. There is a benefit conferred by surgery for the group as a whole which is highly significant statistically (93.5% survivors versus 84.1%, $P = < 0.001$), and this is particularly evident in those with three-vessel disease (94.9% versus 84.9%, $P = < 0.001$). No benefit was shown in two-vessel disease. Although this study was convincing in showing the value of surgery in patients who were selected, it does not provide evidence about the elderly, about women, or about those with compromised left ventricular function. A study in the United States (Coronary Artery Surgery Study — CASS) involving a wider group of patients will be completed in the near future.

In view of the prognostic advantage of surgery, the question arises as to whether, or how, one identifies patients whose symptoms alone do not merit surgery but who might benefit in terms of life expectancy. As yet, no satisfactory study has identified those who are likely to benefit, without undertaking the potentially hazardous and expensive investigation of coronary arteriography, but it seems probable that the majority of such patients could be recognised by their response to an exercise test. Those who develop ST cardiographic changes or angina at a relatively low work load, those whose blood pressure rises by less than 25% on exercise and those who fail to raise the heart rate are likely to have three-vessel or left main vessel disease. It should not be necessary, therefore, to undertake coronary arteriography on all patients with angina in order to determine those who might benefit from surgery, but this investigation can be reserved for those with symptoms or exercise tests suggesting severe disease.

PERCUTANEOUS TRANSLUMINAL ANGIOPLASTY

For some years, techniques have been developed for dilating peripheral arteries with a balloon mounted on the end of a catheter, which can be introduced percutaneously into the femoral or brachial arteries. More recently, Gruntzig et al (1979) have developed a special catheter for use in the coronary arteries. It has been possible to show that atheromatous coronary arteries can be dilated successfully so that, for example, a stenosis that has narrowed the artery by 90% can be reduced to one of 30%. The exact mechanism by which this dilatation occurs is not clear, although some cracking of atheromatous plaques and stretching of media and adventitia probably takes place. Experience is still limited, but there is no doubt of its effectiveness, particularly in single-vessel coronary disease. Cases must be carefully selected and considerable expertise is required. In order to be successful, the lesion to be dilated should be relatively proximal, concentric, uncalcified, and not too close to a major coronary artery branch. The technique has also been found to be effective in some cases of graft narrowing and has been used in a relatively small number of cases of two-vessel coronary disease, but the risks are higher in this context. As yet, the number of cases suitable for this procedure is small but with more experience this may increase.

MYOCARDIAL INFARCTION

Community studies have shown that, of all who die within the first four weeks of the onset of an acute coronary heart attack, some 40% die within the first hour (Armstrong et al 1972). When these observations were made, it was commonly accepted that acute myocardial infarction was the usual cause of death: however, following the work of Cobb et al (1975), it has become increasingly clear that a very high percentage of the sudden deaths are, in fact, not attributable to a recent myocardial infarction but to ventricular fibrillation occurring in the absence of fresh necrosis or coronary occlusion. Consequently, it may be concluded that acute myocardial infarction itself has not such a high early mortality rate as suggested by these studies and that many of the deaths in this condition occur in the succeeding few hours.

Death caused by ventricular fibrillation may occur in the absence of severe left ventricular damage, in patients whose blood pressure and cardiac status appear to be relatively good. Such cases are regarded as examples of 'primary' ventricular fibrillation; the successful correction of such episodes has been the greatest single contribution of coronary care units. The close observation of oscilloscope screens has revealed that many patients have ventricular arrhythmias before ventricular fibrillation and it was assumed that there was a causal relationship. However, continuous ECG monitoring, accompanied by tape-recording to allow detailed analysis subsequently, has shown that so-called 'warning arrhythmias' are as common in those who do not proceed to ventricular fibrillation as in those who do, and that, furthermore, ventricular fibrillation commonly occurs without any preceding arrhythmia at all (Lie et al 1975). Such observations have led to the concept that ventricular fibrillation should be prevented by routine antiarrhythmic therapy. Following the observations of Lie et al (1974), in a controlled study, and of Wyman & Hammersmith (1974) in an uncontrolled study, the routine use of lignocaine in prophylaxis has become widespread, particularly in the United States. This therapy is not always effective and is attended by a moderately high level of neurotoxic and cardiac side effects. As ventricular fibrillation is usually easy to reverse in the coronary care unit, many physicians do not use prophylactic therapy.

Pre-hospital coronary care

Following the initiative of Pantridge, many centres throughout the world have now developed mobile coronary care facilities. In some cities, as in the original Belfast example, special mobile coronary ambulances are used, staffed by medical personnel. Although there is no doubt that these can manage patients effectively outside hospital and have achieved many successful defibrillations, the shortage of medical personnel and the logistic difficulties of running such units has led to the widespread development of vehicles manned by paramedical staff. These generally deal, not only with heart attacks, but with other forms of medical emergency and trauma. It has been shown clearly that many lives may be saved in this way, but a successful service of this kind depends not only upon training the paramedical personnel and equipping them with appropriate apparatus, but also instructing the public in cardiopulmonary resuscitation (Thompson et al 1979).

Home versus hospital treatment

The controversy as to whether patients are better treated at home or in hospital has been revived by studies undertaken in Nottingham (Hill et al 1978). In this study, a junior hospital doctor and a trained nurse in a coronary care unit were sent to patients' homes following a call from the general practitioner. The team gave emergency treatment to all patients except those in whom the diagnosis of infarction was improbable, and stayed in the home for 2 hours. After this period, the patients were allotted at random to home or hospital treatment, unless there were overriding considerations for the choice of one or other place. Two hundred and sixty four cases were included in the study: at 28 days, 11% of those treated in hospital had died, compared with 13% in the home, this difference not being statistically significant. The numbers in the study were so small that it is quite possible that any beneficial effect of hospital treatment may have gone undetected. Eight patients died on the first day at home and only one in hospital: this argues strongly against the concept of patients being 'frightened to death', as had been suggested in previous studies. Although the lack of statistical difference between the home and hospital groups has been used as an argument against hospital admission, it should be pointed out that the home-treated group received better treatment than would have been normally available (including the correction of ventricular fibrillation). Furthermore, the patients were allocated to their groups a very long time after the onset of infarction (a median time of over 5 hours), and the success rate from treating ventricular fibrillation was much lower than that found in other centres. It is, therefore, not possible to draw any valid conclusions from this study.

Management of cardiac failure and shock in myocardial infarction

In recent years there have been substantial increases in our understanding of cardiac failure and shock complicating myocardial infarction, and many new therapies have been introduced. How far these have affected the eventual survival of the patient is not clear. However, there are some important features which should be identified and treated appropriately. One such feature is a reduction in effective blood volume, leading to a low filling pressure, which may be readily corrected by infusion; another is a high venous pressure caused by right ventricular infarction, which may incorrectly suggest left ventricular failure. Although these problems may be suspected on clinical grounds, they are better verified by actual measurements of the pulmonary arterial wedge pressure, right atrial pressure and, when the arterial pressure is low, by intra-arterial pressure recordings. The development of the Swan-Ganz balloon-tipped catheter has been an important advance, enabling haemodynamic studies to be undertaken at the bedside without the need for visualisation of the catheter and the costly radiographic apparatus necessary for this.

Pulmonary congestion is usually best treated with morphine, oxygen, and bedrest, supplemented by intravenous frusemide and possibly intravenous isosorbide dinitrate. If these measures fail, consideration should be given to the use of prazosin or hydrallazine, but it is preferable that the pulmonary arterial wedge pressure should be measured before these drugs are administered. The role of digitalis in acute myocardial infarction is still controversial. Apart from its use for atrial arrhythmias, it is indicated mainly in patients who have well-marked cardiomegaly; the reduction of cardiac size may reduce oxygen requirement.

If a low blood pressure is accompanied by other features of shock, a cause should be sought. In the majority of cases this will be a large infarction, which may be associated with either a raised or normal filling pressure. In the presence of a low filling pressure of the left ventricle, hypovolaemia or right ventricular infarction should be suspected, and the use of intravenous dextran 40 may prove helpful. Dopamine is the drug most often used to increase myocardial contractility in this context, in a dose of 2–5 μg/kg per min but this may be increased up to 30 μg/kg per min. In spite of such measures, shock remains a highly lethal condition.

Intra-aortic balloon pumping has proved effective in improving the clinical condition of patients with shock. In this technique, a catheter with a balloon attached is inserted via the femoral artery into the descending aorta and triggered to inflate during diastole and deflate during systole; this reduces impedance to ventricular contraction while increasing diastolic blood flow and, thereby, coronary blood flow. Patients treated in this way have improved peripheral perfusion, increased urinary output, and often lose their chest pain. However, unless the patient can receive some form of treatment to improve myocardial function, this measure provides only temporary benefit. If, for example, there is a ventricular septal defect or papillary muscle rupture which can effectively be treated surgically, then the insertion of an intra-aortic balloon pump is a most valuable intermediary measure.

Attempts to salvage ischaemic myocardium

Great interest has been evoked in the possibility of limiting the size of infarction by strategies which either diminish myocardial oxygen requirement or increase myocardial blood flow (Opie 1980a). Whether this can be achieved is open to doubt, although animal experiments support the concept.

Beta-adrenergic blocking drugs have been particularly investigated in this context and their relative safety has been demonstrated in a large number of studies. Of particular interest have been the observations of Norris et al (1978), which show that propranolol diminishes creatine kinase (CK) release after infarction, and the findings of Yusuf et al (1980), which suggest that atenolol may reduce infarct size, as judged by ECG and enzymatic criteria.

Vasodilators such as nitroprusside and nitrates have also been advocated in this context, but beneficial effects of their actions are less well substantiated.

Attempts to increase coronary blood flow by surgery have been of questionable benefit. Impressive results have been reported with the use of intracoronary streptokinase (Rentrop et al 1981) but this approach is still experimental. Claims have also been made for hyaluronidase, glucose-insulin and potassium, and for non-steroidal anti-inflammatory agents, but none of these can yet be said to be of proved value.

MEDIUM- AND LONG-TERM PROGNOSIS AFTER MYOCARDIAL INFARCTION

There has been great interest in establishing the prognosis of patients who have recovered from an acute myocardial infarction. Information about prognosis is of value in the management of the patient — for example, in enabling the physician to advise on such matters as retirement and return to work — but may also act as a guide to secondary preventive measures.

Unfortunately, most of the published studies have indicated that the most reliable and potent predictors of death in the months or years after infarction are irremediable (Norris et al 1974, Luria et al 1979), for example age, previous history of infarction, and indices of left ventricular dysfunction. Hypotension, sustained sinus tachycardia, pulmonary oedema, atrial arrhythmias and cardiomegaly at the time of the acute episode, all suggest a poor late prognosis; more elaborate tests of left ventricular function, such as nuclear imaging, echocardiography or angiographic left ventriculography all point to the same conclusion (Schulze et al 1977). The height of the enzyme peak during the acute event is also of prognostic value, but the electrocardiogram is less useful in this context. Thus, although transmural infarctions are more likely to cause death in the acute phase than are subendocardial infarctions, long-term prognosis is not very dissimilar (Madigan et al 1976, Smeets et al 1981). This apparent anomaly seems to result from the fact that subendocardial infarction often occurs in patients with very widespread coronary disease, who may have had previous infarction and have a liability to recurrence.

Clearly, it would be of value if one could identify reversible risk factors in patients after infarction. The most promising factor appears to be the response to exercise during the early weeks after infarction. Théroux et al (1979), who carried out a modified exercise test at approximately 3 weeks, found that the development of ST-segment depression was highly significant in relation to prognosis. Thus, the 1-year mortality rate was 2.1% in patients without ST changes during exercise, and 27% in those with ST-segment depression. It seems probable that exercise tests will be carried out increasingly during the convalescent phase of myocardial infarction — either some 7–21 d after the onset while the patient is still in hospital, or at the first outpatient follow-up. It must be emphasised that the exercise test should be modified so that the heart rate does not exceed 120–130 per minute, and should be discontinued if any adverse features such as angina, hypotension or ventricular arrhythmias are encountered. Furthermore, it should not be undertaken in the presence of cardiac failure or of recent chest pain at rest. Provided that these precautions are observed, there is no reason to suppose that there is any appreciable danger in carrying out an exercise test at this time. Not only does it provide information of prognostic and therapeutic value, but it often gives the patient a good impression of his ability to return to an active life. Those patients who sustain angina and, more particularly, those who develop ST-segment depression, are obviously candidates for therapy. There appears to be a good case for starting to use beta-blocking drugs in this context, provided that they are not contraindicated. However, many of these patients are likely to come to coronary artery bypass surgery in the succeeding months.

There has been a considerable interest in the relationship between ventricular arrhythmias during the convalescent phase (as demonstrated on the electrocardiogram, on exercise testing or by ambulatory monitoring), and subsequent death, especially sudden death. Although several studies have confirmed that such a relationship exists, it is less clear that the two phenomena are *directly* related (Vismara et al 1975, Ruberman et al 1980). Ventricular arrhythmias in the convalescent phase are closely related to the severity of the coronary artery disease and the associated left ventricular damage. They are relatively rare in patients with single-vessel disease or in those with preserved left ventricular function. Furthermore, therapy that patients receive at this time for left ventricular dysfunction, particularly digitalis, may lead to ventricular arrhythmias. It cannot be inferred, therefore, that the presence of ventricular arrhythmias is necessarily an indication for treatment. Nevertheless, there are some patients who, during the convalescent phase following infarction, have repeated ventricular arrhythmias of symptomatic or haemodynamic importance. These may be prolonged attacks of ventricular tachycardia or episodes of ventricular fibrillation. Undoubtedly, these are of prognostic importance and merit treatment.

SECONDARY PREVENTION AFTER MYOCARDIAL INFARCTION

Although there is clearly a limit to what can be achieved in patients with myocardial infarction, as they must already have advanced coronary disease and some degree of left ventricular dysfunction, appropriate treatment and modifications in life-style may achieve an appreciable improvement, not only in well-being but in long-term prognosis.

Anticoagulants

The first major attempt at secondary prevention was the use of long-term anticoagulants in the 1960s. Several studies produced evidence that the long-term use of oral anticoagulants was effective in preventing recurrent myocardial infarction (International Anticoagulant Review Group 1970). Although therapy with long-term anticoagulants was adopted in some countries, notably the Netherlands, it was not taken up enthusiastically in the United States or the United Kingdom because of its hazards, difficulties in compliance and lack of conviction of its value in ordinary clinical practice.

A recent study from the Netherlands suggests that this matter may require further review. In the Sixty Plus Reinfarction Study (1980), patients who had been on long-term anticoagulant therapy following infarction were randomly assigned to withdrawal from the therapy or to continuation. Those who stopped therapy had a significantly higher incidence of reinfarction and death than those who continued. This study calls for two comments. Firstly, it could be argued that the untoward effect of withdrawal does not prove the value of therapy, particularly if a rebound effect might occur. However, the fact that the reinfarctions and deaths occurred over a long period and were not related closely to the time of discontinuation suggests that this objection is not valid. Secondly, the patients on long-term anticoagulant therapy entered into the trial had already demonstrated their ability to take the treatment reliably and without severe toxicity. One cannot, therefore, conclude that anticoagulant treatment is appropriate for all patients, as those who were non-compliant or at high risk of adverse effect were not included.

Platelet active agents

Several drugs which affect platelet aggregation have been tested in patients after infarction.

Aspirin has been widely used over the last few years and results of a number of studies have been published. In several of these there appears to have been a reduction in the incidence of myocardial infarction, but the death rate has not been significantly reduced. In the largest, the aspirin–myocardial infarction study (AMIS), aspirin appeared to exert an unfavourable effect (Aspirin Myocardial Infarction Study Research Group 1980), but it should be pointed out that the drug was not started for months or even years after the acute event and there was some imbalance in the randomisation. The persantin–aspirin reinfarction study (Persantin-Aspirin Reinfarction Study Group (PARIS) 1980) showed a more favourable trend, with some benefit in relation to reinfarction. However, a further similar study is now being undertaken to confirm the apparent trend. In the Anturane Reinfarction Trial, sulfinpyrazone in a dosage of 200 mg q.i.d. was employed 25–35 d after infarction (Anturane Reinfarction Trial (ART) Research Group 1980). Although in two published articles it was claimed that there was a significant reduction in sudden death in sulfinpyrazone-treated patients, further examination of the data has cast doubt on this conclusion. There was not a significant reduction in total mortality or reinfarction (the latter being the primary end-point of the study). A further report is awaited on the validity of the analysis. For the present, it cannot be concluded that sulfinpyrazone is effective in reducing mortality following infarction.

Beta-adrenergic blockade

There have been several trials of the use of β-adrenergic blocking drugs following myocardial infarction. Earlier studies with alprenolol and practolol (Wilhelmsson et al 1974, Multicentre International Study 1977), failed to show an overall effect upon total mortality in the 2 years following infarction, but in both instances there was evidence suggesting a reduction in cardiac death, particularly within the first few hours of a new event. Other studies which were negative with alprenolol and propranolol (Baber et al 1980) concerned relatively small groups of patients. In a study of 1884 patients undertaken by the Norwegian Multicentre Study Group (1981) using timolol 10 mg b.d., a highly significant ($P < 0.01$) effect upon mortality was observed in patients followed for 12 to 32 months after infarction. Reductions were seen not only in total death, but in sudden death and in fatal and non-fatal reinfarction. The patients were stratified before randomisation into three risk groups: risk group I contained patients with previous myocardial infarction with or without adverse factors during the acute event, risk group II represented patients who had adverse factors (such as cardiac failure) during their recent first myocardial infarction, and risk group III were those with first infarction without the adverse factors. Timolol appeared to prevent death and reinfarction in each of these groups.

It can be concluded that the β-blocking drug timolol is effective in secondary prevention in the first 1 to 3 years after infarction. It is not yet certain whether this is a special characteristic of timolol or whether the findings can be extrapolated to other β-blocking agents. If one accepts that the alprenolol, practolol and timolol studies are all indicative of benefit and that alprenolol is a non-selective β-blocker with intrinsic sympathomimetic activity, that practolol is a selective β-blocker with intrinsic sympathomimetic activity and that timolol is a non-selective drug without intrinsic sympathomimetic activity, it is difficult to conclude that this benefit is due to any characteristic of these drugs other than their β-blocking capabilities. The question also arises as to whether one should give a β-adrenergic blocking drug to all patients following myocardial infarction, provided that there are no contraindications. The timolol study itself failed to show any group that did not benefit from the drug but more work is required to define those sub-sets of patients who are or are not benefited by β-blockade.

Other secondary preventive measures

As yet, there are no satisfactory controlled trials to show that control of primary risk factors is beneficial in post-infarction patients. Nevertheless, the evidence from observations on patients who stop or continue smoking is highly suggestive. Reports from a number of centres including Sweden and Dublin (Wilhelmsson et al 1975, Hickey et al 1978). indicate a very substantial reduction in mortality in those who discontinue smoking after infarction, compared with those who continue. Efforts to control lipids are of more doubtful value and the Coronary Drug Project (Coronary Drug Project Research Group 1975) failed to show any significant benefit. There have been no satisfactory studies of the control of hypertension in post-infarction patients.

Rehabilitation programmes have been undertaken energetically in some centres, in certain countries in particular. As yet, there is no evidence that physical rehabilitation is effective in improving prognosis in regard to life, although a sense of well-being is certainly greater in those who exercise.

As yet, no satisfactory controlled trials of the value of coronary artery bypass surgery have been undertaken in the post-infarction period. However, coronary artery surgery can be performed within 3 months of infarction, with a low mortality and satisfactory results, and there is suggestive evidence of improvement in prognosis (Rogers et al 1980).

Because of the relationship between ventricular arrhythmias in the convalescent phase and subsequent sudden death, it would seem logical to use antiarrhythmic drugs prophylactically. However, studies with a number of drugs have proved ineffective (Chamberlain et al 1980). This may be because the available drugs are so toxic that they cannot be given in a dose sufficient to prevent ventricular fibrillation.

REFERENCES

Antman E, Muller J, Goldberg S, MacAlpin R, Rubenfire M, Tabatznik B et al 1980 Nifedipine therapy for coronary-artery spasm. New England Journal of Medicine 302: 1269–1273

Anturane Reinfarction Trial (ART) Research Group 1980 Sulfinpyrazone in the prevention of sudden death after myocardial infarction. New England Journal of Medicine 302: 250–256

Armstrong A, Duncan B, Oliver M F, Julian D G, Donald K W, Fulton M et al 1972 The natural history of acute coronary heart attacks. British Heart Journal 34: 67–80

Aspirin Myocardial Infarction Study Research Group (AMIS) 1980 A randomized, control trial of aspirin in persons recovered from myocardial infarction. Journal of the American Medical Association 243: 661–669

Awan N A, Miller R R, De Maria A N, Maxwell K S, Neumann A, Mason D T 1977 Efficacy of ambulatory systemic vasodilator therapy with oral prazosin in chronic refractory heart failure. Circulation 56: 346–354

Baber N S, Wainwright Evans D, Howitt G, Thomas M, Wilson C, Lewis J A et al 1980 Multicentre post-infarction trial of propranolol in 49 hospitals in the United Kingdom, Italy and Yugoslavia. British Heart Journal 44: 96–100

Bala Subramanian V, Lahiri A, Paramasivan R, Raftery E B 1980 Verapamil in chronic stable angina. Lancet 1: 841–844

Beevers D G, Bannan L T, Jackson S H D 1981 The treatment of mild hypertension. European Heart Journal (In press)

Burdine J A, De Puey E G, Orzan F, Mathur V S, Hall R J 1979 Scintigraphic, electrocardiographic and enzymatic diagnosis of perioperative myocardial infarction in patients undergoing myocardial revascularization. Journal of Nuclear Medicine 20: 711–714

Chamberlain D A, Jewitt D E, Julian D G, Campbell R W F, Boyle D McC, Shanks R G et al 1980 Oral mexiletine in high-risk patients after myocardial infarction. Lancet 2: 1324–1327

Cobb L A, Baum R S, Alvarez H, Schaffer W A 1975 Resuscitation from out-of-hospital ventricular fibrillation: 4-year follow-up. Circulation 51/52 (suppl III): 223–228

Cohn J N, Burke L P 1979 Nitroprusside. Annals of Internal Medicine 91: 752–757

Committee of Principal Investigators 1978 A co-operative trial in the primary prevention of ischaemic heart disease using clofibrate. British Heart Journal 40: 1069–1118

Coronary Drug Project Research Group 1975 Clofibrate and niacin in coronary heart disease. Journal of the American Medical Association 231: 360–381

Dayton S, Pearce M L, Hashimoto S, Dixon W J, Zomiyasu U 1969 A controlled clinical trial of a diet high in unsaturated fat. Circulation 40 (supplement II): 1–63

Ekelund L G, Orö L 1979 Antianginal efficiency of nifedipine with and without a beta-blocker, studied with exercise test. A double-blind, randomized subacute study. Clinical Cardiology 2: 203–211

European Coronary Surgery Study Group 1980 Prospective randomised study of coronary artery bypass surgery in stable angina pectoris. Lancet 2: 491–495

Fitchett D H, Marin Neto J A, Oakley C M, Goodwin J F 1979 Hydralazine in the management of left ventricular failure. American Journal of Cardiology 44: 303–309

Gruntzig A R, Senning A, Siegenthaler W E 1979 Nonoperative dilatation of coronary artery stenosis — percutaneous transluminal coronary angioplasty. New England Journal of Medicine 301: 61–68

Guazzi M D, Fiorentini C, Olivari M T, Bartorelli A, Necchi G, Polese A 1980 Short- and long-term efficacy of a calcium antagonistic agent (nifedipine) combined with methyldopa in the treatment of severe hypertension. Circulation 61: 913–919

Hickey N, Mulcahy R, Graham I, MacKenzie G 1978 The effect of smoking on prognosis after myocardial infarction. In: Hjalmarson A, Wilhelmsen L (eds) Acute and long-term management of myocardial ischaemia. Astra, Sweden, p 274–278

Hill J D, Hampton J R, Mitchell J R A 1978 A randomised trial of home-versus-hospital management for patients with suspected myocardial infarction. Lancet 1: 837–841

Hypertension Detection and Follow-up Program Co-operative Group 1979 Five-year findings of the hypertension detection follow-up program. Journal of the American Medical Association 242: 2562–2577

International Anticoagulant Review Group 1970 Collaborative analysis of long-term anticoagulant administration after myocardial infarction. Lancet 1: 203–209

Kirklin J W 1981 The replacement of cardiac valves. New England Journal of Medicine 304: 291–292

Koch-Weser J 1976 Drug therapy: hydralazine. New England Journal of Medicine 295: 370–373

Lie K I, Wellens H J J, von Capelle F J, Durrer D 1974 Lidocaine in the prevention of primary ventricular fibrillation. New England Journal of Medicine 291: 1324–1326

Lie K I, Wellens H J J, Downar E, Durrer D 1975 Observations of patients with primary ventricular fibrillation complicating acute myocardial infarction. Circulation 52: 755–759

Luria M H, Knoke J D, Wachs J S, Luria M A 1979 Survival after recovery from acute myocardial infarction. American Journal of Medicine 67: 7–14

Lynch P, Dargie H, Krikler S, Krikler D 1980 Objective assessment of antianginal treatment: a double-blind comparison of propranolol, nifedipine, and their combination. British Medical Journal 2: 184–187

Madigan N P, Rutherford B D, Frye R L 1976 The clinical course, early prognosis and coronary anatomy of subendocardial infarction. American Journal of Medicine 60: 634–641

Management Committee 1980 The Australian therapeutic trial in mild hypertension. Lancet 1: 1261–1267

Miettinen M, Turpeinen O, Karvonen M J, Elosuo R, Paavilainen E 1972 Effect of cholesterol-lowering diet on mortality from coronary heart disease and other causes. A 12-year clinical trial in men and women. Lancet 2: 835–838

Multicentre International Study 1977 Reduction in mortality after myocardial infarction with long-term beta-adrenoceptor blockade. British Medical Journal 2: 419–421

Norris R M, Caughey D E, Mercer C J 1974 Prognosis after myocardial infarction: 6-year follow-up. British Heart Journal 36: 786–790

Norris R M, Clarke E D, Sammel N L, Smith W M 1978 Protective effect of propranolol in threatened myocardial infarction. Lancet 2: 907–909

Norwegian Multicentre Study Group 1981 Timolol-induced reduction in mortality and reinfarction in patients surviving acute myocardial infarction. New England Journal of Medicine 304: 801–807

Oakley C M, Darrell J H 1980 Infective endocarditis. Prescribers' Journal 20: 98–106

Opie L H 1980a Myocardial infarct size. American Heart Journal 100: 355–372, 531–552

Opie L H 1980b Calcium antagonists. Lancet 1: 806–809

Persantin-Aspirin Reinfarction Study Group (PARIS) 1980 Persantin and aspirin in coronary heart disease. Circulation 63: 449–461

Pluth J R 1981 Prosthetic valve replacement. In: Hamer J, Rowlands D J (eds) Recent advances in cardiology 8. Churchill Livingstone, Edinburgh, ch 4. p 93

Rentrop A B, Blanke H, Karsch K R, Kaiser H, Köstering H, Leitz K 1981 Selective intracoronary thrombolysis in acute myocardial infarction and unstable angina pectoris. Circulation 63: 307–316

Ritchie J L, Albro P C, Caldwell J H, Trobaugh G B, Hamilton G W 1979 Thallium-201 myocardial imaging: a comparison of the redistribution and rest images. Journal of Nuclear Medicine 20: 477–483

Rogers W J, Smith L R, Oberman A, Kouchoukos N T, Mantle J A, Russell R O Jr et al 1980 Surgical vs non-surgical management of patients after myocardial infarction. Circulation 62 (supplement I): 67–74

Rose G 1981 Impact of primary prevention programmes on ischaemic heart disease. In: Hamer J, Rowlands D J (eds) Recent advances in cardiology 8. Churchill Livingstone, Edinburgh, ch 9, p 181

Royal College of Physicians 1977 Third Report: Smoking or health. Pitman Medical, Tunbridge Wells

Ruberman W, Weinblatt E, Goldberg J D, Frank C W, Shapiro S, Chaudhary B S 1980 Ventricular premature complexes in prognosis of angina. Circulation 61: 1172–1178

Rubin S A, Chatterjee K, Gelberg H J et al 1979 Paradox of improved exercise but not resting hemodynamics with short-term prazosin in chronic heart failure. American Journal of Cardiology 43: 810–815

Schultze R A, Strauss H W, Pitt B 1977 Sudden death in the year following myocardial infarction. American Journal of Medicine 62: 192–199

Simoons M L, Taams M, Lubsen J, Hugenholtz P G 1980 Treatment of stable angina pectoris with verapamil hydrochloride: a double-blind cross-over study. European Heart Journal 1: 269–274

Singh B N, Ellrodt C, Peter C T 1978 Verapamil, a review of its pharmacological properties and therapeutic use. Drugs 15: 169–197

Sixty Plus Reinfarction Study Group 1980 A double-blind trial to assess long-term oral anticoagulant therapy in elderly patients after myocardial infarction. Lancet 2: 989–993

Smeets J P, Legrand V, Rigo P, Demoulin J-C, Boland J, de Landsheere C et al 1981 Subendocardial myocardial infarction: a follow-up study of 55 cases. European Heart Journal 2: 57–63

Smith R H, Radford D J, Clark R A, Julian D G 1976 Infectious endocarditis: a survey of cases in the south-east region of Scotland between 1969–1972. Thorax 31: 373–379

Starr A, Grunkenmeier G L, Lambert L E, Thomas D R, Sugimura S, Lefrak E A 1977 Aortic valve replacement: a 10 year follow-up on non-cloth-covered vs cloth-covered caged-ball prostheses. Circulation 56 (part II): 133

Théroux P, Waters D D, Halphin C, Debaisieux J-C, Mizgala H F 1979 Prognostic value of exercise testing soon after myocardial infarction. New England Journal of Medicine 301: 341–345

Thompson R G, Hallstrom A P, Cobb L A 1979 Bystander-initiated cardiopulmonary resuscitation in the management of ventricular fibrillation. Annals of Internal Medicine 90: 737–740

Turini G A, Brunner H R, Gribic M, Waeber B, Gavras H 1979 Improvement of chronic congestive heart failure by oral captopril. Lancet 1: 1213–1215

Vismara L A, Amsterdam E A, Mason D T 1975 Relation of ventricular arrhythmias in the late hospital phase of acute myocardial infarction to sudden death after hospital discharge. American Journal of Medicine 59: 6–12

Wackers F J, Schoot J B, Sohole E B, Samson G, Niftrik G J C V, Lie K I et al 1975 Non-invasive visualization of acute myocardial infarction in man with thallium-201. British Heart Journal 37: 741–744

Walker W J 1977 Changing United States life-style and declining vascular mortality: cause or coincidence. New England Journal of Medicine 297: 163–165

Walton S, Kafetzakis E, Shields R A, Testa H J, Rowlands D J 1978 Use of ^{129}caesium, ^{99}Tc^{m}-stannous pyrophosphate and a combination of the two in the assessment of myocardial infarction. British Heart Journal 40: 874–882

Wilhelmsson C, Vedin J A, Elmfeldt E, Tibblin G, Wilhelmsen L 1975 Smoking and myocardial infarction. Lancet 1: 415–419

Wilhelmsson C, Vedin J A, Wilhelmsen L, Tibblin G, Werko L 1974 Reduction of sudden deaths after myocardial infarction by treatment with alprenolol. Lancet 2: 1157–1159

Willerson J T, Parkey R W, Bonte F J, Meyer S L, Stokeley E M 1975a Acute subendocardial myocardial infarction in patients: its detection by technetium-99m stannous pyrophosphate myocardial scintigrams. Circulation 51: 436–441

Willerson J T, Parkey R W, Bonte F J, Meyer S L, Atkins J M, Stokeley E M 1975b Technetium stannous pyrophosphate myocardial scintigrams in patients with chest pain of varying aetiology. Circulation 51: 1042–1046

Wyman M G, Hammersmith L 1974 Comprehensive treatment plan for the prevention of primary ventricular fibrillation in acute myocardial infarction. American Journal of Cardiology 33: 661–667

Yusuf S, Ramsdale D, Peto R, Furse L, Bennett D, Bray C et al 1980 Early intravenous atenolol treatment in suspected acute myocardial infarction. Lancet 2: 273–276

5

Respiratory disease

T. B. Stretton

FIBREOPTIC BRONCHOSCOPY

In the past decade there has been a progressive increase in the use of fibreoptic instruments for endoscopic examination of the bronchial tree and the alimentary tract. Although the fibreoptic bronchoscope has several advantages over the older, rigid instrument which it has largely superseded for much routine diagnostic bronchoscopy, it cannot replace this altogether and the rigid bronchoscope remains essential for certain purposes.

Fibreoptic bronchoscopy is usually performed under local anaesthesia with the subject in the fasting state, and it is well tolerated by the majority of patients. Most operators insert the instrument through the anaesthetised nose; if it is passed through the mouth a guard is inserted between the patient's teeth to protect the bronchoscope. The examination can be done with the patient in his bed, seated in a chair, or semirecumbent on a couch or X-ray table. Premedication with atropine is given half an hour beforehand and is usually combined with a sedative, although this is not essential (Pearce 1980).

There is one absolute contraindication to fibreoptic bronchoscopy used in this way: an inadequate airway. Fortunately, because of the small diameter of the instrument this is rarely a problem. Even in a patient with, for instance, severe tracheal stenosis it is possible to inspect the lesion from above and to assess the disease in this way. In patients with respiratory failure, oxygen therapy can be given or continued during the procedure to lessen the fall in arterial P_{O_2} which would otherwise occur during the period of intubation with the bronchoscope; oxygen is given by an Edinburgh mask or Ventimask® and the bronchoscope is inserted through the plastic face-piece. When faced with the urgent need to bronchoscope a patient with acute ventilatory failure and a rising P_{CO_2}, it is wise first to insert an endotracheal tube and ventilate the patient by IPPV; this can be maintained through the side arm of a ⊢ shaped connector while the bronchoscope is passed through a hole in a rubber membrane occluding the proximal end of the connector. Alternatively, a rigid instrument should be used for bronchoscopy in these circumstances, to secure an airway through which the patient's ventilation can be maintained.

The indications for bronchoscopy have expanded since the advent of the fibreoptic bronchoscope. The use of flexible instruments has also greatly extended the visual range of the bronchoscopist to the subsegmental bronchi. Of course, the major role is still in the investigation of suspected malignancy, whether this presents with haemoptysis, collapsed lung, 'unresolved pneumonia', localised wheezing, or phrenic or recurrent laryngeal nerve palsy. The diagnosis can be established and the suitability of the patient for surgical treatment assessed using either a flexible or rigid bronchoscope. One potential problem with the fibreoptic instrument is the size of biopsy samples, which are tiny compared with those obtained by the much larger forceps used in conjunction with a rigid bronchoscope. The sample may be unrepresentative of the bulk of the tumour and may at times pose some difficulty in interpretation for the histopathologist.

Bronchoscopy is indicated whenever there is the possibility of a foreign body in the bronchial tree; this includes patients with recurrent pneumonia (which may 'flit' from one lung segment to another) or atelectasis, and some with recurring lower respiratory tract infections without evident consolidation. Such patients do not necessarily remember, and may not have had, an acute episode of choking when the foreign material entered the tracheobronchial tree. Although the fibreoptic bronchoscope has been used for the removal of foreign bodies, this is properly the province of a skilled operator using a rigid bronchoscope, so that the offending object can be grasped with strong forceps and removed through the bronchoscope or together with this instrument as it is withdrawn; this can be a difficult task, especially with an irregular object such as a piece of bone which may have been present for a long time and has become embedded in the bronchial wall. However, patients who might harbour a foreign body can be very conveniently assessed first by fibreoptic endoscopy and submitted to rigid bronchoscopy under full anaesthesia if required.

Patients with a bronchial adenoma are rare and they present, often in early adult life, with recurrent haemoptysis or features of local bronchial obstruction, similar to those caused by a foreign body. They, too, may first be recognised at fibreoptic bronchoscopy and must then be referred to a thoracic surgeon for treatment.

The fibreoptic bronchoscope has been used increasingly in the investigation of patients with diffuse lung disease. In patients with obscure pneumonitis, especially those who are immunosuppressed and may have an opportunistic infection, it is possible to obtain diagnostic information from material obtained by transbronchial lung biopsy, bronchial brushings, aspirated bronchial secretions, or alveolar lavage. Alternatively, such patients may require percutaneous needle or drill biopsy of their lungs, or open biopsy through a limited thoracotomy incision to achieve a definite diagnosis. Although the most certain means of reaching a histological diagnosis is by thoracotomy, transbronchial biopsy is successful in about 70% of cases (Mitchell et al 1980).

Bronchoalveolar lavage with saline through the fibreoptic bronchoscope is a safe and convenient way of obtaining cells and other material from the alveoli for further study. The tip of the instrument is impacted in a subsegmental bronchus and 60–100 ml saline are injected through the bronchoscope. The saline is then aspirated and collected for investigation. This technique has excited considerable interest and may prove useful in the management as well as the diagnosis of patients with widespread alveolar disease, although at present it is essentially a research procedure. Electron-microscopic examination of the contents aspirated from alveoli may permit the diagnosis of rare diseases such as alveolar proteinosis and histiocytosis X. More important, this technique yields living cells, predominantly macrophages, the behaviour of which can then be studied in vitro. These cells are especially abundant in cigarette smokers. The proportions of different types of cells in the alveolar fluid may also be instructive: lymphocyte counts, low in normal subjects, are increased in sarcoidosis and allergic pneumonitis; they may also be of prognostic value in patients with fibrosing alveolitis, in whom those with predominant lymphocytes appear to respond to corticosteroid treatment, while the majority, in whom the numbers of neutrophils or eosinophils are increased, respond less well or deteriorate (Haslam et al 1980). This fascinating field of progress in respiratory medicine has been well reviewed by Gee & Fick (1980).

The technique just described must not be confused with therapeutic bronchopulmonary lavage in which the objective is to wash out and clear secretions from the lung. This cannot be done by fibreoptic bronchoscopy on any useful scale, although simple aspiration of secretions from major air passages is both feasible and effective through the fibrescope. Therapeutic lavage has been used mainly in asthma and alveolar proteinosis, and may be curative in the latter condition. A major bronchopulmonary lavage can be performed on only one lung at a time and is achieved under general anaesthesia via a cuffed, dual-lumen endotracheal tube. This is placed at the bifurcation of the trachea so that each lung is isolated from the other. The patient is then oxygenated and ventilated on one lung while the oxygen in the other is replaced with warmed, buffered saline and the lung is washed at its functional residual capacity with tidal volumes of saline. Up to 20 l of liquid may be used in this process. At a subsequent session the other lung is similarly treated. In alveolar proteinosis the treatment is repeated at intervals until the lungs are clear. Although benefit from this kind of procedure has been claimed in patients with severe, intractable asthma, its use is both controversial and hazardous. However, a limited form of lavage may be beneficial during IPPV treatment of status asthmaticus: 20–30 ml aliquots of isotonic saline or bicarbonate solution are squirted down the endotracheal tube and are aspirated after a minute or two, together with strings of mucus and cellular bronchial casts. This is repeated until a litre or more of solution has been used. It is a slow process and demands continous care and attention. In the meantime the patient is ventilated, oxygenated, rehydrated and given bronchodilator drugs and steroids in the usual way. In neither of these forms of treatment is a fibreoptic bronchoscope required, although there are many other occasions when it can be used with advantage to clear secretions from the bronchial tree of enfeebled and seriously ill patients, both in the general ward and in the intensive care unit.

Complications of fibreoptic bronchoscopy are rare (Credle et al 1974). They include reactions to the drugs used for premedication and the topical anaesthetic. Laryngospasm may occur in an inadequately prepared patient. Transient hypoxia can be anticipated. Infection might be expected to be more common as the instrumentation procedure cannot be sterile; in practice, infection is most unusual. Cross-infection should not occur. Transbronchial biopsy is, on occasions, inevitably associated with bleeding or the production of a pneumothorax, but the incidence of these complications is very low (5–10%).

GRANULOMATOUS DISEASES OF THE LUNGS

Granuloma formation occurs in the lungs in a wide variety of diseases, some of known aetiology, some unknown. It is a notable feature of certain infections, such as *tuberculosis* and *histoplasmosis,* and is seen in *allergic pneumonitis* caused by repeated exposure to mouldy hay, avian and other antigens. It may be a response to inhalation of a chemical, as in *berylliosis,* or to infestation with parasites, as in *tropical pulmonary eosinophilia.* Often it is not possible to ascertain a cause, although the identity of the disease may not be in doubt, as with *eosinophilic granuloma, allergic granulomatosis, Wegener's granulomatosis* and *sarcoidosis.*

Allergic and Wegener's granulomatoses

These conditions have features in common with one another and with polyarteritis nodosa, and disturbed immunological mechanisms are thought to be implicated in their pathogenesis. Necrotising vasculitis is an essential feature in them all. In the two variants, allergic granulomatosis and Wegener's granulomatosis, the respiratory tract is a major 'target organ' for the disease process and the damage thus caused may be extensive. There is, at times, sufficient overlap of clinical features for it to be difficult to categorise a patient's disease precisely. However, the management is in principle the same.

Allergic granulomatosis appears to be a form of polyarteritis nodosa in which the main brunt of the pathology is borne by the lungs. The patient, who is often atopic, may have severe asthma with marked peripheral blood eosinophilia ($> 1.5 \times 10^9$ eosinophils/litre), or may present with patchy pneumonitis and consolidation or cavitation of the lungs. The isolation from the sputum of pathogens such as *Staphylococcus aureus,* which may themselves be responsible for a necrotising pneumonia, easily diverts attention from the true nature of the lung pathology in these circumstances, and may delay the introduction of appropriate treatment.

Histopathological examination shows that, in addition to nodular polyarteritis, there is a granulomatous reaction and eosinophil infiltration of the tissues. Repeated careful examination of patients with allergic granulomatosis may reveal papulonodular cutaneous lesions of allergic vasculitis, especially over the elbows and knees, and ulcerating lesions in the mouth. Polyarthritis may occur and there may be renal damage, mononeuritis multiplex, or other manifestations of polyarteritis nodosa.

In 'classic' polyarteritis nodosa a history of allergy is uncommon, and eosinophilia and lung involvement are less prominent features. Cutaneous evidence of disease may occasionally be found in the form of livedo reticularis and, rarely, palpable subcutaneous nodules. Hypertension attributable to renal involvement is common and visceral lesions may cause episodes of abdominal pain or frank intestinal infarction. The disease causes segmental necrotising vasculitis of small and medium-sized arteries with secondary damage due to varying degrees of thrombosis, ischaemia, and tissue infarction. Small aneurysmal dilatations (< 1 cm) are formed on medium-sized arteries and these may be demonstrated by renal, hepatic and mesenteric angiography. Although such lesions may be characteristic of polyarteritis nodosa they are not pathognomonic (Fauci et al 1978) and it would be difficult to justify angiographic studies solely for this purpose.

Although *Wegener's granulomatosis* usually has well-defined clinical and pathological features which readily distinguish it from allergic granulomatosis and polyarteritis nodosa, this is not invariably the case. The presence of necrotising granulomatous vasculitis in the upper respiratory tract causes obstruction and secondary bacterial infection in the nasal sinuses and nasopharynx, resulting in pain in the face and head with nasal obstruction and a purulent or blood-stained discharge. Nasal mucosal ulceration may be followed by erosion of bone and perforation of the nasal septum. Chronic serous otitis media is common, causing pain and deafness. Laryngeal involvement causes hoarseness, pain and dyspnoea with stridor due to subglottic stenosis. Major intrathoracic airways may be similarly obstructed. Parenchymal lung involvement causes consolidation, sometimes in the form of bilateral rounded, solid lesions which may cavitate, or as irregular segmental pneumonitis. Evidence of a necrotising glomerulonephritis usually completes the clinical picture of Wegener's granulomatosis, in which the major sites of pathology are the upper respiratory tract, the lungs and the kidneys. However, neurological lesions, polyarthritis and skin manifestations occur in a proportion of patients, as in allergic granulomatosis.

Treatment

The response to corticosteroid and immunosuppressive treatment is consistent with the hypothesis that, in these diseases, the tissue damage is attributable to immunopathological processes. It has been recognised for over 40 years that hypersensitivity may play a part in the genesis of polyarteritis nodosa (Rich 1942), and the demonstration of an association between this disease and hepatitis B antigenaemia (Gocke et al 1970) lent support to the view that allergic mechanisms are involved. The current idea is that, if circulating immune complexes are not efficiently cleared by the reticuloendothial system, they may be deposited in blood vessel walls, activate complement and evoke an inflammatory response. Recently it has been shown that relapses in Wegener's granulomatosis may be provoked by bacterial or viral infections (Pinching et al 1980) and that such relapses are accompanied by the presence of circulating immune complexes; moreover, with intercurrent infections which do not provoke a relapse, immune complexes are rarely detectable. While these observations are in keeping with the proposed immunopathogenesis of Wegener's granulomatosis, their detailed significance remains to be elucidated.

The outlook in Wegener's granulomatosis has been transformed by immunosuppressive treatment, cyclophosphamide being the current drug of choice. This disease, once almost invariably fatal, can now be arrested in a high proportion of cases by daily doses of 150–200 mg. This is usually combined with prednisolone, at least initially, and especially in patients who are febrile and toxic. The dose of cyclophosphamide is cautiously reduced when a remission has been induced, and may be stopped if the remission can be maintained for 18 months to 2 years.

Sarcoidosis

Although sarcoidosis continues to attract considerable attention, the aetiology of this enigmatic disease also remains elusive. Much of the research activity directed towards sarcoidosis in recent years appears to have explored epiphenomena of the disease and profits us little in the management of patients with the condition. Nevertheless, the fund of knowledge relating to sarcoidosis continues to grow.

The definition of sarcoidosis as a multisystem granulomatous disease of unknown aetiology requires no modification. A diagnosis of sarcoidosis should, strictly, include the demonstration of non-caseating epithelioid granulomata in tissue biopsy;

favoured sites for biopsy are the skin, lymph nodes, lungs and liver. The availability of a tested, validated and potent Kveim reagent for skin testing is of considerable value in confirming a presumptive clinical diagnosis of sarcoidosis without subjecting the patient to rather unpleasant and even potentially risky procedures to obtain a tissue biopsy. We are fortunate in having such material available in Britain. The Kveim-Siltzbach test is positive in 70–80% of patients wih active sarcoidosis.

The altered immunological state of patients with sarcoidosis is well known. Hyperglobulinaemia because of increased B cell activity is common. Circulating immune complexes have been found in some patients, as many as 58% in one study (Johnson et al 1980). Skin tests of cell-mediated hypersensitivity using tuberculin, fungal and other antigens are negative more often than in control subjects, and in vitro tests with cultured lymphocytes also show impaired T-cell responsiveness. However, the clinical relevance of these observations is still uncertain. The risk of intercurrent infection in patients with sarcoidosis, which might be supposed to be enhanced in the face of impaired cell-mediated immunity, is not increased, with the possible exception of cryptococcal and aspergillus infections in the USA (Winterbauer & Kraemer 1976).

Sarcoidosis usually affects young adults of either sex, and is much more florid, aggressive and indolent in black subjects than in white. Evidence of intrathoracic disease is found in 90% of patients at some stage. Lymph-node enlargement, splenomegaly, skin and ocular involvement are all common modes of presentation. Sarcoidosis of bones, the heart or the nervous system is uncommon.

Intrathoracic disease includes hilar lymphadenopathy and pulmonary disease. Pleural effusions are rare (Nicholls et al 1980). The high frequency of lung involvement has encouraged the use of transbronchial biopsy to obtain histological confirmation of the diagnosis, and the yield of positive results may be as high as 82% (Mitchell et al 1980). The study of alveolar cells 'harvested' by lavage of the lungs at the time of bronchoscopy has shown that lymphocytes are present in abundance, that these are largely active T cells and that there may be lymphocyte–macrophage rosettes in the lavage fluid (Hunninghake et al 1979, Gee & Fick 1980). The contrast between the cells obtained from the alveoli and the lymphocytes in the peripheral blood of patients with sarcoidosis is at once evident and has led to the observation that the depletion of T cells from the blood reflects their sequestration in the lungs and at other sites of active disease (Hunninghake & Crystal 1981).

Bone involvement in sarcoidosis (Fig. 5.1) causes focal cystic, 'permeative' or destructive changes, usually in the hands or feet, but occasionally in the nasal bones, palate or temporal bones (Neville et al 1977). Radiographically evident disease occurs in approximately 5% of patients overall, the prevalence ranging from 1–13% in different series. Routine X-rays of the hands and skull are only worthwhile in the presence of chronic skin lesions and in the few patients with sarcoidosis of the mucosa of the upper respiratory tract. In general, bone sarcoidosis occurs in patients with intractable disease elsewhere, and the increased mortality of these patients is mainly due to associated and severe lung involvement.

Hypercalcaemia is also an uncommon, although well-recognised, complication of sarcoidosis. It very occasionally accompanies focal bone disease. Although in some studies hypercalcaemia has been reported in well over 10% of patients, personal experience and that of others in Britain suggests that here it occurs in less than 2%.

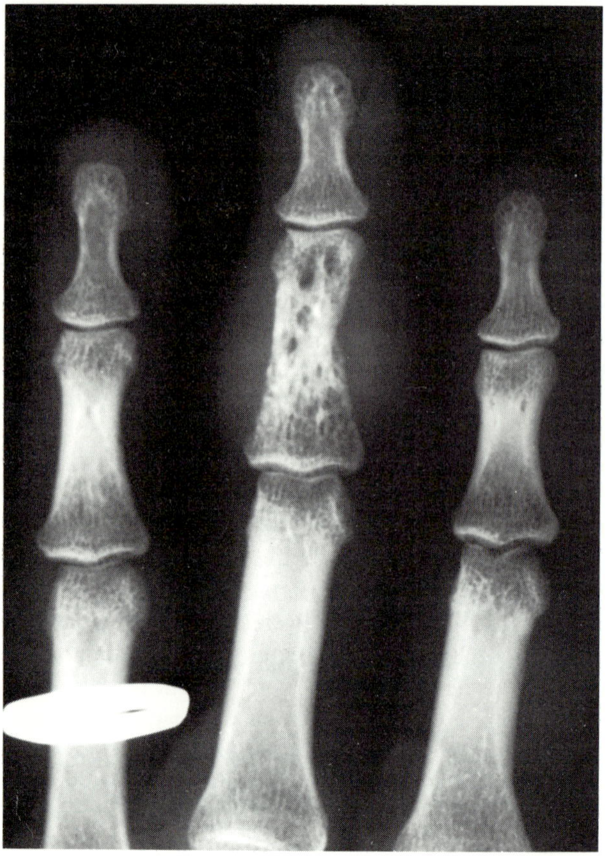

Fig. 5.1 Radiographic appearances of sarcoidosis of bone. Note the surrounding digital soft-tissue swelling

When hypercalcaemia is found, the possibility of causes other than sarcoidosis should be entertained. In particular, if hypercalcaemia fails to respond to corticosteroid therapy, the possibility of coincidental hyperparathyroidism must be investigated (Rømer 1980). In an occasional patient hypercalcaemia may be a seasonal (summer) event and is associated with a rise in 1, 25-dihydroxy-cholecalciferol, presumably because of overproduction of this hormonal form of vitamin D (Papapoulos et al 1979). Although hypercalcaemia is infrequent in sarcoidosis, abnormal calcium metabolism is a common occurrence (Reiner et al 1976, Handslip et al 1981), as shown by an increase in urinary calcium excretion and alimentary absorption, with increased bone turnover (Reiner et al 1976). The mechanism of these changes is unknown but as they appear to have no harmful implications for the majority of patients with sarcoidosis, and need no treatment, their routine investigation is unnecessary. However, it is important to measure the serum calcium and check renal function, particularly in young males within the first 2 years of the onset of sarcoidosis, in whom the risk of renal damage is greatest (Rømer 1980).

The recognition of an increase in serum angiotensin-converting enzyme (ACE) in sarcoidosis (Lieberman 1975) attracted attention to this substance as a possible biochemical marker of the disease. ACE is present in normal pulmonary vascular tissue and catalyses the conversion of angiotensin I to the pressor agent, angiotensin II. In sarcoidosis the high serum ACE concentrations are believed to reflect activity of granulomatous tissue in lymph nodes and elsewhere. High levels of serum ACE have been reported in about 50% of patients with active sarcoidosis, but also in patients with other diseases, notably primary biliary cirrhosis, tuberculosis, silicosis, asbestosis and idiopathic pulmonary fibrosis (Studdy et al 1978, Gronhagen-Riska et al 1979, Lieberman et al 1979, Editorial, Lancet 1980). Thus, although measurement of serum ACE may help to assess the response to treatment of patients known to have sarcoidosis, and to detect relapse of those with chronic disease, it is of less value as a diagnostic test.

Finally, studies of histocompatibility locus antigens (HLA) in sarcoidosis have suggested that host factors may influence the clinical manifestation or course of the disease. Thus, an increase in HLA-B8 has been reported in patients with acute sarcoidosis with erythema nodosum or arthritis or both of these features (Neville 1977). In addition, more recently, it has been shown that patients whose intrathoracic sarcoidosis (bilateral hilar lymphadenopathy with or without pulmonary mottling) undergoes complete resolution, have a higher frequency of HLA-B8 than those developing lung fibrosis, in whom the frequency was the same as that in a control group (Smith et al 1981).

LEGIONNAIRES' DISEASE

Legionnaires' disease (Balows & Fraser 1979) is an acute pneumonic illness which is now known to be due to infection by a motile Gram-negative bacterium. The disease first achieved recognition, a name, and considerable notoriety as a result of an outbreak of severe respiratory infection among members of the American Legion attending a convention in Philadelphia in 1976, when 15% of those affected died.

This 'new' and alarming disease attracted wide publicity and, as a result of intense study, the responsible organism was isolated within a matter of months. The causative bacillus has since been named *Legionella pneumophila*. However, although hitherto unrecognised, *L. pneumophila* was apparently isolated in 1947 from a guinea-pig inoculated with blood from a patient with pneumonia (McDade et al 1979), when it was thought to be rickettsial and of guinea-pig origin.

It seems probable that legionnaires' disease escaped recognition for so long because *L. pneumophila* is difficult to culture, being nutritionally fastidious, and also difficult to detect microscopically in tissue unless special silver staining techniques are used. In a few instances the organism has been isolated from pleural fluid or blood, or recognised in a smear of aspirated bronchial secretion; most positive cultures have come from lung tissue at autopsy. Serological diagnostic techniques could, of course, be developed and exploited only after the organism had been isolated. Such techniques were rapidly introduced after the 1976 outbreak and confirmation of the diagnosis in presumed cases of legionnaires' disease then became possible. The majority of diagnoses are thus retrospective and are based on a fourfold rise in antibody titre or a single titre $\geqslant 256$. Six serotypes of *L. pneumophila* have been identified and, of these, type 1 has been the major cause of disease; four other species of *Legionella* have also been recognised (Editorial, Lancet 1981).

Retrospective investigation has shown that there had been previous outbreaks of legionnaires' disease in the USA during the 1960s and early 1970s. This was clearly not a new disease. Nor was legionnaires' disease confined to the USA: cases were soon identified in many other countries of the world. In Britain it was first recognised in holiday-makers who had been to Spain and then in others who had been abroad, usually to a Mediterranean resort. Indigenously acquired, sporadic infections were diagnosed in Nottingham and elsewhere. Finally, small clusters of cases have arisen in hospitals in Cardiff, Oxford and elsewhere (Tobin et al 1980).

Thus, different epidemiological patterns of infection with *L. pneumophila* have been established: geographically localised epidemics in healthy subjects visiting a particular place, even perhaps a single hotel; sporadic illness occurring either in travellers who have been abroad or in members of the community; and in hospital patients, particularly those who are immunodepressed by virtue of another disease or its treatment. Case-to-case transmission of infection is evidently rare, if it occurs at all. It seems probable that the disease is acquired as an airborne infection and there is strong circumstantial evidence to suggest that this has originated in air-conditioning units or showers, where the organism may have survived in the water in conjunction with algae or amoebae and from which it is sprayed into the atmosphere as an aerosol. Although a common origin of infection may be identified in an outbreak of legionnaires' disease, the source is seldom evident in sporadic cases. The true prevalence of the disease is unknown, although it is interesting to note that in the Nottingham area between 1.5 and 4.7% of different groups of subjects are sero-positive against *L. pneumophila* (Macrae et al 1979).

The spectrum of illness caused by *L. pneumophila* is wide, ranging from a mild febrile reaction to a fulminating pneumonia. Asymptomatic infections may also occur. There is a seasonal incidence of legionnaires' disease with a peak in late summer. About two-thirds of the diagnosed cases are male and almost a third are over the age of 60 years. Increased awareness of the condition has shown that the overall mortality rate is considerably lower than that of the original Philadelphia epidemic in 1976.

After an incubation period of 2–10 d, legionnaires' disease begins with prodromal symptoms of malaise, myalgia and fever. Abdominal symptoms (nausea, vomiting, distension and diarrhoea) are reported in approximately half the patients during the first few days of their illness. Confusion and clouding of consciousness are common and seem out of proportion to the height of the fever. The patient has a dry cough or one productive of a little mucoid, purulent or blood-stained sputum. There is a confluent bronchopneumonia which may spread to assume a lobar or multilobar distribution, with appropriate physical and radiographic signs, and there may be a small pleural effusion. Cavitation is rare and is more likely to occur in immunodepressed patients than in those who were previously healthy. Resolution of the X-ray changes tends to be slow and may take several months.

Laboratory investigation shows a normal white cell count or a moderate polymorphonuclear leucocytosis. The sputum is purulent but fails to grow pathogens on culture. Hyponatraemia is commonly reported. Other findings include a rise in the serum level of liver enzymes and there is evidence of renal damage in some patients.

Treatment of these patients includes general or intensive supportive measures and an appropriate antibiotic regimen. As the diagnosis is usually not known at first, the initially prescribed antibiotic combination may need to be adjusted according to the patient's clinical response. In a seriously ill, perhaps elderly or immunocompromised patient with an undiagnosed lobular or lobar pneumonia, initial treatment is likely to include a penicillin and an aminoglycoside. To this combination it is recommended that erythromycin be added in a dose of 1 g 6-hourly. If the diagnosis can be established, the other antibiotics are discontinued. Treatment with erythromycin may be given intravenously at first and is continued by mouth for 3 weeks. Rifampicin has been advocated for the treatment of legionnaires' disease and its use should be seriously considered in the very ill. There is an understandable and very proper reluctance to use this drug for non-tuberculous disease but this is one circumstance in which the addition of 100–200 mg rifampicin 8-hourly could be lifesaving.

ASBESTOS-INDUCED DISEASE

Inhalation of asbestos fibre can cause intra- or extrapulmonary pathology: the former includes asbestosis and carcinoma of the bronchus; the latter may be seen as pleural plaques, diffuse pleural thickening, pleural effusion or mesothelioma.

The term asbestosis refers specifically to the condition of diffuse pulmonary fibrosis caused by inhaling asbestos and should not be used loosely to describe other manifestations of exposure to this substance. To do this may cause confusion and even misery to someone afflicted by nothing more sinister than fibrous or calcified pleural plaques. Such lesions may be recognised on a routine chest radiograph done as part of an industrial survey or for some other reason in an individual without evident respiratory disease, or in a patient with chest symptoms quite unrelated to any past occupational hazard. In these circumstances, careless explanation of the nature of the problem may create immense anxiety, may intentionally or otherwise encourage the patient, possibly unwisely, to embark on a protracted process of litigation, or may raise the spectre of malignant disease now or in the future. Thus, it is important to be precise when using diagnostic labels in subjects with asbestos-induced pathology and also to understand the implications of the different manifestations.

Asbestos and its uses

Asbestos is the name given to a group of fibrous silicate minerals. Chief among these is chrysotile — white asbestos — a magnesium silicate with flexible fibres which is the most abundant and commercially used form of asbestos. Chrysotile is mined principally in Canada, southern Africa and the USSR. The other forms of asbestos, the amphiboles, are iron silicates and have short straight brittle fibres. They include amosite, anthophyllite and crocidolite or blue asbestos, and are mined in Finland, S. Africa, Australia and Bolivia.

Asbestos has acquired its unique importance in industry and commerce because of its special physical and chemical properties. These include fire resistance, mechanical strength and chemical stability, as well as the fibrous structure which makes some types of asbestos suitable for spinning into yarn. Asbestos yarn can be used to make rope, or woven into cloth to make fireproof blankets, curtains or protective garments. Asbestos has been used extensively in conjunction with other materials such as cement, rubber and synthetic resins, to act as a filler or binder, or to provide them with reinforcement. The materials thus formed have been used in the manufacture of weather-resistant roof and wall sheeting, insulation board, gutters, pipes, linoleum and floor tiles, roofing compounds, clutch and brake linings, and many other products.

Asbestos presents a respiratory hazard wherever it is processed or handled in such a way that a dust is created and respirable fibres are released into the atmosphere. This occurs (1) where the mineral is mined and crushed, (2) in asbestos factories where the raw material is spun or manufactured into various products and (3) where the end product is trimmed, sawn or used in some other way which liberates dust. Because asbestos products are, or have been, so widely used, a workman may have been exposed in any of a wide variety of industrial activities: these include building construction and demolition, light and heavy engineering, electrical engineering, the motor trade, railway locomotive, aircraft and shipbuilding. A notoriously high incidence of asbestos-induced disease has occurred in laggers who in the past commonly prepared by hand the mixture to be used on site, at times contaminating the atmosphere sufficiently to cause disease in other workers in the vicinity who were not directly handling the asbestos. Although substitutes such as glass fibre are now used instead, the widespread use of asbestos in the past to insulate furnaces, boilers and pipes in steelworks, power stations, factories and ships, has left a hazardous legacy for those whose job it is to strip down and replace the old material.

From the foregoing it is apparent how detailed an occupational history may be necessary to identify the job responsible for a man's disease, especially as this may have been undertaken many years earlier and perhaps for only a relatively short time. Moreover, although rarely, disease has been known to occur in the spouse of an asbestos worker. In such a case it is assumed that the husband has carried the asbestos-containing dust home in his clothing. Shaking the dust-impregnated overalls before washing them, repeated perhaps over a period of years, has released the dust and this has been sufficient to cause the wife's disease.

In areas of Turkey, certain forms of asbestos-induced disease appear to be endemic. Pleural thickening and calcification were found in 6.5% of a sample of the adult population around Cermik in the south-east of the country (Yazicioglu et al 1980) and, of these, more than one in every five had evidence of interstitial pulmonary fibrosis. There was also an increased incidence of mesotheliomas in the locality. The cause of the disease seemed to be the use of whitewash and stucco on the walls of the houses. These materials were quarried from outcrops of asbestiform minerals containing the amphibole, tremolite and other materials. The quarrying was done by the men and the grinding and application by women, so that both sexes suffered the consequences. Disease in the form of calcified pleural plaques, fibrosing pleurisy and mesothelioma is also endemic in Karain, a village in Anatolia (Baris et al 1978). Although a source of asbestos in the local water supply was suspected, the cause of the disease in Karain was obscure and no asbestos was identified in the local soil or rock, nor was any handled in the village.

Fate of inhaled asbestos fibres

The distance which asbestos fibres travel down the airways probably depends on their aerodynamic properties. Although they are relatively long, the fibres are light and become aligned with the airstream, thus penetrating far into the lung. Short straight amphibole fibres may possibly reach the alveoli more readily than the curly fibres of chrysotile, which impinge on the walls of the air passages; fibres which are trapped in the mucous blanket will be cleared from the airways by ciliary activity. Of those reaching the alveoli, some are engulfed by macrophages and removed. Others remain and are transformed into the well-known drumstick-shaped asbestos bodies; these are coated with a layer of protein which is impregnated with iron, thus giving rise to the typical golden-brown colour seen in light microscopy. Some fibres penetrate to the interstitial layer of the lung where, with the aid of the electron microscope, they may be found in greater numbers than are evident using the ordinary optical microscope. Uncoated amphibole fibres may persist in the tissues indefinitely while the chrysotile disintegrates as magnesium is leached out.

It is not clear how asbestos reaches the pleura to cause pathological changes there. Fibres may not be evident in the pleura or even in the lung, suggesting that some product of the dissolution of asbestos may have reached the pleura by way of the lymphatics.

In asbestosis there is alveolitis, bronchiolitis at the level of the respiratory bronchioles, and diffuse interstitial fibrosis. How these effects are mediated by asbestos is uncertain, although immune mechanisms, possibly triggered by the alveolar macrophages, may be implicated. Although the significance of circulating autoantibodies is not known, antinuclear factor is found in the serum of about 25% of patients with asbestosis. The possibility that constitutional factors may influence the risk of contracting asbestosis has led to a number of studies of HLA phenotypes in asbestos workers. A small but definite increase in the frequency of HLA-B27 has been found in subjects who have asbestosis, in comparison with unaffected workers and with volunteers not exposed to asbestos. There is also a suggestion that B5 may be associated with a protective factor, as the frequency of B5 is reduced in individuals showing radiographic progression of their disease. However, these differences in HLA frequencies are too small to be useful as a screening procedure in an attempt to identify workers who might be more or less susceptible to asbestosis (Gregor et al 1979).

Manifestations of asbestos-induced pathology

Pleural plaques

These involve the parietal rather than visceral pleura. They are usually bilateral and may be best demonstrated radiographically in the posterolateral region of the middle and lower chest wall. Oblique, as well as posteroanterior (PA) and lateral radiographs may be required to detect hyaline plaques, although calcified lesions may be abundantly evident on the PA film (Fig. 5.2). These lesions are the radiographic hallmark of past exposure to asbestos, in contrast to the other radiographic abnormalities found in subjects with either pleural or intrapulmonary disease attributable to asbestos, which lack specificity. However, they appear to be entirely benign and do not interfere with lung function.

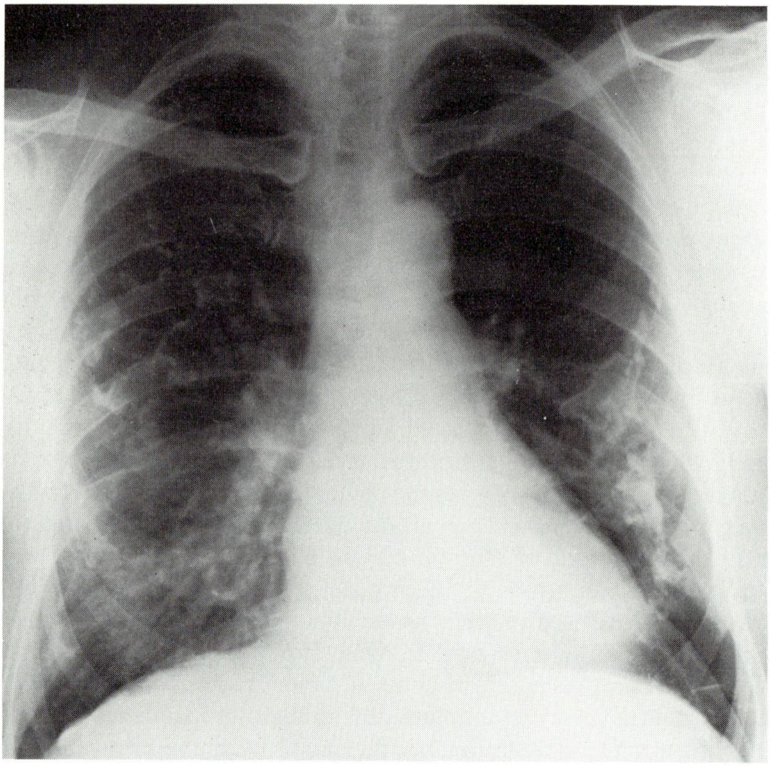

Fig. 5.2 Bilateral irregular opacities due to calcified pleural plaques, also seen in tangential view on each dome of the diaphragm

Diffuse pleural thickening

Diffuse pleural thickening, of no particular clinical significance, often accompanies asbestosis or may occur alone. Occasionally, however, there is a dense fibrous adhesive pleurisy which restricts the movement of the lungs, causing a reduction in the vital capacity independent of any intrapulmonary disease; this may be sufficient to cause severe breathlessness on exertion (Fig. 5.3).

Pleural effusions

Pleural effusions may be benign or malignant, and distinguishing one from the other can be difficult. Non-malignant effusions may be bilateral; the fluid is an exudate and is often haemorrhagic. Expert cytopathological examination of the fluid is most useful, but the nature of the disease may become apparent only after careful follow-up observation of the patient. It is, of course, important not to overlook other causes of pleural effusions occurring coincidentally in these patients.

Mesothelioma

The clinical features of mesotheliomas, based on a review of 327 cases confirmed by autopsy, have been reviewed by Elmes & Simpson (1976). Eighteen per cent of their

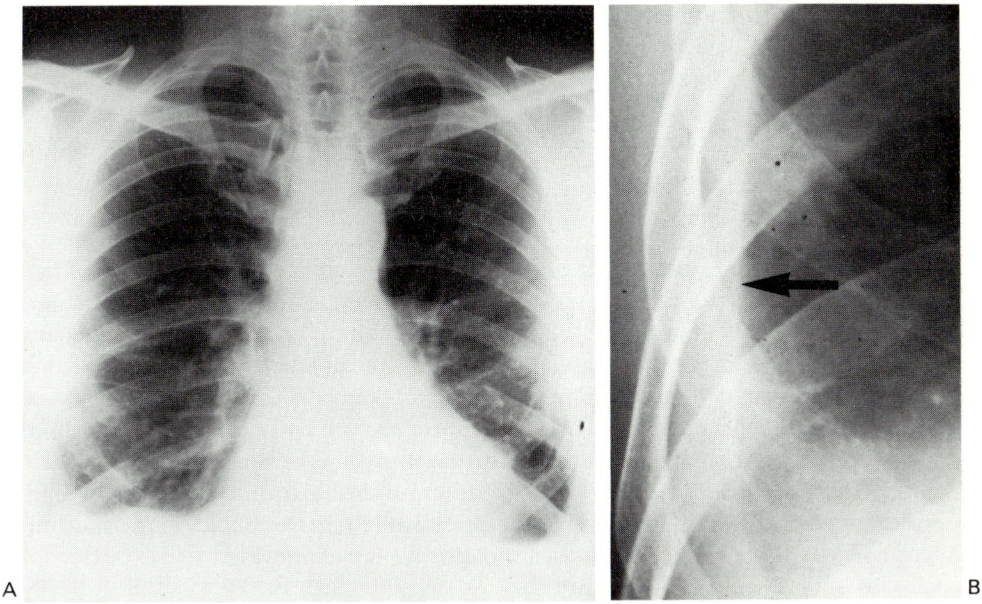

Fig. 5.3 A. Bilateral restrictive pleural thickening due to asbestos
B. More penetrating radiograph showing the thickness of the cuirass of pleural fibrosis

patients were women. The disease was nearly always insidious in onset and the dominant early symptom was chest pain, sometimes beginning simply as a feeling of 'heaviness'. Breathlessness as an initial symptom was marked only in those with a large associated effusion but became common as the tumour spread. The general health of the patient was often undisturbed in the early stages. Associated signs of asbestosis and clubbing of the fingers were rare. Bilateral calcified pleural plaques and obvious changes due to asbestosis were seen in only 12% of the chest radiographs available for study.

Peritoneal mesotheliomas occurred in 60 of the subjects and in 23 of these there was also a pleural tumour. The earliest symptoms were vague abdominal discomfort, loss of appetite, constipation and abdominal fullness or distension. Physical signs were uncommon until late in the evolution of the disease, which often defied diagnosis during life, despite detailed investigation, even including laparotomy.

At present no treatment seems to influence the outcome of a malignant mesothelioma. The mean duration of illness from onset of symptoms to death was approximately 16 months for pleural and 10 months for peritoneal tumours in the series described by Elmes & Simpson (1976).

Mesotheliomas appear to be increasing in frequency. This may be attributable, in part, to greater awareness of the condition. In England and Wales about 120 new cases a year are notified to the Medical Advisory Service (Greenberg & Lloyd Davies 1974). Occupational exposure to asbestos is established in only 68% of cases. The intensity of exposure is very variable, and the latent interval before the malignancy makes its presence felt is long — over 25 years in 85% of cases, the average being 40 years. One subject, with a recorded duration of exposure to asbestos of only three weeks, died of a mesothelioma more than 50 years later. At the other extreme, a mesothelioma can develop within 3 or 4 years of first exposure (Greenberg & Lloyd Davies 1974). Although these tumours appear to be caused chiefly by amphibole forms of asbestos, especially crocidolite, the question of the relative 'safety' of chrysotile in this respect, and indeed of other natural or synthetic respirable fibres, still requires an answer (Peto 1978, Elmes 1980).

Asbestosis

Asbestosis has clinical features similar to those found in fibrosing alveolitis: increasing breathlessness on exertion, leading to breathlessness at rest; inspiratory crackles best heard at the base of the lungs; clubbing of the fingers; reticular, reticulonodular or linear radiographic shadows most marked in the lower zones of the lungs; and impaired lung function with a reduction in diffusing capacity and a restrictive ventilatory defect, leading to hypoxic respiratory failure without carbon dioxide retention (although this may occur terminally). Given a history of exposure to asbestos, a combination of any two of these sets of clinical features is sufficient for a presumptive diagnosis of asbestosis. The detection of asbestos bodies in the sputum does not contribute to the diagnosis, although they are clear evidence of exposure to asbestos.

No treatment influences the natural history of asbestosis, although oxygen therapy is of help to the patient in respiratory failure. The prognosis is influenced by the risk of associated malignancy and by the rate of decline of lung function. Although this may be slow, each patient with asbestosis is unique and only repeated reassessment will make it possible to determine the individual's rate of progression. Whereas the risk of lung cancer is increased by asbestosis, it is the interaction of cigarette smoking and asbestos which causes the very high incidence of lung cancer in these subjects (Selikoff & Hammond 1979). Accordingly, asbestos workers and all those known to have been exposed to asbestos in the past should be urged not to smoke.

CHRONIC AIRFLOW OBSTRUCTION

Chronic airflow obstruction may be the result of stenosis of a major airway or widespread disease of the lower respiratory tract. The possibility that localised pathological changes ('upper airway obstruction') are the cause of a patient's dyspnoea and wheezing, must not be overlooked, although such localised changes are rare in comparison with diffuse obstructive bronchial disease. Severe stenosis of the larynx, trachea or a major bronchus causes frank stridor, but in the earlier stages the noise generated during inspiration and expiration may not be obvious when the patient is breathing quietly. Forced inspiratory and expiratory manoeuvres help to identify the nature of the problem and, if suitable recording apparatus is available, to distinguish between extrathoracic and intrathoracic sites of obstruction. The simplest recording apparatus is a spirometer and, with this, forced expiratory and inspiratory vital capacity manoeuvres can be compared. From the records thus made the FEV_1 is noted and so is the volume inspired in the first second of a forced inspiratory vital capacity (FIV_1). In health the FEV_1 is less than the FIV_1, the normal ratio of FEV_1/FIV_1 being about 0.8. Upper airway obstruction may be 'fixed' or 'variable'. A fixed obstruction impairs airflow as much in expiration as in inspiration and, although FEV_1 and FIV_1 are both reduced, their ratio is close to normal. In the presence of variable extrathoracic obstruction the FIV_1 is impaired more than the FEV_1. This is because structures in the neck are exposed to surrounding atmospheric pressure which compresses the airway more during inspiration, when the pressure within the trachea is subatmospheric, than during expiration when the pressure within the airway is raised above atmospheric. The ratio of FEV_1/FIV_1 may be doubled in these circumstances. In contrast, in the presence of a variable intrathoracic tracheal obstruction the ratio of FEV_1/FIV_1 falls, because of the (reversed) effects of changes in *intrathoracic* pressure on the airway during expiration and inspiration: during forced expiration the raised intrathoracic pressure around the lungs and airways compresses the already stenosed airway, whereas during forced inspiration the fall in intrathoracic pressure leads to widening of the airway. However, if the pathological changes responsible cause a rigid stenosis which is not influenced by these dynamic changes in airway calibre, a fixed obstruction ensues.

If it is available, the more sophisticated technique of recording flow–volume loops

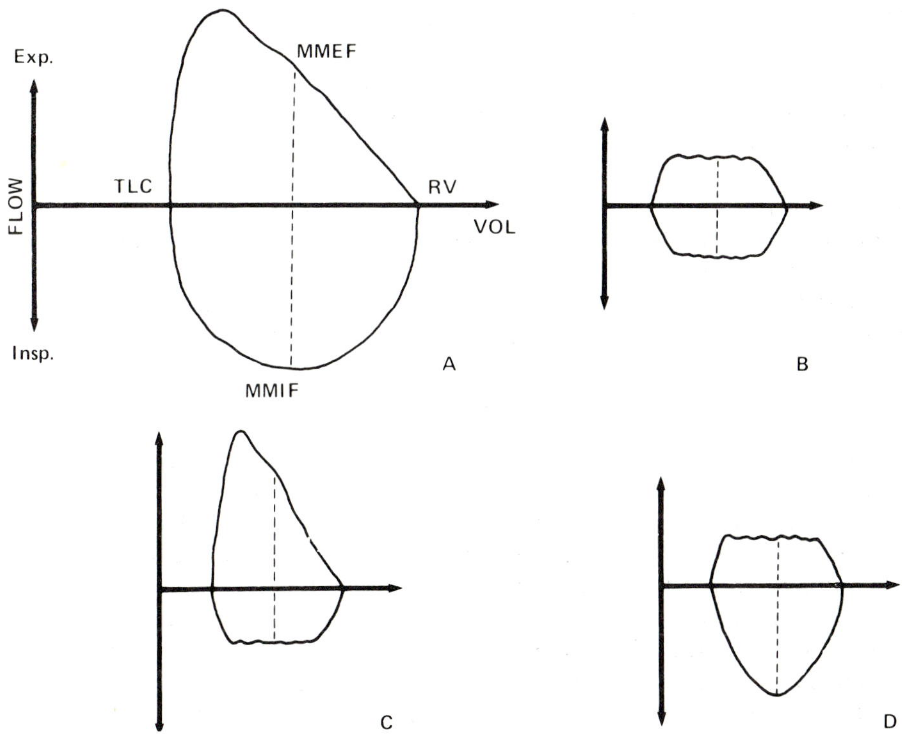

Fig. 5.4 Flow–volume loop facsimiles. Respiratory airflow (*y* axis) and volume (*x* axis) are recorded simultaneously during a complete forced inspiratory and expiratory cycle, from residual volume (RV) to total lung capacity (TLC) and back to RV. Inspiration (Insp.) is down and expiration (Exp.) is upwards. Maximum mid-inspiratory flow (MMIF) and maximum mid-expiratory flow (MMEF) are measured at the mid-point of the forced vital capacity. The ratio of MMEF/MMIF in a normal flow–volume loop (A) is approximately 0.9 Examples are seen of flow–volume loops in patients with fixed upper airway obstruction (B), variable extrathoracic (C) and variable intrathoracic (D) upper airway obstruction (*see text*)

during the assessment of forced expiratory/inspiratory vital capacities is desirable in patients suspected of having upper airway obstruction (Harrison 1976, Kryger et al 1976). On such recordings (Fig. 5.4) the ratio of expired to inspired flow rate is measured at the midpoint of the vital capacity. In normal subjects this is about 0.9. With variable extrathoracic obstruction the ratio increases and with intrathoracic obstruction it falls, for the same reasons as the changes in FEV_1/FIV_1 described above. With fixed upper airway obstruction both mid-expiratory and mid-inspiratory flow rates are equally reduced and the ratio is unaltered. Sequential documentation of flow–volume loops is particularly useful in following the progress of an obstruction in the upper airway.

The commonest cause of variable extrathoracic obstruction is vocal cord paralysis: tumours are responsible for the majority of variable intrathoracic obstructions. The most frequent cause of a fixed obstruction is a stricture attributable to a previous tracheostomy and prolonged endotracheal intubation. Other causes of chronic upper airway obstruction are: a goitre; lymphatic and other tumours compressing the airway; post-traumatic stricture (from chemical or thermal burns, or penetrating injuries); Wegener's granulomatosis; vascular malformations; amyloid disease; relapsing polychondritis, and other rare disorders.

The direct way to investigate a suspected upper airway obstruction is by bronchoscopy. If a fibreoptic instrument is used, care must be taken not to jeopardise the patient's airway during the procedure. It is usually possible to inspect the lesion from above only, and any other sites of stenosis below the proximal lesion will be overlooked. Tomography is the most convenient alternative means of assessing the length and calibre of a stenotic lesion. Treatment is usually surgical, although radiotherapy may be required for inoperable malignant obstruction: in rare instances medical treatment may be curative, as for example with a granulomatous stenosis.

Diffuse airflow obstruction

Chronic diffuse airflow obstruction is usually attributable to chronic bronchitis, with or without emphysema, and is then often termed obstructive airways disease (OAD) or chronic obstructive lung disease (COLD). These terms and other equivalent acronyms must not be applied indiscriminately to all patients merely because they have chronic airflow obstruction, as this can lead to the misdiagnosis of patients with upper airway obstruction and those with other diseases causing diffuse airflow obstruction. The most important of these other diseases is asthma, but conditions such as bronchiectasis, cystic fibrosis, bronchiolitis, byssinosis and the immotile cilia syndrome should not be overlooked. It is usually possible to distinguish these by careful attention to the history and by appropriate investigations.

With asthma of late onset, the differentiation from chronic bronchitis can at times be difficult and the two may coexist. An abrupt and sustained increase or marked variability in airflow obstruction, with episodes of wheezing at rest causing the patient to wake during the night, suggest the possibility of asthma. So does a history that the patient is a non-smoker, although of course cigarette smoking does not exclude a diagnosis of asthma. Nasal irritability with bouts of sneezing and rhinorrhoea is common in asthma and rare in chronic bronchitis. The presence of eosinophilia in blood and sputum supports a diagnosis of asthma, as does a good bronchodilator response to a β-sympathetic agonist. When asthma is thought to be responsible for severe, unrelenting chronic airflow obstruction, a therapeutic trial of corticosteroids is indicated. Such a trial must be done with care and should ideally be placebo-controlled, although this is not always possible in practice; however, it is important to obtain adequate baseline tests of pulmonary function, such as peak flow recordings, with which changes caused by treatment can be compared.

There are two notable clinical features in patients with chronic bronchitis: hypersecretion of mucus and diffuse airflow obstruction. Hypersecretion is an essential feature whereas airflow obstruction may or may not be present to an extent which is clinically important. Both are manifestations of pathological change in the air passages but the degree to which they are expressed varies from patient to patient. Thus, some patients have chronic expectoration with little, if any, airflow obstruction and some have chronic airflow obstruction with little evidence of hypersecretion of mucus. While both features are strongly linked aetiologically with cigarette smoking, it appears that the development of progressive and disabling airflow obstruction may be influenced by other factors in the host and his environment. What seems evident is that mucous hypersecretion is not, in itself, responsible for the development or progression of airflow obstruction. Indeed, some chronic bronchitic patients who discontinue smoking notice a marked reduction in the amount of sputum they produce, yet their airflow obstruction continues to deteriorate. Nevertheless, there is some evidence that stopping smoking will halt or reduce the rate of progression of airflow obstruction and every attempt should be made to persuade patients to do this.

The pathology of 'chronic obstructive lung disease' and the relationship of this to disabling airflow obstruction have attracted great interest in recent years. The seminal observations of Hogg et al (1968) focussed attention on the importance of disease in small, peripheral airways ($<$2 mm diameter), although it should not be forgotten that the air passages form a continuum and there may be important abnormalities in airways of all diameters. Structural changes which may be responsible for chronic airflow obstruction have been summarised by Thurlbeck (1980) as follows:

1. *Disease in large airways:* mucous gland enlargement; bronchial wall thickening; increased muscle; atrophy of cartilage; mucus within the lumen. Abnormal collapsibility of large airways imposes severe limitation in the rate of airflow during forced expiration when there is dynamic compression of the air passages.
2. *Disease in small airways:* inflammation; goblet cell metaplasia; increased muscle; mucus within the lumen; and bronchiolar narrowing, collapse, obliteration or tortuosity.
3. *Loss of elastic recoil of the surrounding lung,* as in emphysema. This leads to a reduction in the tractional force or negative pressure exerted on the airways by the surrounding lung tissue which normally helps to maintain the airways' calibre: thus they become narrower. As the emphysematous lung distends the airways will widen, but at any given lung volume their diameter tends to be less than normal. During expiration they close and obstruct the flow of air from the alveoli.

Whatever the mechanism of the airflow obstruction, and this may vary from patient to patient, there can be no doubt that the difficulty in breathing which this causes is responsible for the progressive disability, with the patient's subsequent death from respiratory failure, cor pulmonale or both. Hypoxia is a key issue in these patients and is attributable in most to a combination of mismatching of ventilation and perfusion in the lungs, with or without hypoventilation and a rise in P_{CO_2}. The severity of the hypoxia may be aggravated by exercise and by exacerbations of chronic bronchitis. There may also be transient episodes of profound hypoxaemia during sleep.

It has long been known that minor falls in P_{O_2} and a rise in P_{CO_2} can occur in normal subjects during sleep, and in recent years various clinical syndromes associated with sleep apnoea have been recognised (Guilleminault et al 1976). It is now realised that episodes of apnoea during sleep may be caused by upper airway obstruction (obstructive apnoea) or cessation of respiratory movements ('central apnoea'), or to both of these events combined. Studies during sleep in patients with chronic bronchitis and emphysema have shown that the periods of profound nocturnal hypoxaemia which befall the 'blue and bloated' type of patient are attributable to a combination of hypoventilation and impaired ventilation/perfusion relationships (Douglas et al 1979).

The diurnal and nocturnal hypoxia in these patients is believed to be responsible for vasoconstrictive pulmonary hypertension and secondary polycythaemia, which are amenable to improvement by long-term oxygen therapy. The results of a controlled trial of such treatment have been reported by a working party of the British Medical Research Council (Medical Research Council Working Party Report 1981). In this, patients who were in respiratory failure because of chronic obstructive bronchitis or emphysema and who had a history of congestive cardiac failure were allocated at random to a treatment group and a control group. The former received oxygen by nasal insufflation at a rate of 2 l/min for 15 h a day, including their period of sleep, while the control group did not. Patients from both groups received bronchodilator drugs, diuretics, antibiotics and digoxin at the discretion of their attendant physician. All patients were followed up until death or 5 years' survival. In men, the mortality during the first 500 d was no different in the treated and control groups; thereafter, the group receiving oxygen therapy had a reduced mortality rate (11.9% per annum compared with 29.4% of the control group). In women the prognosis was improved from the start of treatment (5.7% of the treatment group died per annum and 36.5% of the controls). As only 21 women were studied and only nine received oxygen therapy, an analysis of the individual factors influencing their prognosis was not attempted. However, prognosis in the female controls was particularly poor, eight of the 12 being dead in 3 years. Prognosis in the men was difficult to predict from the various observations made at entry to the study, although a combination of the Pa_{CO_2} and red cell mass was an indicator of early mortality. Disappointingly, despite improved survival, neither the work attendance nor the time these patients spent in hospital because of exacerbations of their disease was altered by long-term oxygen therapy. However, the patients being studied were already very ill at the time of entry to the trial.

In the USA, it has been shown that a group of patients receiving oxygen therapy for 24 h a day survived longer than a matched group who received oxygen for 12 h at night (Nocturnal Oxygen Therapy Trial Group 1980). In this study the continuous-treatment group began to show benefit from the outset: there was no delay before the survival curves of the two groups began to diverge, such as was seen in men in the British investigation. A possible explanation for the British experience is that a proportion of male patients who entered the trial were already very ill and their disease was too advanced to be capable of deriving benefit from oxygen treatment; their fate was thus already sealed, so that only when these individuals had succumbed could any statistical advantage from long-term oxygen begin to appear. The corollary to such an explanation, if correct, is that treatment with oxygen should be started earlier in the natural history of these patients' disease.

With deaths in the UK from chronic bronchitis and emphysema approaching 30000 per annum, the financial implications are awesome. Not all these patients would derive benefit from long-term oxygen treatment and it is now a matter of some urgency to establish clear criteria to identify those who should be offered this treatment and when it should start. It is also important to find out whether treatment improves the quality of life as well as prolonging its duration. In this context the effects on the patient's family as well as the patient himself deserve careful consideration.

At present the only generally available method of providing long-term domiciliary oxygen therapy under the National Health Service in Britain is by a regular supply of oxygen cylinders, costing up to £3500 per patient per annum. An economic appraisal of the cost of alternative methods shows that an oxygen concentrator is the cheapest for all but a very small number of patients (Lowson et al 1981). Oxygen concentrators are electrically operated devices which act as a 'molecular sieve' and separate oxygen from other gases in the air. They cost approximately £1000 to buy and about half this sum per annum to run. Although they are easily installed they do require servicing and maintenance facilities.

However, it should not be forgotten that much can be done for these patients without the widespread introduction of long-term oxygen therapy (Editorial, Lancet 1981): stopping smoking, weight reduction, regular exercise, and appropriate treatment with bronchodilator drugs, diuretics, antibiotics, and venesection for polycythaemia, can all be of benefit. Ultimately, prevention must be the key to the

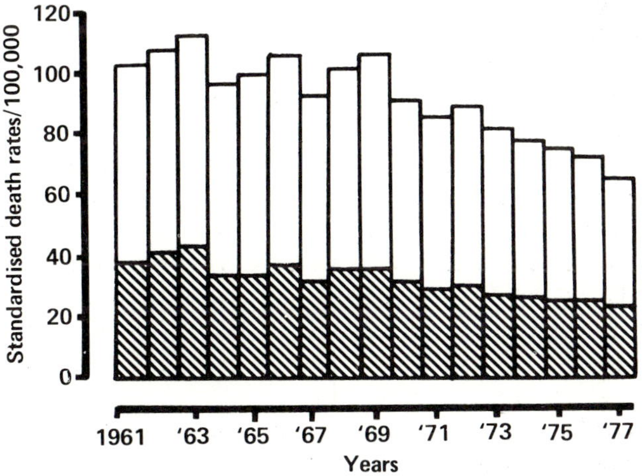

Fig. 5.5 Approximate age-standardised death rates from bronchitis, emphysema and asthma in England and Wales, using 1968 as the base year. Superimposed on the columns for mortality in men are hatched columns giving the death rates in women. Compiled from statistics kindly provided by Professor Ian Leck

control of chronic bronchitis and it is encouraging to note the present downward trend in mortality from this and allied diseases (Fig. 5.5) which suggests that preventive and therapeutic measures already in operation are having a beneficial effect.

REFERENCES

Fibreoptic bronchoscopy

Credle W F, Smiddy J F, Elliott R C 1974 Complications of fibreoptic bronchoscopy. American Review of Respiratory Diseases 109: 67–72

Gee J B L, Fick R B Jr 1980 Bronchoalveolar lavage. Thorax 35: 1–8

Haslam P L, Turton C W G, Lukoszek A, Salsbury A J, Dewar A, Collins J V et al 1980 Bronchoalveolar lavage fluid cell counts in cryptogenic fibrosing alveolitis and their relation to therapy. Thorax 35: 328–339

Mitchell D M, Emerson C J, Collyer J, Collins J V 1980 Fibreoptic bronchoscopy: 10 years on. British Medical Journal 281: 360–363

Pearce S J 1980 Fibreoptic bronchoscopy: is sedation necessary? British Medical Journal 281: 779–780

Granulomatous diseases of the lungs

Editorial 1980 ACE in sarcoidosis. Lancet 1: 804–805

Fauci A S, Haynes B F, Katz P 1978 The spectrum of vasculitis: clinical, pathologic, immunologic, and therapeutic considerations. Annals of Internal Medicine 89: 660–676

Gee J B L, Fick R B Jr 1980 Bronchoalveolar lavage. Thorax 35: 1–8

Gocke D J, Hsu K, Morgan C, Bombardieri S, Lockshin M, Christian C L 1970 Association between polyarteritis and Australia antigen. Lancet 2: 1149–1153

Gronhagen-Riska C, Selroos O, Wager G, Fyhriquist F 1979 Angiotensin-converting enzyme. Scandinavian Journal of Respiratory Diseases 60 (2): 94–101

Handslip P D, Bone M, Woodhead J S, Davies B H 1981 Calcium and phosphate metabolism in sarcoidosis with particular reference to parathyroid function. British Journal of Diseases of the Chest 75: 55–60

Hunninghake G W, Crystal R G 1981 Pulmonary sarcoidosis; a disorder mediated by excess helper T-lymphocyte activity at sites of disease activity. New England Journal of Medicine 305: 429–434

Hunninghake G W, Fulmer J D, Young R C Jr, Gadek J E, Crystal R G 1979 Localization of the immune response in sarcoidosis. American Review of Respiratory Disease 120 (1): 49–57

Johnson N Mc I, McNicol M W, Burton-Kee J E, Mowbray J F 1980 Circulating immune complexes in sarcoidosis. Thorax 35: 286–289

Lieberman J 1975 Elevation of serum angiotensin converting enzyme (ACE) level in sarcoidosis. American Journal of Medicine 59: 365–372

Lieberman J, Nosal A, Schlessner L A, Sastre-Foken A 1979 A serum angiotensin converting enzyme for diagnosis and therapeutic evaluation of sarcoidosis. American Revue of Respiratory Disease 120: 329–335

Mitchell D M, Emerson C J, Collyer J, Collins J V 1980 Fibreoptic bronchoscopy: 10 years on. British Medical Journal 2: 360–363

Neville E 1977 HLA antigens and disease. Mount Sinai Journal of Medicine 44: 772–777

Neville E, Carstairs L S, James D G 1977 Sarcoidosis of bone. Quarterly Journal of Medicine, New Series 46: 215–227

Nicholls A J, Friend J A R, Legge J S 1980 Sarcoid pleural effusion: three cases and review of the literature. Thorax 35: 277–281

Papapoulos S E, Clemens T L, Fraher L J, Lewin I G, Sandler L M, O'Riordan J L H 1979 1,25-Dihydroxycholecalciferol in the pathogenesis of the hypercalcaemia of sarcoidosis. Lancet 1: 627–630

Pinching A J, Rees A J, Pussell B A, Lockwood C M, Mitchison R S, Peters D K 1980 Relapses in Wegener's granulomatosis: the role of infection. British Medical Journal 281: 836–838

Reiner M, Sigurdsson G, Nunziata V, Malik M A, Poole G W, Joplin G F 1976 Abnormal calcium metabolism in normocalcaemic sarcoidosis. British Medical Journal 2: 1473–1476

Rich A R 1942 Role of hypersensitivity in periarteritis nodosa as indicated by 7 cases developing during serum sickness and sulfonamide therapy. Bulletin of the Johns Hopkins Hospital 71: 123–140

Rømer F K 1980 Renal manifestations and abnormal calcium metabolism in sarcoidosis. Quarterly Journal of Medicine, New Series 49: 233–247

Smith M J, Turton C W G, Mitchell D N, Turner-Warwick M, Morris L M, Lawler S D 1981 Association of HLA B8 with spontaneous resolution in sarcoidosis. Thorax 36: 296–298

Studdy P, Bird R, James D G, Sherlock S 1978 Serum angiotensin-converting enzyme (ACE) in sarcoidosis and other granulomatous disorders. Lancet 2: 1331–1334

Winterbauer R H, Kraemer K G 1976 The infectious complications of sarcoidosis. Archives of Internal Medicine 136: 1356–1362

Legionnaires' disease

Balows A, Fraser D W (eds) 1979 International symposium on legionnaires' disease. Annals of Internal Medicine 90: 489–703

Editorial 1981 Legionella and amoebae. Lancet 1: 703–704

McDade J E, Brenner D J, Bozeman F M 1979 Legionnaires' disease bacterium isolated in 1947. Annals of Internal Medicine 90: 659–661

Macrae A D, Appleton P N, Laverick A 1979 Legionnaires' disease in Nottingham, England. Annals of Internal Medicine 90: 580–583

Tobin J O'H, Beare J, Dunnill M S, Fisher-Hoch S, French M, Mitchell R G et al 1980 Legionnaires' disease in a transplant unit: isolation of the causative agent from shower baths. Lancet 2: 118–121

Asbestos-induced disease

Baris Y I, Sahin A A, Ozesmi M, Kerse I, Ozen E, Kolacan B et al 1978 An outbreak of pleural mesothelioma and chronic fibrosing pleurisy in the village of Karain/Ürgüp in Anatolia. Thorax 33: 181–192

Elmes P C 1980 Mesotheliomas, minerals, and man-made fibres. Thorax 35: 561–563

Elmes P C, Simpson M J C 1976 The clinical aspects of meseothelioma. Quarterly Journal of Medicine, New Series 45: 427–449

Greenberg M, Lloyd Davies T A 1974 Mesothelioma Register 1967–1968. British Journal of Industrial Medicine 31: 91–104

Gregor A, Singh S, Turner-Warwick M, Lawler S, Parkes W R 1979 The role of histocompatibility (HLA) antigens in asbestosis. British Journal of Diseases of the Chest 73: 245–252

Peto J 1978 The hygiene standard for chrysotile asbestos. Lancet 1: 484–489

Selikoff I J, Hammond E C 1979 Asbestos and smoking. Journal of the American Medical Association 242 (5): 458–459

Yazicioglu S, Ilcayto R, Balci K, Sayli B S, Yorulmaz B 1980 Pleural calcification, pleural mesotheliomas, and bronchial cancers caused by tremolite dust. Thorax 35: 564–569

Chronic airflow obstruction

Douglas N J, Calverley P M A, Leggett R J E, Brash H M, Flenley D C, Brezinova V 1979 Transient hypoxaemia during sleep in chronic bronchitis and emphysema. Lancet 1: 1–4

Editorial 1981 Long-term oxygen and advanced chronic bronchitis. Lancet 1: 701–702

Guilleminault C G, Tilkian A, Dement W C 1976 The sleep apnoea syndromes. Annual Review of Medicine 27: 465–483

Harrison B D W 1976 Upper airway obstruction — a report on 16 patients. Quarterly Journal of Medicine, New Series 45: 625–645

Hogg J C, Macklem P T, Thurlbeck W M 1968 Site and nature of airway obstruction in chronic obstructive lung disease. New England Journal of Medicine 278: 1355–1360

Kryger M, Bode F, Antic R, Anthonisen N 1976 Diagnosis of obstruction of the upper and central airways. American Journal of Medicine 61: 85–93

Lowson K, Drummond M F, Bishop J M 1981 Costing new services: Long-term domiciliary oxygen therapy. Lancet 1: 1146–1149

Medical Research Council Working Party Report 1981 Long-term domiciliary oxygen therapy in chronic hypoxic cor pulmonale complicating chronic bronchitis and emphysema. Lancet 1: 681–685

Nocturnal Oxygen Therapy Trial Group 1980 Continuous or nocturnal oxygen therapy in hypoxaemic chronic obstructive lung disease: a clinical trial. Annals of Internal Medicine 93: 391–398

Thurlbeck W M 1980 Smoking, airflow limitation, and the pulmonary circulation. American Review of Respiratory Disease 122: 183–186

6

Neurology

J. B. Foster

FACIAL NERVE

Since Charles Bell's description of idiopathic palsy of the facial nerve, there has been controversy concerning the pathogenesis of this, the most common mononeuropathy. Recently, discussion has been centred on the determination of how the prognosis can best be estimated and, in patients thought to have a poor prognosis what treatment should be considered. Physicians who are presented with a case of lower motor neurone palsy of sudden onset must be aware of structural pathology other than that of the idiopathic variety and must consider in particular the possibility of the nerve being compromised by pathological conditions of the middle ear cleft, such as otitis media, acute and chronic tuberculous lesions, trauma and tumours. Most infections seen today occur in association with a congenital dehiscence of the facial canal, exposing the nerve to compression by a swollen and infected mucous membrane, and calling for antibiotic therapy. Where cholesteatoma is responsible, aspiration of the middle ear cleft is urgently required. In the neonate, a unilateral palsy may follow forceps delivery or may present initially in children during the course of leukaemia or nephritis. Therefore, while Bell's palsy remains the commonest cause of unilateral facial weakness, hypertension, renal disease and haemorrhage in patients with thrombocytopenia should be considered.

Facial nerve involvement in herpes zoster is well recognised and well described: there is a vesicular eruption either of the pinna or of the soft palate. It is generally accepted that such cases carry a worse prognosis than the idiopathic variety. Unilateral facial palsy of more gradual onset may indicate a lesion of the cerebral hemisphere where the upper face is spared, or may be a false localising sign of tumour in the supratentorial compartment or even of benign intracranial hypertension, but more commonly indicates a lesion of the nucleus in the pons, the intrapontine facial fibres, or the nerve in its course in the subarachnoid space and facial canal. Pontine gliomas and multiple sclerosis may first present with facial weakness and, where the nerve is affected in the subarachnoid space, tuberculous and neoplastic meningitis must be considered in addition to the more acute pyococcal meningitides. Occasionally, lower motor neurone palsy of the face occurs as a presenting feature of post-infective polyradiculopathy (Guillain-Barré syndrome), but usually the weakness is bilateral, as in those cases where mononucleosis is the underlying cause. In the cerebello-pontine angle an acoustic neuroma may grow to sufficient size to compress the facial nerve before the loss of auditory acuity is noted by the patient or his adviser and similarly, other angle lesions such as meningioma, aneurysm or even an eccentrically placed chordoma may produce initial and isolated facial nerve compression. Poliomyelitis, so rarely seen in the Western World, must always be considered in a patient who is systemically ill with evidence of meningism at the onset of the facial weakness.

Bilateral weakness of the face may be mimicked by depressive illness or the facial immobility of early Parkinson's disease, but more commonly is seen in myasthenia where the fatiguability, diplopia, ptosis and the other clinical phenomena of the condition should be recognised. Bilateral weakness may form part of a more generalised myopathic process, be this a metabolic myopathy, a pure muscular dystrophy or autoimmune myositis.

Fortunately, most cases of facial palsy of acute onset are idiopathic and carry a good prognosis. Clinical examination, electrophysiological studies and the practice of exploration of the facial canal have confirmed that, in the majority of cases, the lesion lies below the geniculate ganglion and in some 50% will lie distal to the entry of the chorda tympani into the main trunk of the nerve. Patients are therefore seen, with partial or total facial weakness, who have retained taste on the anterior tongue with a distal lesion, lost taste with a more proximal lesion or lost taste and lacrimation with an even more proximal lesion. The majority of patients complain of pain in and behind the ear at the onset of the paralysis.

There have been many reviews of possible pathogenetic mechanisms (Frew & Diamond 1979). For the proponents of the viral theory, no inflammatory reaction has yet been identified except in those cases where a viral pathogenesis is undoubted, for example in herpes or other polioclastic virus infections. There are protagonists of the vascular or ischaemic theory and others who feel that idiopathic Bell's palsy is a cell-mediated autoimmune disorder and draw analogies between it and postinfective radiculopathy. The acute onset of the disease, the association with pain and the generally good prognosis bear some relation to the clinical pattern of neuralgic amyotrophy, paralysis of the long thoracic nerve of Bell and paralysis of the laryngeal nerve, all of which have been suggested as having an autoimmune pathogenesis.

The basic pathology is one of demyelination and distal Wallerian degeneration. Whatever the theories considered, there are certain clinical imponderables. Why should the condition almost always be unilateral? How do we explain recurrences which tend to be more common in the female? How do we explain the more common occurrence of idiopathic facial palsy in pregnancy and how do we explain apparent epidemics of facial palsy? Safman (1971) and Ardour (1976), have suggested that idiopathic Bell's palsy is part of a generalised polyneuritis cranialis and they quote evidence of clinical involvement of the opposite side of the face in 14 out of 18 patients, involvement of the motor division of the fifth cranial nerve in 3% of 200 patients, and involvement of the afferent arc of the gag reflex in 35% of patients.

The clinical importance and resolution of these problems of pathogenesis must involve the possibility of early and successful prevention of total denervation, a hitherto poor prognostic feature. Age influences prognosis: the older the patient, the more likely is there to be permanent denervation. Although pain was at one time thought to be associated with a poor prognosis, this is not necessarily so. Prognosis is not influenced by the precise site of the lesion in the fallopian canal and, in particular, loss of taste on the anterior tongue has no prognostic significance. It is generally accepted, however, that a dry eye is a bad prognostic sign. It is certainly true that denervation is more likely in cases where the paralysis is complete, but denervation can become complete some days after the onset of the paralysis. The reported studies of groups of cases indicate that some 85% of patients in whom incomplete paralysis is seen at the initial examination will recover completely, and where paralysis is never complete, then complete recovery is the rule. As it is not possible to determine, by clinical or electrophysiological means, in which cases incomplete paralysis seen at the onset might lead to total denervation with its attendant bad prognosis, then is it not reasonable to treat all patients, if we believe that an effective treatment exists? The majority of patients with idiopathic Bell's palsy recover spontaneously. It is difficult properly to evaluate the natural history of the condition, because patients with pain will attend early but may well have a good prognosis. Patients who are beginning to recover may fail to attend the general practitioner and are not likely to be referred to hospital. Perhaps the prognosis is better than the published series indicate and the quoted natural history is necessarily influenced by such case selection. As far as neurophysiological studies are concerned, Matthews (1982) in a recent review has suggested that the finding of an inexcitable nerve indicates that it is too late for treatment to be planned, but a rising threshold to stimulation is not necessarily an indication of impending denervation. He quotes various inconclusive results in the literature which indicate that an inexcitable nerve does not necessarily imply total denervation and full recovery is possible even when the denervation has occurred. Thus, because electrophysiological studies do not necessarily help to determine the prognosis for patients with an incomplete paralysis, many departments have given up referring patients with Bell's palsy for electrophysiological studies and treat their patients on an ad hoc basis which has existed since the time of Charles Bell.

Surgical decompression of the facial nerve has never been shown to be effective in Great Britain and such operations are no longer undertaken. The majority of practising clinicians will treat their patients with corticosteroids either as prednisolone or perhaps dexamethasone in high doses for the first few days, if they are fortunate enough to see the patients within 24h of the onset of the palsy. This necessarily implies that the treatment of Bell's palsy devolves upon the general practitioner and fewer patients are being referred to hospital clinics for evaluation and treatment. Patients who fail to recover will suffer partial paralysis, evident ectopic reinnervation with synkinetic movements around the eye and mouth and often the very disabling condition of crocodile tears. In patients with severe facial paralysis there are reconstructive operative techniques such as hypoglossal anastomosis which will improve the appearance of the face in repose and often bring benefit in terms of more symmetrical voluntary movement.

Involuntary facial movement

Movement in the face which is apparently spontaneous may indicate a simple habit spasm or tic, that is, a movement under volitional control. Movement may also occur in the half face as part of a focal or partial seizure and so-called epilepsia partialis continua may involve the lower face, particularly in the elderly following cortical infarction.

A more disabling chronic twitching of the muscles of the face, i.e. hemi-facial spasm or clonic facial spasm, must be differentiated from the benign facial myokymia which occurs in the lower lids of many people following heavy work and protracted periods of reading. Hemi-facial spasm, although usually seen in late middle life, may occur at any age and recently the author has seen a 15-year-old girl who was significantly disabled by hemi-facial spasm and cured by posterior fossa surgery. The disorder is characteristically unilateral, mild at its inception, usually affecting one or other eye with slight twitching in the orbicularis oculi muscle but becoming more severe and widespread, eventually involving all the muscles of facial expression including the platysma. The patients are usually extremely embarrassed by the uncontrollable winking and twitching of the side of the face which may affect their ability to eat; the profound social embarrassment has caused many sufferers to become reclusive and many even to contemplate suicide. The disorder is not common and indeed much less common than the tic involving the trigeminal nerve, i.e. trigeminal neuralgia. Many causes have been suggested and many abortive attempts at treatment have been devised, most of which have involved section of the facial nerve trunk, its main branches anterior to the parotid or, more recently, a distal selective neurectomy in the substance of the muscles affected by the twitching. However, the overall effect of such surgery is towards facial paralysis and diminution in the twitching is quantitative rather than qualitative.

Following the work of Jannetta (1980) it has been recognised that the pathogenesis of this condition may lie in the posterior fossa. Jannetta has described 85 patients whose age ranged from 20 to 75 years whose posterior fossa he explored on the ipsilateral side and in 66 of whom he found an aberrant single artery irritating or influencing the facial nerve in the cerebello-pontine angle. In 13, multiple arteries were involved; in two a vein was implicated. In all, using microsurgical dissection techniques, he was able to decompress the facial exit zone and by mobilising the nerve, maintain separation of nerve and artery with a small piece of muscle taken from the incision wound. Although his initial results were critically received he has described excellent results in 74 of his 85 patients and a complicating facial weakness in six only, all but one of whom eventually recovered. More recently Kaye & Adams (1981) described their experience with 16 patients who had severe hemi-facial spasm and were similarly explored. Excellent results were reported in 14 of 16 cases, seven of whom had been followed up for four years or longer. Their technique is to wrap sponge around the facial nerve for, in only four of their 16 patients did they find the definable vascular compression so frequently described by Jannetta. They feel that the trauma of the wrapping of the nerve with non-absorbable sponge is sufficient to relieve the condition.

Experience in the Newcastle Department of Neurology (Sengupta, personal communication) suggests that we now have a successful and relatively safe operative treatment for a condition which hitherto was totally intractable. Although posterior fossa exploration must not be lightly entertained, it should be stressed that the technical difficulties in the majority of such exposures reflect the underlying pathology, for example, aneurysm, tumour or abscess. In patients with hemi-facial spasm the posterior fossa is anatomically normal without distortion and, with the use of an operating microscope, such operations should carry a nil mortality and little morbidity.

TRIGEMINAL NEURALGIA

There has been a similar change in the surgical approach to the management of patients with trigeminal neuralgia or tic douloureux. Because this disease usually affects people in later life, many of the neurosurgical techniques, such as extradural or intradural approaches for trigeminal root section, have carried a considerable morbidity. The medical treatment of this condition involves the use of carbamazepine and some 80% of patients will obtain relief from the pain if they are given sufficient carbamazepine during a 24 h period. However, in those patients who are unable to tolerate this compound or whose pain is not relieved sufficiently, neurosurgical procedures should always be considered. Phenol injection of the trigeminal (gasserian) ganglion and direct root section are now rarely practised. A form of controlled thermocoagulation of the gasserian ganglion, which was introduced by Sweet & Wespic in 1974, is now practised by many neurosurgeons. Essentially the technique involves percutaneous puncture and placing of a needle in the ganglion via the foramen ovale under radiological control. Pain fibres are more susceptible to the heat generated by a radio-frequency generator and it is hoped that trigeminal neuralgia will be relieved thereby without reduction of sensitivity in the face. Many large series are reported. The technique is ideally suitable for the elderly and initial failure can be followed by a second operation. Jannetta (1975) has evaluated a posterior fossa approach similar to that used for patients with hemi-facial spasm and has found arterial loops distorting, indenting and compressing the fifth cranial nerve at the root entry zone. Many neurosurgeons have now corroborated Jannetta's work and a posterior fossa approach offers an alternative to medical treatment or thermocoagulation in those patients fit for neurosurgical anaesthesia. The great advantage of the posterior fossa approach is that the patients have no numbness in areas served by the trigeminal nerve, after the procedure.

PARKINSON'S DISEASE

In the last edition of *Progress in Clinical Medicine,* recent understanding of the pathogenesis of Parkinson's disease and of its treatment was discussed. Over the last 4 years it has become increasingly apparent, to those responsible for the care of many patients with Parkinson's disease, that the early euphoria brought about by the advent of levadopa and its analogues in pure and compound forms, has not been maintained. Many patients showing an initial dramatic response to treatment are now becoming increasingly incapacitated, not only physically but intellectually, and it is becoming clear that parkinsonism can be, and often is, associated with progressive dementia. It has been suggested that these drugs have not significantly altered life expectation.

Before treatment with L-dopa, the dementia was almost certainly masked by the physical disability and the poor prognosis but now, with the longer survival of incapacitated and elderly patients, marked dementia may become apparent. Lieberman et al (1979) have described 372 patients of whom 32% showed evidence of clinical dementia after a minimum follow-up period of 4 years. They concluded that the frequency in their series was such that a chance association between Parkinson's disease and Alzheimer's disease could no longer be sustained but they concluded that the association was not related to the treatment with L-dopa, although others have thought that the early use of L-dopa may be responsible for dementia in Parkinson's disease. Surveys are being undertaken in units with experience of dementia scoring and expertise in cortical cell counting in order to determine the relationship or otherwise between the evident dementia of Parkinson's disease and the early use of L-dopa.

Unfortunately, the on-off phenomenon remains as difficult to control as it was at the time of the last edition and there is no evidence that bromocriptine either alone, in small or large doses, or in combination, is more effective than L-dopa alone in relieving this troublesome complication of treatment.

Although stereotaxic surgery in Parkinson's disease is less frequently used, there are still patients with principally unilateral tremor, who are normotensive and have no significant involvement of central structures, who would benefit from such surgery; many who are unable to eat because of the extensive tremor of their hands can be helped by a unilateral thalamotomy.

PERIODIC MIGRAINOUS NEURALGIA

Migraine is usually classified into three groups, (1) common migraine, (2) classic migraine and (3) complicated migraine. In order to satisfy the diagnostic criteria for migraine a patient should be suffering from the characteristic paroxysmal disturbance, of which headache is the most constant element and where nausea may accompany the headache or some sensory abnormality may precede or coincide with the headache. There are, however, many patients whose migraine does not follow such a typical or recognisable pattern. These include those whose headaches are associated with a dense hemiplegia with or without dysphasia, where the condition may be familial, i.e. familial hemiplegic migraine, or those with more complicated migraine where ocular complications are evident, for example ocular motor palsy or persisting scotoma or hemianopic defect, and cases of basilar or ophthalmoplegic migraine.

An ill-understood and frequently misdiagnosed migraine variant is so-called periodic migrainous neuralgia. This was initially described by Wilfred Harris in 1926 and elegantly assessed by Symonds (1951) in his paper on migrainous variants. The condition is well known to neurologists and is almost certainly a nosological entity, although confusingly referred to as ciliary neuralgia, Horton's cephalgia, sphenopalatine neuralgia, autonomic facial neuralgia, histamine headache, Sluder's headache, or in the USA, cluster headache. This last term is certainly descriptive of the inclination of the headaches to recur frequently over a period of weeks or months, only to subside and recur in a second or another cluster. There are certain characteristic features of this peculiar form of migraine for it almost invariably affects the male and usually begins in middle life, unlike common or classic migraine. The pain is almost invariably unilateral, situated in and around the orbit or behind the eye and relatively short-lived, lasting 1 to 2h. Although paroxysms of pain may recur in a 24-h period, frequently they occur at the same time each day and often will occur in the night, waking the patient from sleep with a disturbing regularity, almost to the point of the timing being predictable. Having begun, a cycle or cluster of headaches will persist for weeks or months then abruptly cease, only to begin again, perhaps with a seasonal tendency. Sometimes the pain is referred from the orbit into the cheek or temple on the affected side and the patient describes it as a dull aching pain which is often extremely severe and frequently is associated with lacrimation of the ipsilateral eye and stuffiness of the ipsilateral nostril. Occasionally a myotic pupil is seen at the height of the ache and after many attacks this may become permanent. Frequently the eye appears puffy and the forehead red, but curiously, and again in contrast to common and classic migraine, there is very rarely a family history and very rarely are there dietetic or emotional precipitants although it is my own feeling that heavy cigarette and cigar smoking often precipitate attacks in predisposed individuals.

No pathophysiological explanation exists for this, perhaps the most severe of the migraine syndromes, and diagnosis is often missed or delayed. Treatment has proved extraordinarily difficult. Symonds has suggested ergotamine tartrate 0.25 mg by subcutaneous injection three times a day until the cluster of headaches subsides but frequently it is not possible for the patient to undertake this injection regime and often it fails. Of the serotonin antagonists, pizotifen and methysergide are sometimes effective. Because of their emotional reaction to the debilitating effect of the daily headache, many patients will claim some benefit from tricyclic drugs although the headaches, in the author's experience, are not directly relieved. In the past, stellate ganglion block and even stellate ganglionectomy have been advised but the results are very uncertain. The use of β-blockers, i.e. propranolol 40 mg 6-hourly has helped some patients. More recently lithium carbonate has been suggested and in some patients has proved extremely effective (Peatfield 1981). The drug is essentially useful in the treatment and prevention of acute mania and also valuable in the prophylaxis of recurrent depressive episodes: it was the cyclical variation in manic depressive illness which suggested to Ekbom (1977) that lithium might help in the prophylaxis of cluster headache. Peatfield has described his experience with 48 patients with cluster headache seen at the Princess Margaret Migraine Clinic at Charing Cross Hospital. He treated 31 of these with lithium carbonate and claimed that 14 patients showed a marked improvement in the first week of receiving 800 mg of the drug at night. Personal experience confirms the usefulness of lithium in this condition and certainly a controlled trial should be initiated.

Oral steroids, prednisone in particular, have been claimed to be effective (Russell 1979). More recently it has been suggested that a non-steroid anti-inflammatory compound (indomethacin) may be effective in some patients, given by mouth or by suppository. This is an unusual effect, for indomethacin is well recognised to produce severe headache in some sensitive patients when used in the treatment of rheumatic and other acute musculoskeletal disorders.

The importance of this uncommon variety of migraine is that very often it is unrecognised, so that patients are subjected to expensive and at times potentially hazardous investigation. Relief with one or other of the suggested drugs can be very dramatic.

TRANSIENT ISCHAEMIC ATTACKS

Transient episodes of neurological dysfunction. visual, motor or sensory, may be induced by tumour or subdural haematomas, form part of a focal seizure, or precede the headache of classic migraine. Much more frequently however they represent the transient impairment of function in an area of neural tissue rendered ischaemic by microemboli or impairment of blood flow; transient cerebral ischaemia or transient ischaemic attacks (TIA).

During the past 35 years TIA have been defined, studied and treated but their natural history, pathogenesis and prognosis are still controversial. How frequently do these attacks presage a major stroke? What is the most effective means of their identification and how can they be treated? They have been defined by the World Health Organisation (1978) as 'episodes of temporary and focal cerebral dysfunction of vascular origin leaving no permanent neurological deficit and lasting less than 24 hours' (WHO, 1978) and by an ad hoc committee for the classification of cerebrovascular diseases, thus: 'A TIA is a temporary and focal episode of neurological disturbance of presumed vascular origin which typically lasts for 2 to 15 minutes: it should not last longer than 24 hours nor leave any neurological deficit'. This second definition appreciates the transience of the TIA, and both allow a definition upon which studies of prognosis may be based. Both appreciate that a TIA is symptomatic and that signs do not persist, i.e. there is no permanent evidence of infarction. It was originally suggested that TIAs resulted from reversible cerebrovascular insufficiency related to posturally induced changes in cerebral perfusion in those with anomalous or inadequate intracranial collateral circulation (Denny-Brown 1951). However, after the importance of atheromatous disease in the extracranial arteries was appreciated, it became generally agreed that the majority of TIAs result from microemboli from atheromatous plaques in the carotid and vertebral systems. Nevertheless such symptomatic episodes can result from aneurysm hypoglycaemia or intracranial small vessel disease. Lacunae and haemodynamic factors may still be important in some patients, for the commonest presenting feature in patients with carotid occlusion is a transient ischaemic attack.

Some 40% of patients suffering from cerebral hemisphere TIAs or from amaurosis fugax will have demonstrable carotid artery disease and in these it is assumed that microemboli of atheromatous material or platelets and fibrin are responsible. Such emboli can be seen in pial vessels at autopsy or frequently in the retinal circulation during or after episodes of amaurosis fugax. There has been considerable discussion about the source of emboli in patients in whom radiological investigations of the carotid artery have shown no evidence of occlusion or atheroma. Are there still radiologically invisible lesions in the carotid territory, either extracranial or intracranial, or has the material come from the aortic arch or innominate artery? Cardiac lesions may be responsible which, in themselves, are not significant, e.g. mural or valvular thrombosis, or thrombosis from a mitral leaflet prolapse in the young patient (Geyer & Franzini 1979, Barnett et al 1980). What part does a fluctuating systemic blood pressure play in the pathogenesis, especially fluctuations induced by cardiac dysrhythmia? Fisher (1978) has commented that TIA patients very rarely have a significant dysrhythmia and a study of TIA patients by ambulatory ECG monitoring has confirmed this (de Bono & Warlow 1981) and yet if cerebral infarction follows acute hypotension, why not transient ischaemia?

The assessment of treatment has been foiled by poor understanding of the natural history of TIAs with an estimated incidence varying between 0.3–1.3 per 1000 adults per year in western communities (Friedman et al 1969, Joint Committee for Stroke

Facilities 1974). Estimates of infarction rates after follow-up range from less than 2% to 53% (Marshall 1964, Acheson & Hutchinson 1971). Such factors as the patient's recall, his age, blood pressure and the probability of 'treatment' will influence both of these estimates, as well as inevitable patient selection. However, it has been pointed out that the commonest cause of death in TIA patient is 'cardiac' and not cerebral infarction (Warlow 1982) and that a reasonable estimate of the risk of stroke after TIAs is 5% per annum and that of death, 10% per annum (Baker et al 1968). It is agreed that the risk of infarction is highest in the first weeks following the TIA (Cartlidge et al 1977) and carotid TIAs are considered to carry a higher risk of subsequent 'stroke' than those from the hind-brain circulation (Marshall 1964).

Management

The purpose of the investigation of patients suffering TIAs must be to determine pathological changes which will respond to medical and/or surgical treatment, thus reducing the risk of infarction or stroke and, if possible, reducing the risk of cardiac death. In this regard the TIA itself is not important but simply indicates the possibility of potentially lethal pathological changes.

It is essential to exclude diabetes, significant anaemia or polycythaemia and cardiac dysrhythmias. Most investigators will carry out echocardiography and will attempt to define any pathological changes in the carotid by direct or indirect carotid angiography. Real-time and also pulsed Döppler ultrasonic imaging (Sumner et al 1979) provides a non-invasive alternative to angiography, but in most centres engaged in research into TIAs indirect four-vessel angiography of the neck arteries is the definitive investigation. However, in some 25% of patients no lesion will be defined, in the neck or elsewhere.

When a well-defined carotid lesion is present, carotid endarterectomy has been the popular prophylactic treatment. However its effectiveness in preventing stroke remains controversial, for, as yet, no acceptable trial has demonstrated its benefit and a peri-operative stroke rate of 5.7% with an operative mortality rate of 3.4% has been quoted (West et al 1979). The American Joint Study (Fields et al 1970) did not demonstrate any benefit from carotid endarterectomy superior to the best available medical treatment.

The successful prophylaxis of TIAs will depend upon the elimination of atheroma and, until degenerative arterial disease is better understood, the medical treatment of TIAs will be directed at reducing the incidence of embolism. Conventional anticoagulant treatment has been largely discarded after enjoying popularity over many years and it is now unlikely that any prospective randomised trial will be mounted to justify such treatment.

In recent years, drugs which influence platelet behaviour have been in vogue, in particular aspirin, sulphinpyrazone and dipyridamole. Aspirin inhibits platelet aggregation and has been shown clinically to reduce the frequency of TIAs (Dyken et al 1973). The 'aspirin in transient ischaemic attack study' was prospective, randomised and double-blind, comparing 650 mg of aspirin given twice daily, with placebo; the study involved patients who were considered to be unsuitable for, or who had successfully undergone, carotid endarterectomy (Fields et al 1977, 1978). In the Canadian Co-operative Study Group (1978) trial of aspirin and sulphinpyrazone in threatened stroke, 649 patients with carotid or vertebrobasilar TIAs were randomly allocated. The trial was analysed after 18 months and finally at its conclusion. Aspirin was shown to reduce the rate of stroke and/or death in the men by 48% but not in the women. There was an overall 31% reduction in the rates of stroke and/or death from all causes in the aspirin group as against the 'no-aspirin' patients. There was no statistically significant difference between the aspirin and the sulphinpyrazone groups. No adequate trials of dipyridamole in TIA patients have yet been published but they are in progress, comparing aspirin with aspirin plus dipyridamole. Current clinical practice appears to be towards the use of the two drugs in combination (1200 mg of aspirin per day with 100 mg of dipyridamole three times daily).

External carotid–internal carotid anastomosis (ECIC)

This procedure is now under trial for selected patients with carotid occlusion and/or stenosis and in neurosurgical situations where direct attack on large aneurysms in the carotid sinus is judged to be risky and anastomosis is recommended. The technique involves microsurgical anastomosis of a branch of the superficial temporal artery with a branch of the middle cerebral artery in an attempt to improve flow in the latter. The technique is well established and improved flow and subsequent patency and enlargement of the middle cerebral arterial end of the anastomosis, demonstrable by angiography, has been confirmed. The results of the multicentre collaborative study are awaited.

ACUTE NECROTIC ENCEPHALITIS

More than 40 viruses can act neurotropically and produce symptomatic injury to the central nervous system. The infection may involve principally the meninges, spinal cord or brain, either selectively or collectively; enteroviruses are capable of inducing one or all three patterns of clinical illness, i.e. meningitis, myelitis or encephalitis.

It is generally accepted that the majority of cases of fatal acute encephalitis in the Western world are caused by the herpes simplex virus type 1 (HS). The pathology of the acute encephalitis is well documented. Focal necrotic lesions coalesce in the temporal lobes and are associated with haemorrhagic infarction and diffuse brain swelling, reflected in a haemorrhagic and inflammatory CSF. Selective vulnerability of the temporal lobes, in particular the hippocampal gyri and the orbital plates, may derive from the origin of the virus in the olfactory mucosa (Davis & Johnson 1978, Dinn 1980). The histology is characteristically that of a viral encephalitis, with inclusion bodies in the neurones and oligodendroglia of the cells adjacent to the patchy non-laminar areas of cortical necrosis. The clinical evolution of the disease is often over many days, with behavioural abnormalities prominent, together with hallucinations, seizures, aphasia and hemiparesis, indicating early involvement of the temporal lobes.

An antecedent illness, pyrexia and meningism suggest an infective pathology. The main differentiation is between acute necrotic encephalitis and a temporal lobe abscess, either intrinsic or lying in the middle intracranial fossa.

The significance and possible specificity of the EEG in herpes simplex encephalitis was first recognised in the late 1950s (Upton & Gumpert 1970, Illis & Taylor 1972). The changes are typically a disruption and slowing of the background activity with the appearance from the 2nd to the 15th day of the illness of repetitive, almost stereotyped slow-wave discharges from one or other of the temporal lobes. Towards the termination of the disease the repetitive features become less evident and the amplitude of the background slow activity diminished. Such EEG changes are seen in more than 50% of patients with HS encephalitis but may be mimicked by temporal lobe pyococcal abscess. The CSF pressure is usually moderately raised and a lymphocytosis of between 50 and 100 cells per mm^3 is seen. Red blood cells are seen in up to 40% of cases. Unfortunately the CSF is by no means specific and many centres rely on brain biopsy and subsequent specific immunofluorescent techniques to establish the diagnosis. Recently Klapper et al (1981) have described a specific radio-immune absorbent assay technique for serum and CSF IgG antibodies against herpes simplex. They comment that an accurate diagnostic index was obtained in 23 out of 26 patients, and out of 10 patients tested before the 10th day of the neurological illness, five had positive diagnostic indices. They comment that their technique may allow an early diagnosis. The method is non-invasive and, if positive, will preclude the need for brain biopsy.

The CT scan has proved very helpful in the early identification of the temporal lobe involvement in this condition, with the appearance of ill-defined low-density areas in one or other of the temporal lobes producing a space-occupying effect.

Considerable argument has raged over the treatment of HS encephalitis, particularly over the use of steroids to reduce cerebral oedema (Rappel 1971, Upton et al 1971) and more recently over the combination of steroid with antiviral agents.

A reduction of the mortality rate from 70 to 50% has been achieved by modern intensive care techniques, respiratory support and more aggressive control of cerebral oedema (Rappel 1973). However, there has been no formal trial of steroid against placebo although 'medical decompression' by dexamethasone is practised by most neurologists. Herpes virus replication can be arrested by a number of potentially useful antiviral compounds and the advent of these agents during the 1960s led to several trials and the first use of idoxuridine. However, despite claims for the drug's usefulness, side effects were common. Cytosine arabinoside was considered to be a less toxic but less effective drug than idoxuridine. A multicentre trial of adenosine arabinoside was reported by Whitley et al (1977) but unfortunately the usefulness of the drug has yet to be confirmed.

Acycloguanosine is a guanine derivative which apparently is absorbed preferentially by herpes-infected cells. It has been said to be some 10–30 times more active against viral than cellular DNA polymerase (Editorial, Lancet 1981) and strains of herpes simplex virus have been found to be very sensitive to it in tissue culture. Already the drug has been found to be active when used topically in labial and genital herpes and the Lancet editorial mentions reports about the intravenous use of the drug in immune-compromised patients, apparently without the previously recorded devastating effects of idoxuridine and cytosine. The value of this new drug in the management of herpes zoster infection has been documented (Peterslund et al 1981) and a multicentre trial testing acyclovir versus dexamethasone has been mounted in the United Kingdom. Hitherto, only isolated case reports of the use of acyclovir in herpes infections of the brain have appeared (New England Journal of Medicine 1979). It is hoped that acyclovir will prove to be effective and non-toxic, but the use of such drugs will require early diagnosis before active cellular necrosis has produced irreparable temporal lobe damage.

BRAIN IMAGING

The advent of computerised tomography (CT scanning) produced a very significant change in the investigation of structural disease of the brain and upper spinal cord; it has been the experience of all major Departments of Neurology that the numbers of patients undergoing ventriculography and air encephalography have fallen to something of the order of 1% of those before CT was available (Foster 1981). CT of the brain, and indeed of the whole body, is now well-established throughout the world and the effect on clinical neurological practice has been profound.

Other forms of brain imaging such as scintigraphy have been further developed with the advantage over CT that the gamma camera is speedy and there is a possibility of undertaking dynamic studies. However, the scintigram is less specific than the CT scan.

Emission tomography

A further refinement of isotope scanning is emission tomography; a ring of detectors around the head detect the radioactive emission from the injected isotope and the information is fed to a computer to build up an image of the radioactive emission from a slice of brain. The advantage of this technique is that the interaction of the radioactive tracer coupled to a chemical substrate allows data to be recorded which are not related to the physical properties of the tissue being investigated, but to its metabolic function.

Digital radiography

The purpose of digital radiography is to remove interfering shadows by means of some form of subtraction so that clinically significant details can be displaced with enhanced visibility. The term 'digital radiography' generally encompasses a broad spectrum of activities within diagnostic imaging. In its early form, standard radiographic films were digitalised and a computer was used in an attempt to enhance and redisplay the information contained. Currently, X-ray signals are detected electronically and are converted to a digital form and processed before being recorded and displayed. Film can be used for the final storage or the images can be stored on magnetic tape.

Two methods of subtraction have been developed. The first is temporal subtraction, in which images are required before and after the intravenous as opposed to intra-arterial injection of contrast medium. These images are then subtracted and enhanced in a digital processor to yield an image of the arteries, which of course are only very faintly seen on the original image. The arteries are then visualised, enhanced and devoid of overlying shadows such as bone and soft tissue.

Energy subtraction is based on the fact that X-ray attenuation is energy-dependent and the energy dependence varies for materials having different atomic numbers. In energy subtraction, images are acquired using different X-ray spectra. These are then digitalised and combined in a processor to suppress signals from some materials or to enhance signals from others. For example, using this technique the bone shadows can largely be eliminated from a chest radiograph leaving only the heart and pulmonary vessels visible.

The full clinical potential of digital radiography has yet to be defined. However, it does provide a simpler and less risky method of defining vascular tissues than that currently involved in conventional arteriography. For example, carotid stenosis may be demonstrated by means of an intravenous injection without the need for direct or indirect angiography. In addition it is possible to store X-ray images without the use of film, with the obvious financial advantage of this both in terms of space and the use of expensive radiography materials.

Nuclear magnetic resonance

The major recent advance in the field of brain imaging has been the development of nuclear magnetic resonance (NMR) employing magnetic fields and radio-frequency radiation. If a strong magnetic field is applied to a body containing hydrogen nuclei they tend to polarise in a north–south direction while continuing their normal spinning movement. A second magnetic field at an angle to the first will tilt some of the nuclei while they continue to rotate. If a pulse of radio frequency is then applied at the same resonant frequency as the tilted hydrogen nuclei they absorb some of the energy and are further tilted. On stopping the radio wave they return to their resting state emitting the absorbed energy in another pulse of radio-frequency radiation. This can be detected and a measure of the density of hydrogen nuclei can be obtained. If the strength of the second magnetic field is varied across the body, the hydrogen nuclei absorb and emit different levels of energy and so the plane of the emission within the body can be determined. These signals are collected from the various planes, and digitally processed to form an image. Thus an image of the distribution as well as of the overall density of hydrogen nuclei can be visualised. Furthermore the behaviour of hydrogen nuclei varies with how loosely or closely they are bound to other atoms, so that free fluid may be distinguished from closely bound hydrogen nuclei.

Images can be made of planes taken at any angle through the object, which is an advantage over CT. 'Three dimensional' information can be obtained from a single scan and any tomographic view can be constructed *after* the conclusion of the study. The abundance of the hydrogen proton in living tissue and its simplicity have made it the nucleus of choice in NMR. However, the future use of phosphorus-31 may allow NMR imaging of the physiological rather than the anatomical state of tissue. Radio-frequency radiation is employed with the patient lying in a uniform magnetic field, modified by shaping coils generating gradient fields subject to radio-frequency wide-band excitation pulses generated by the coil. One further advantage of NMR is the absence of moving parts in the apparatus, and yet the body in any plane can be imaged after electronic selection. The advantages in head scanning are evident, for here there is very little movement and no problem of artefact production by visceral pulsation or movement, as there may be in other parts of the body. Since there is no ionising radiation, repeated studies can readily be undertaken without risk to the patient. It is probable that NMR will eventually prove to be cheaper, safer and much more versatile than conventional CT but, as yet, the scanning cannot be executed more rapidly than CT.

This challenge to CT, with many centres in the UK already undertaking NMR imaging, is well recognised in radiological circles and the published reports are beginning to confirm the initial enthusiasm. White matter and basal ganglia can be clearly demarcated and structures in the posterior fossa are visualised with much less artefact than in CT scanning. The cerebellar connections are better visualised and the pathological appearances of intrinsic lesions, tumour, infarct and aneurysm are demonstrably more clear than with CT (Doyle et al 1981). Thus not only would NMR appear to show anatomical variation more clearly than CT, but small pathological abnormalities are seen. In certain disease processes hitherto not particularly well visualised by CT, NMR may have its greatest value. For example, Young and colleagues (1981) have shown that in multiple sclerosis, a disease notoriously difficult to demonstrate with CT, NMR has a distinct advantage. They quote their experience with 10 patients suffering from multiple sclerosis, who were submitted to CT with and without contrast enhancement. In these patients 19 periventricular lesions were visualised by CT. With NMR a further 112 lesions were demonstrated in addition to these 19 abnormalities. The lesions varied in size from 4 mm × 3 mm to 12 mm × 7 mm and the authors comment that this resolution is capable of demonstrating abnormalities in MS on a scale not previously seen even at necropsy. The enormous potential of this new technique in brain imaging is well established.

BRAIN DEATH

Despite the carefully considered and detailed statement issued by the Honorary Secretary of the Conference of Medical Royal Colleges and their Faculties in the United Kingdom on the 11th October 1976 (published in full in the *British Medical Journal* of that year), there has recently been considerable acrimonious debate on what constitutes brain death and at what stage organs should be removed for transplant patients. It is essential that not only those working in intensive care units in the hospital service, but also others associated with the management of brain death, should fully understand the agreed diagnostic criteria acceptable in the United Kingdom.

The adverse publicity given to the subject by the British Broadcasting Corporation has led to considerable misunderstanding among the public about our attitude to ventilation and 'life support' and the requirement of the transplant doctors to obtain kidneys from potential donors. The publicity following the programme led to a decline in the availability of kidneys for transplantation over the ensuing months.

Before the advent of intensive care techniques the diagnosis of death was usually considered to be straightforward. When the patient ceased to breathe and the heart ceased to beat then the patient was judged to be dead, not only the body but the person. Now, however, situations commonly arise where a patient, brain-damaged by trauma, haemorrhage or other pathological factors, is maintained on a mechanical ventilator and can be so maintained even after irreversible death of the brain stem. It was the intention of the Medical Royal Colleges 'to distinguish between those patients who retain the functional capacity to have a chance of even partial recovery and those where no such possibility exists'. The criteria demand a clear diagnosis of an irreversible disorder responsible for the patient being in coma, together with a careful clinical examination of brain stem function, without necessary recourse to EEG or other ancillary investigation. It was agreed that permanent functional death of the brain stem constituted *brain death,* suggesting that the death of the brain stem would always be followed by arrest of the heart beat and death of any surviving cells in the cerebral hemisphere or elsewhere. The assumption was that after brain stem death, the death of all cells is an inevitable sequel.

In 1981 a composite review of the experience of three neurosurgical units was published in the *British Medical Journal* (Jennett et al 1981). The authors considered a total of 447 published cases in addition to their own experience in Cambridge, Glasgow and Swansea. Six hundred and nine patients diagnosed clinically as brain-dead were studied; 326 had final cardiac asystole while still being ventilated and ventilation was discontinued in the remainder. No patient recovered. Prospective data on 1003 survivors from severe head injury showed that not one of these patients would have been suspected of being 'brain-dead'. The authors comment that recovery after supposed brain death has been alleged in patients who were thought to be brain-dead but in fact were not, and in cases where reflex movements in the limbs were mistaken for signs of life. They maintain that the safeguards in diagnosing brain death include establishing that there is irreversible structural brain damage (excluding the effects of drugs) and that enough time has been allowed to establish the diagnosis beyond doubt. Jennett and his colleagues, in their review, stress the overriding importance of thus justifying the proposed clinical criteria for the diagnosis of brain death, emphasising that such criteria remain the only reliable means of diagnosing brain death until some other confirmatory test becomes available.

The subject is of such importance that the conditions for considering a diagnosis of brain death should be re-stated. It was suggested by the Colleges that all of the following should co-exist:

1. That the patient should be in deep coma. It is essential that the possibility of this coma being drug-induced should be excluded. Depressant drugs such as narcotics, hypnotics and tranquillisers may have an extremely prolonged action, especially when associated with hypothermia, and attention should be given to the cumulative effect of benzodiazepines, especially when these have been used as anticonvulsants or to assist patients on mechanical ventilators. It is essential, therefore, that an adequate and detailed drug history should be reviewed before a decision on brain death is made, and that the possible time during which drug effects would persist is exceeded. The possibility of primary hypothermia should have been excluded; endocrine and metabolic disturbances, which may be contributory to coma, should also be considered and thereby excluded. The recommendation is that serum electrolyte levels, acid-base balance and blood glucose concentration should not be profoundly abnormal.

2. The patients should require assisted respiration (i.e. be maintained on a ventilator) because spontaneous respiration had previously become inadequate or had ceased altogether. In this context, neuromuscular blocking agents should be excluded as a cause of the respiratory deficiency or failure and, therefore, it should be established that there is adequate neuromuscular conduction.

3. There should be no doubt that the patient's condition is due to irremediable structural brain damage. It is essential that the cause of the brain damage is fully established: for example, primary intracranial haemorrhage, severe head injury or brain damage after neurosurgery should be carefully assessed and a decision made that the condition is irremediable. When the cause of the coma is anoxia from cardiac

arrest, then the Colleges consider that it may take longer to establish the diagnosis and to be confident of the prognosis. This is especially true in cases of suspected fat embolism. Thus, to establish absolutely the nature of the disorder which has led to brain death may take a long period of clinical investigation.

Tests for confirming brain death

The Colleges recommend that the following tests should be undertaken:

1. Tests of brain stem reflexes: it should be confirmed that all brain stem reflexes are absent, which includes the pupils being fixed in diameter and unresponsive to sharp changes in the intensity of incident light.
2. There should be no corneal reflex.
3. The vestibular ocular reflexes should be absent i.e. no spontaneous eye movements should occur during or after slow injection of 20 ml of ice-cold water into each external auditory meatus in turn, and in patients where access to the tympanic membrane is seen to be clear.
4. There should be no motor responses elicitable within the cranial nerve distribution by adequate stimulation and the patient should show no gag reflex or reaction to bronchial stimulation.
5. When the patient is disconnected from his ventilator there should be no spontaneous respiratory movement where the Pa_{CO_2} has reached 6.7 kPa (50 mmHg). This ideally calls for the measurement of blood gases. The Colleges suggest that, in the absence of facilities for blood gas analysis, then the ventilator should be supplied with pure oxygen for 10 minutes and then 5% CO_2 and oxygen for 5 minutes, followed by disconnection of the ventilator for 10 minutes while delivering oxygen at 6l/min by catheter into the trachea.

Once brain death has been established by such criteria, it is not considered necessary for the EEG to be used to confirm the clinical evidence of brain death. However, the recommendation is firmly made that these tests should be repeated to ensure that there is no observer error, and the recommendation is that the interval between testing should be 24 h. It is recommended that the body temperature should be above 35°C before the diagnostic tests are carried out and it is clearly recommended that the clinician undertaking the tests should be experienced and senior. Before the decision is made to withdraw artificial support, the patient should have been examined, preferably by a consultant in charge of the case with one other doctor or, if the consultant is not available, then his deputy, who should have been registered for 5 years or more and should be experienced in such cases, and one other doctor. It has now been established that no single case has been reported in which the British criteria were met and yet the patient survived. It is generally stated that an iseolectric EEG record cannot by itself increase the reliability of these criteria and indeed it has been argued that an iseolectric EEG may be positively misleading, because such a trace is occasionally found in patients who ultimately recover (that is, patients who do not fulfil the above criteria). This is especially the case after narcosis and/or extreme hypothermia (Hughes 1978). In addition, it has been shown by Powner & Fromm (1979) that electrical activity may be recorded in patients diagnosed as clinically brain-dead who, despite continuing ventilation, have all ultimately died. The Department of Health in a letter to all Medical Officers drew attention to a letter in the *British Medical Journal* from the Honorary Secretary of the Conference of Medical Royal Colleges and their Faculties in the UK dated 15 August 1981, confirming that, following further meetings of College, it had been decided that there was no requirement to reconvene the Expert Working Parties which had formerly drawn up the Conference statement.

The following recommendations were made:

1. The diagnosis of brain death should be made by two medical practitioners who have expertise in this field. One should be a consultant, the other should be a consultant or senior registrar who should assure him/herself that the pre-conditions have been met before testing is carried out. The length of time required before the pre-conditions can be satisfied varies according to the circumstances; although it may be less than 24 h it may extend to several days.

2. The two doctors may carry out the tests separately or together. If the tests confirm brain death they should nevertheless be repeated. It is for the two doctors to decide how long the interval between tests should be, so that the time should be adequate for the reassurance of all those directly concerned.

3. There may be circumstances in which it is impossible or inappropriate to carry out every one of the tests. The criteria published by the Conference give recommended guidelines rather than rigid rules and it is for the doctors at the bedside to decide when the patient is dead. It was suggested that new entrants to medical practice in the NHS should be provided with a copy of the Code of Practice and that this should be made readily available in the relevant hospital units.

It is hoped that these clearly defined guidelines will quieten the apprehension of the Colleges' critics and allow doctors in intensive care units to use straightforward protocols, sensibly and confidently to explain decisions of management to the relatives and, by carefully considering the criteria, to re-kindle the hope of the many patients awaiting renal transplantations.

REFERENCES

Facial Nerve

Ardour K K 1976 Cranial polyneuritis and Bell's palsy. Archives of Otolaryngology 102: 262–267

Frew I, Diamond C 1979 The facial nerve. Oxford University Press, Oxford, ch 4, p 136–148

Jannetta P J 1980 Hemifacial spasm. In: Wilson C B, Hoff J T (eds) Current surgical management of neurologic disease. Churchill Livingstone, Edinburgh, ch 23, p 300–306.

Kaye A H, Adams C B T 1981 Hemifacial spasm: a long-term follow-up of patients treated by posterior fossa surgery or facial nerve wrapping. Journal of Neurology, Neurosurgery and Psychiatry 44: 1100–1103

Matthews W B 1982 The treatment of Bell's palsy. In: Matthews W B, Glaser G H (eds) Recent advances in clinical neurology, 3rd edn. Churchill Livingstone, Edinburgh, ch 12, p 239–247

Safman B L 1971 Bilateral pathology in Bell's palsy. Archives of Otolaryngology 93: 55–59

Trigeminal neuralgia

Jannetta P J 1975 Microsurgical approach to the trigeminal nerve for tic douloureux. In: Krayenbühl H, Maspes P E, Sweet W H (eds) Progress in neurological surgery. S Karger, Basel, ch 7, p 180–200

Sweet W H, Wespic J G 1974 Controlled thermocoagulation of trigeminal ganglion and rootlets for differential destruction of pain fibres. 1. Trigeminal ganglion. Journal of Neurosurgery 39: 143–156

Parkinson's disease

Lieberman A, Dziatolowski M, Kupersmith M 1979 Dementia in Parkinson's disease. Annals of Neurology 6: 355–359

Periodic migrainous neuralgia

Ekbom K 1977 Studies on cluster heacaches. Headache 17: 39–40
Harris W 1926 Neuritis and neuralgia. Oxford University Press, London
Peatfield R C 1981 Lithium in migraine and cluster headache: a review. Journal of the Royal Society of Medicine 74: 432–436
Russell D 1979 Cluster headache: trial of a combined histamine H1 and H2 antagonist treatment. Journal of Neurology, Neurosurgery and Psychiatry 42: 668
Symonds C P 1951 Migrainous variants. Transactions of the Medical Society of London 67: 237–245

Transient ischaemic attacks

Acheson J, Hutchinson E C 1971 The natural history of 'focal' cerebral vascular disease. Quarterly Journal of Medicine 40: 15–23
Baker R N, Ramsey J C, Schwartz W S 1968 Prognosis in patients with transient cerebral ischaemic attacks. Neurology 18: 1157–1165
Barnett A J M, Boughter D R, Taylor W, Cooper P E, Kostuk W J, Nichol P M 1980 Further evidence relating mitral-valve prolapse to cerebral ischaemic events. New England Journal of Medicine 302: 139–144
Canadian Co-operative Study Group 1978 A randomised trial of aspirin and sulphinpyrazone in threatened stroke. New England Journal of Medicine 229: 53–59
Cartlidge N E F, Whisnant J P, Elvebach L R 1977 Carotid and vertebral-basilar transient cerebral ischaemic attacks. A community study. Rochester Minnesota Proceedings of the Mayo Clinic 52: 117–120
Committee on Cerebrovascular Diseases 1975 Stroke 5: 277–281
De Bono D P, Warlow C P 1981 Potential sources of emboli in patients with presumed transient cerebral or retinal ischaemia. Lancet 1: 343–346
Denny-Brown D 1951 The treatment of recurrent cerebrovascular symptoms and the question of vasospasm. Medical Clinics of North America 35: 1457–1474
Dyken M L, Kolar O J, Jones F H, 1973 Differences in the occurrence of carotid transient ischaemia attacks associated with anti-platelet aggregation therapy. Stroke 4: 732–736
Fields W S, Lernak N A, Frankowski R F, Hardy R J 1977 Controlled trial of aspirin in cerebral ischaemia. Stroke 8: 301–315
Fields W S, Lernak N A, Frankowski R F, Hardy R J 1978 Controlled trial of aspirin in cerebral ischaemia. II. Surgical group. Stroke 9: 309–318
Fields W S, Maclenikov V, Meyer J S, Hass W K, Remington R D, MacDonald M 1970 Joint study of extracranial arterial occlusion. Progress report of prognosis following surgery or non-surgical treatment for transient cerebral ischaemic attacks and cervical carotid artery lesions. Journal of the American Medical Association 211: 1993–2003
Fisher M 1978 Holter monitoring in patients with transient focal cerebral ischaemia. Stroke 9: 514–516
Friedman G D, Wilson S, Mosier J M, Colandrea M A, Nichaman M Z 1969 Transient ischaemic attacks in a community. Journal of the American Medical Association 210: 1428–1434
Gayer S J, Franzini D A 1979 Myxomatous degeneration of the mitral valve complicated by non-factorial endocarditis with systemic embolisation. American Journal of Clinical Pathology 72: 489–492
Joint Committee for Stroke Facilities 1974 Stroke 6: 563–570
Marshall J 1964 The natural history of transient ischaemic cerebro vascular attacks. Quarterly Journal of Medicine 33: 309–324
Sumner D S, Russel J B, Ramsey D E, Hajjar W M, Milos R D 1979 Non-invasive diagnosis of extracranial carotid arterial disease. Archives of Surgery 114: 1222–1229
Warlow C 1982 In: Matthews W B, Glaser G H (eds) Recent advances in clinical neurology, 3rd edn. Churchill Livingstone, Edinburgh, ch 9, p 192
West H, Burton R, Roon A J, Malone J M, Gouldstone J, Moore W S 1979 Comparative risk of operation and expectant management for carotid artery disease. Stroke 10: 117–121
World Health Organisation 1978 Cerebrovascular disease: a clinical and research classification. World Health Organisation, Offset Publications, Geneva, No 43

Acute necrotic encephalitis

Davis L E, Johnson R T 1978 An explanation of the localisation of herpes simplex encephalitis. Annals of Neurology 5: 2–5

Dinn J J 1980 Transolfactory spread of virus in herpes simplex encephalitis. British Medical Journal 2: 1392

Editorial 1981 Acyclovir. Lancet 2: 845–846

Illis L S, Taylor F M 1972 The electroencephalogram in herpes simplex encephalitis. Lancet 1: 718–721

Klapper P E, Laing I, Longson M 1981 Rapid non-invasive diagnosis of herpes encephalitis. Lancet 2: 607–608

Letter to the Editor 1979 Diagnosis of herpes simplex encephalitis. Lancet 2: 1181–1182

Massachusetts General Hospital – Case Records 1979 Case 44. New England Journal of Medicine 301: 987–994

Peterslund N A, Ipsen J, Schonheyder H, Seyer-Hansen K, Esmann V, Juhl H 1981 Acyclovir in herpes zoster. Lancet 2: 827–830

Rappel M 1971 Treatment of herpes encephalitis. Lancet 1: 971

Rappel M 1973 The management of acute necrotizing encephalitis: a review of 369 cases. Postgraduate Medical Journal 49: 419–421

Selby P J, Jameson B, Watons J G, Morgenstern G, McElwain T J, Powles, R L et al 1979 Parenteral acyclovir therapy for herpes virus infections in man. Lancet 2: 1267–1270

Upton A R M, Gumpert J 1970 Electroencephalography in the diagnosis of herpes simplex encephalitis. Lancet 1: 650–653

Upton A R M, Barwick D D, Foster J B 1971 Dexamethasone treatment in herpes simplex encephalitis. Lancet 1: 290–291

Whitley R J, Seng-Jaw Soong, Dolin R, Galasso G J, Ch'ien L T, Alford C A and the Collaborative Study Group 1977 Adenine arabinoside therapy of biopsy proved herpes simplex encephalitis. New England Journal of Medicine 297: 289–294

Williams B B, Lerner A M 1980 Some previously unrecognised features of herpes simplex virus encephalitis. Neurology 28: 1193–1196

Brain imaging

Doyle F H, Gore P C, Pennock J M, Bydder G M, Orr J S, Steiner R E et al 1981 Imaging of the brain by nuclear magnetic resonance. Lancet 2: 53–57

Foster J B 1981 Brain imaging. In: Tunbridge W M G (ed) Advanced medicine. Pitman Medical, Tunbridge Wells, p 184–196

Young I R, Hall A S, Pallis C A, Legg N J, Bydder G M, Steiner R E 1981 Nuclear magnetic resonance imaging of the brain in multiple sclerosis. Lancet 2: 1063–1066

Brain death

Conference of Medical Royal Colleges and their Faculties in the United Kingdom 1976 Diagnosis of brain death. British Medical Journal 2: 1187–1188

Conference of Medical Royal Colleges and their Faculties in the United Kingdom 1976 Diagnosis of brain death. Lancet 2: 1069–1070

Conference of Medical Royal Colleges and their Faculties in the United Kingdom 1979 Diagnosis of death. British Medical Journal 2: 332

Hughes J R 1978 Limitations of the EEG in coma and brain death. Annals of the New York Academy of Sciences 315: 126–136

Jennett B, Gleave J, Wilson P 1981 Brain death in three neurosurgical units. British Medical Journal 2: 533–539

Powner D J, Fromm G H 1979 The electroencephalogram in the determination of brain death. New England Journal of Medicine 300: 502–506

7

Haematology

A. R. Horler

DISORDERS OF THE HAEMOSTATIC MECHANISM

Platelets

Platelets play an essential part in the arrest of haemorrhage by their threefold function of adhesion and aggregation, initiation of blood coagulation and release of vasospastic substances. They are formed in the bone marrow from the cytoplasm of megakaryocytes with which they share many chemical and antigenic properties. Megakaryocytes are themselves derived from pluripotent haematopoietic stem cells. These develop into intermediate committed diploid precursor cells under the influence of thrombopoietin, and further nuclear replication results in the recognisable polyploid megakaryocyte. Cytoplasmic maturation and platelet formation do not proceed simultaneously with nuclear replication — in fact the process does not start until DNA synthesis is complete. Thus the capacity of a megakaryocyte to produce platelets is dependent upon size rather than ploidy.

Platelets are, in effect, cytoplasmic fragments of their parent megakaryocyte produced by a process of membrane demarcation. Platelet zones or territories are formed by invagination of the membrane and by fusion-fission reorganisation. The majority of megakaryocytes have 8–16 nuclei and are capable of producing 4000–8000 platelets. They can be shown by electron microscopy to be located in the subendothelial region of the vascular sinuses of the marrow; by transendothelial penetration, segments of megakaryocytic cytoplasm can enter the lumen of a sinus and be detached as proplatelets into the general circulation. Further fragmentation into platelets occurs at such extramedullary sites as the pulmonary circulation where proplatelet segments are trapped, thus accounting for the greater platelet content of blood leaving the lungs than of that entering. It is possible also that whole megakaryocytes may enter the circulation in this way, as they are to be found in various organs including lungs, spleen, liver and kidneys. This megakaryocyte–endothelial relationship would allow regulatory information such as oxygen tension and thrombopoietin activity to govern the rate of proplatelet release and the resultant level of circulating platelets (Tavassoli 1980).

The site of thrombopoietin production is likely to be the kidney, and some degree of thrombocytopenia is common in chronic renal disease. A thrombocytopoietic factor obtained from the culture of mouse kidney cells has been shown to stimulate megakaryocytopoiesis in the experimental animal (McDonald 1981).

Platelets adhere to injured epithelium and subendothelial structures such as collagen, basement membrane and microfibrils, facilitated in some way by the von Willebrand factor. There follows the release of the contents of platelet granules and the activation of the arachidonate pathway. The discharge of ADP and prostaglandin products results in further aggregation of platelets at the site of injury and propagation of the platelet plug. The availability of platelet factor 3 promotes the formation of thrombin by the coagulation cascade, leading to further aggregation and release. Fibrin formation results in stabilisation of the platelet mass and further platelet adhesion (Packham & Mustard 1977). During the process of aggregation and release, platelets undergo a change in shape to a more rounded form with pseudopodia. It is likely that they have specific receptors to the aggregating agents they encounter in vivo — ADP, collagen, thrombin, serotonin, adrenalin, immune complexes, antibodies, viruses and bacteria. Activation of the arachidonate pathway involves the conversion of arachidonate to the endoperoxides PG G_2 and PG H_2 and thence to thromboxane A_2, products which are themselves both aggregating and release-inducing. In contrast the vessel wall is capable of forming PG I_2 (prostacyclin) from the prostaglandin endoperoxides and this has an inhibiting effect upon platelet aggregation (Malmsten 1979, Marcus 1979).

The relationship between platelets and factor VIII is of great interest. Platelet adhesion to subendothelial tissues is dependent upon von Willebrand factor, a component of the factor VIII molecule, and the ristocetin reaction involves its binding to the platelet surface where glycoproteins in the membrane act as receptor sites. Although the site of production of factor VIII remains obscure, its presence in cultured endothelial cells and circulating platelets is demonstrable by immunofluorescent techniques. This intrinsic platelet factor VIII does not exchange with plasma factor and presumably is derived from the megakaryocyte. It is located in the secretory pool and released with other factors in response to collagen and ADP, thus accounting for the high level of factor VIII Ag found at the site of vascular damage (Koutts et al 1979).

Platelet abnormalities

Diseases involving platelets can result from both functional and numerical deficiencies and are both congenital and acquired. They may be primary or associated with some other disorder, haematological or otherwise.

Thrombocytopenia

Adequate haemostasis depends upon a platelet count above $100 \times 10^9/l$, below which clinical purpura appears and, in so far as this bleeding tendency is measurable by the skin bleeding time, it bears a direct linear relationship to the decrease in circulating platelets. Reduction to below $40 \times 10^9/l$ usually results in significant clinical symptoms with the well-recognised features of capillary bleeding such as petechiae and ecchymoses, epistaxis, gum bleeding and buccal mucosal blisters and the risk of gastrointestinal and intracranial haemorrhage.

Autoimmune thrombocytopenic purpura. In this condition, antibodies against platelets are produced in response to some environmental event such as a viral infection. These are IgG immunoglobulins which bind to a platelet Fc receptor in the presence of complement (C_3 also being demonstrable on the platelet surface). Such antibody-coated platelets are rapidly removed by reticuloendothelial cells, particularly in the spleen, resulting in a marked shortening of their survival time to less than a tenth of the normal 10d, and a two- to five-fold increase in platelet turnover. Megakaryocytes are increased in number, size and immaturity and there is no evidence to suggest either ineffective thrombocytopoiesis or impaired megakaryocytopoiesis. The platelets themselves are reduced in number and increased in size, so that the mean diameter is 1.6 times normal. Megathrombocytes can be regarded as 'stress platelets' and are still detectable in up to 50% of patients in remission, as also are platelets bound with IgG immunoglobulin. There is evidence of thrombocytopathia also in the presence of demonstrable antibody, even when the numerical count is not significantly reduced; this suggests that the same immune mechanism is responsible both for thrombocytopenia and thrombocytopathia and could account for some examples of the easy-bruising syndrome. There is a genetic predisposition to ATP with a strong association with the DR_W2 alloantigen. This is present in 75% as opposed to 23% in matched controls. SLE is associated with DR_W2 and 3 and between 3 and 16% of cases have thrombocytopenia as an early manifestation.

Clinical features allow classification into acute, intermittent and chronic varieties. The acute illness occurs more commonly in childhood and frequently follows a viral infection. It affects the sexes equally and is usually self-limiting with an average duration of 1–2 months. Seven to 28% may progress to the chronic disorder. In the chronic variety, females predominate in a ratio of 2–4 to 1. Remissions, when they occur, are clinical only without recovery of thrombocytopenia and the duration of the condition is prolonged or indefinite. In the less severe intermittent disorder, both clinical and haematological remissions are encountered. In establishing the diagnosis of autoimmune thrombocytopenic purpura, it is necessary to exclude all primary disorders in which thrombocytopenia is a feature, such as lymphoma, SLE, disseminated intravascular coagulation and drug intoxication. Clinically detectable splenomegaly is a rare feature and, when present, tends to discount the diagnosis. The treatment of autoimmune thrombocytopenic purpura is palliative and not curative in view of the demonstrable abnormalities that persist even after haematological remission. Corticosteroids inhibit the sequestration by the spleen of antibody-coated platelets and are effective within a few days of starting treatment. Prednisone, in a dose of 1 mg/kg body weight, will produce an effective response in 36–44% of subjects, causing a rise of platelets to over 100×10^9/l. A higher dose of 1.5–2 mg/kg will improve the platelet count, although not always to haemostatic levels, in 70–80%. All patients who respond to the lower dose of corticosteroid can expect a remission after splenectomy, although 10–12% of these may subsequently relapse, possibly because of an increase in hepatic sequestration. The platelet count usually starts to rise immediately, reaching a peak between the first and second week. Splenectomy is indicated in all patients with autoimmune thrombocytopenic purpura of longer than 6 months' duration, who cannot be maintained free of significant purpura on a daily dose of prednisone which is less than 15 mg. For patients still refractory to treatment, immunosuppressive drugs may be tried but they have not proved to be very effective. Azathioprine is unlikely to produce much significant benefit in under 2 months, although vincristine, when successful, acts within 7–10d (Karpatkin 1980). Immune thrombocytopenia can also occur in lymphoproliferative diseases such as chronic lymphatic leukaemia, lymphoma and Hodgkin's disease. Kaden et al (1979) studied a series of such patients in whom IgG platelet-bound antibody was demonstrable.

Drug-induced thrombocytopenia. Thrombocytopenia is an integral feature of bone marrow aplasia, whether idiopathic or drug-induced, and the development of haemorrhagic complications may well be the presenting feature of this condition. Drugs that produce aplastic anaemia are all capable of depressing platelet production, and the example of mustine and its derivatives indicates that one mechanism involved is a toxic effect on the megakaryocytes. Nevertheless, many instances of fulminating thrombocytopenic purpura after brief exposure to drugs, resemble acute episodes of autoimmune thrombocytopenic purpura and suggest an immunological mechanism for the rapid destruction of circulating platelets. It has long been known that apronal and quinidine behave in this way; patients' serum is found to agglutinate and lyse platelets in the presence of the drug and complement. An increasing number of drugs have since been implicated and include acetazolamide, hydrochlorothiazide, digitoxin, methyldopa, PAS, rifampicin, imipramine, sulphonamides, phenytoin, meprobamate, spironolactone, carbamazepine, heparin and paracetamol.

It is likely that the immune mechanisms involved in the production of thrombocytopenia by drugs resemble those of haemolytic anaemia of similar aetiology. Immune complex thrombocytopenia is exemplified by quinine, quinidine and apronal, where the antibody is an IgG immunoglobulin which binds complement. This is analogous to haemolytic anaemia induced by stibophen, apart from the antibody which is IgM. The second mechanism, that of passive agglutination, involves the combination of drug and target cell against which antibodies are directed, and which is recognised in penicillin-induced haemolytic anaemia. This seems to operate in thrombocytopenia due to trimethoprim and cephalothin. Thirdly, the drug may induce an autoimmune reaction without being involved itself in the combination, as in haemolytic anaemia due to methyldopa; where thrombocytopenia occurs with this drug, platelet antibodies are likely to be similar, namely, IgG non-complement-binding.

In immune thrombocytopenia, withdrawal of the implicated drug is usually followed by rapid remission, in contrast with thrombocytopenia of myelotoxic origin when remission is slow and often incomplete (Miescher & Graf 1980).

Post-transfusion thrombocytopenia. This rare form of thrombocytopenic purpura occurs predominantly in women and arises acutely and often fulminantly approximately 1 week after a blood transfusion. Sensitisation against a platelet antigen, by a previous transfusion or pregnancy, results in the presence of alloantibodies in the plasma of the recipient. Further transfusion with platelets carrying that antigen results not only in the destruction of donor platelets but further destruction of the patient's own platelets by reaction with the resulting immune complexes. In a recent study the platelet-specific alloantibodies were shown to be anti Zw^a and the patients' platelets were Zw^a negative (Pegels et al 1981).

Defects of platelet function

Qualitative platelet disorders are characterised by a demonstrable functional defect, occasionally accompanied by a prolonged bleeding time, in the face of a numerically normal platelet count. Such conditions, collectively described as 'thrombocytopathy', are either hereditary, drug-induced or associated with another acquired disease.

Inherited defects

Von Willebrand's disease has an autosomal dominant inheritance. The characteristics of this condition and deficiencies of various activities of factor VIII were discussed in the last edition of this book. Factor VIII R: Wf, which is probably the same as Factor VIII R: Ag, represents all factor VIII activities influencing platelet function, including skin bleeding time, ristocetin co-factor activity and glass bead adhesion. The platelets in this disorder are intrinsically normal and on restoration of factor VIII (specifically factor VIII R: Wf) tests of platelet function all revert to normal (Koutts et al 1979).

Bernard-Soulier giant platelet syndrome. This condition is inherited as an autosomal recessive. There is strikingly abnormal platelet morphology with some platelets greater than 4 μm in diameter, and dense central granulation giving a pseudonucleated appearance. Similar but milder changes may be found in the heterozygote carriers. The abnormality of function is concerned with adhesion to subendothelial tissues, glass bead adhesion and ristocetin aggregation, all of which are defective. Factor VIII R: Wf is normal and does not correct these defects. It is postulated that Bernard-Soulier platelets have, on their surface membranes, abnormal glycoproteins that fail to act as receptors for factor VIII R: Wf necessary for platelet adhesion.

Glanzmann's disease or hereditary thrombasthenia, was a name at one time used to cover all varieties of hereditary platelet defect, and first appeared in 1917 with a report of several families with differing bleeding disorders. It is now reserved for a haemorrhagic disease inherited as an autosomal recessive, where there is a defect of platelet aggregation in response to ADP, in spite of an ability to undergo viscous metamorphosis and produce normal release with collagen and thrombin. There is also a deficiency of clot retraction, indicating less surface contractile protein, and probably deficiency of other platelet proteins and clotting factors. More recently it has been shown that there is a deficiency of glycoprotein receptors on the platelet surface with an inability to bind fibrinogen. In addition, the heterogeneity of these glycoproteins indicates the likelihood of further subclassification of this condition (Holahan & White 1981, Lee et al 1981).

Defects of release reaction. These can be due to deficiency of the storage pool or to actual abnormalities of the release mechanism of platelets. There may thus be abnormal platelet adhesion and abnormal aggregation with collagen and ADP. There is frequently deficient PF3 availability and prostaglandin production. Adenosine nucleotides are deficient in storage pool disorders and normal in defects of release mechanism. An example of storage pool deficiency is the Hermansky-Pudlak syndrome, an autosomal recessive disorder where a bleeding disease is associated with albinism (Stuart 1975).

Modification of platelet function by drugs. There has been a renewal of interest in the treatment and prevention of arterial and venous thrombosis by the use of drugs that modify platelet function.

Venous thrombosis is a hazard in the elderly and recumbent and is of increased incidence in women taking a steroid contraceptive pill or oestrogen replacement therapy for menopausal symptoms. Established treatment is by anticoagulant drugs, essentially intravenous heparin followed by warfarin for a variable period, and prevention of venous thromboembolism is attempted by the use of low-dose subcutaneous heparin per-operatively for surgical patients at risk. Prevention of arterial thrombosis is directed mainly at strokes and myocardial infarction, and this requires the identification of those at risk. To the clinical indicators of accelerating angina, transient cerebral ischaemic attacks and amaurosis fugax are added the known risk factors of hypertension, obesity, diabetes, hyperlipidaemia, an adverse family history and cigarette smoking. Although, at present, detection of a prethrombotic state by blood investigation has not been very successful, there are certain pointers to increased platelet activity and hypercoagulability that might aid in the selection of patients for prophylactic treatment.

Patients with arterial disease show an increase of platelet activity measured by response to aggregating factors and by prostaglandin production, but this is of little prognostic value. More promising is the assessment of platelet release by the estimation of platelet factor 4 and β-thromboglobulin, for which radioimmune assays are available. These two factors, whose levels correlate well, are found to be raised in acute thrombotic states such as deep venous thrombosis and disseminated intravascular coagulation. They are also found to be raised in peripheral arterial disease and coronary artery disease and may therefore have value in the prediction of arterial thrombosis. Tests of coagulation are unlikely to be specific indicators and factor VIII, for example, is found to be raised in several stressful conditions. However, a raised level of fibrinopeptide A may be an indication of thrombin–fibrinogen interaction and reduced antithrombin III may suggest an increased tendency to thrombosis. While all these remain theoretical and are of limited predictive value, a combination of results may be found which could be used to discriminate those at risk (Sixma 1980).

Various aspects of platelet function are modified by drugs and this has led to their use in the prevention of thromboembolism. Theoretically they should be effective but their therapeutic value has still to be proved conclusively. Aspirin and the non-steroidal anti-inflammatory drugs, indomethacin, phenylbutazone and sulphinpyrazone, as well as the pyrimido-pyrimidine derivatives such as dipyridimole, inhibit collagen-induced aggregation and the second phase of ADP aggregation. They also block the conversion of arachidonate to prostaglandin endoperoxides and thus inhibit the synthesis of thromboxane A_2 (Packham & Mustard 1977, Marcus 1979).

While aspirin may reduce the incidence of strokes in men with transient cerebral ischaemic attacks, it has probably not been used to optimal effect in existing therapeutic trials. By its action on cyclo oxygenase it prevents synthesis of thromboxane A_2 by the platelets, but by the same action it also inhibits the formation of prostacyclin (PG I_2) by the vessel wall and this is likely to neutralise any possible benefit. The inhibiting effect upon the platelet will persist throughout its lifespan, while the endothelium of the vessel wall is capable of producing cyclo oxygenase when the aspirin effect lapses, and thus to resume synthesis of prostacyclin. It is more logical, therefore, to administer aspirin in small doses intermittently (100 mg every third day) to allow selective depression of thromboxane A_2 synthesis without blocking the formation of prostacyclin (Mitchell 1981).

Thrombotic thrombocytopenic purpura. This is a rare form of thrombocytopenia where there is widespread consumption of platelets in a process of disseminated intravascular coagulation, and a microangiopathic haemolytic anaemia with fragmentation of red cells by fibrin deposited in the micro-circulation. There is a risk of neurological, cardiac and renal complications. It has much in common with haemolytic-uraemic syndrome of childhood and with other examples of DIC with demonstrable primary pathology which have been reviewed previously. It has carried a high mortality — 77% before 1960 and 48% in more recent surveys. Cuttner (1980) recently reported 20 patients who had attended Mount Sinai Hospital over 10 years. Fourteen were female, suggesting a role for oestrogenic and progestational hormones in the aetiology. Possible inciting causes were pregnancy, oral contraception and surgery. One patient in whom the condition arose after surgical operation recovered only to relapse after further surgery. The treatment employed was splenectomy and corticosteroids to which antiplatelet agents have recently been added — dipyridamole, aspirin or dextran 70. On this regime an 80% survival rate has been achieved.

Disorders of blood coagulation

Factor VIII

The factor VIII molecule consists of a large protein part, representing the factor VIII related antigen and von Willebrand factor component (VIII R: Ag, VIII R: Wf), and a small labile part representing the procoagulant activity (VIII C). In classic haemophilia A, procoagulant activity is deficient owing to absence of the smaller labile portion of the molecule, but factor VIII R: Ag is relatively unimpaired. This allows detection of female carriers of the disease when, although both components of factor VIII are within normal limits, the ratio of procoagulant activity to immunologically detectable factor VIII produces a figure significantly below the normal line.

In von Willebrand's disease there is also a variable deficiency of factor VIII: Ag with consequent abnormality of platelet function detectable by skin bleeding time, glass bead adhesion and ristocetin agglutination (as previously discussed). However, the complete picture, including procoagulant deficiency and a dominant inheritance, is by no means the rule, although understandably found in the homozygotes. There are 16 possible combinations of findings and each such variant has been recorded. Furthermore, phenotypic variations occur within families and results vary in individuals (Abildgaard et al 1980). Miller et al (1979) studied two large families with von Willebrand's disease and confirmed the phenotypic variability. They concluded that although each member of a kindred was expressing the same abnormal allele, the penetrance of the gene was frequently incomplete. This was particularly evident in the heterozygotes where as many as 50% of known transmitters were found to be normal by the standard tests. Nevertheless, the majority could be identified by discriminant analysis. These findings could well explain some cases of von Willebrand's disease where evidence of inheritance is lacking.

The treatment of haemophilia A. The availability of factor VIII concentrates and cryoprecipitate has revolutionised the management of haemophilia A and has allowed the early control of bleeding episodes and the undertaking of both urgent and planned surgery without undue hazard. Prompt administration of factor VIII preparations intravenously will limit the extent of dangerous haemorrhage in sites such as the neck, retroperitoneal tissues or intracranial region and the minimisation of joint haemorrhage will prevent permanent damage to the articular surfaces and the crippling effects of haemophilic arthropathy. With proper management joint destruction and pseudotumours should become increasingly rare. The widespread use of a home therapy programme where patients or parents are sufficiently skilled and intelligent to administer treatment as soon as symptoms of bleeding are encountered, has greatly facilitated this end. In hospital there is no necessary surgical procedure that cannot be undertaken provided that there is adequate cover with factor VIII aided occasionally by antifibrinolytic substances such as epsilon aminocaproic acid or tranexamic acid. Because of its half-life factor VIII must be given at intervals of 12h with careful monitoring of the plasma levels so that at no time does it fall below the minimum for surgical haemostasis, namely 30%.

The complication of such treatment, however, is the development by the patient of antibodies (inhibitors) to administered factor VIII, thus making him resistant to standard therapy. These antibodies are directed against the procoagulant part of the molecule (factor VIII CAg). Emergencies must then be managed by the administration of human factor VIII in high dosage, by animal preparations of factor VIII which are antigenic and unsuitable for repeated use or by concentrates of activated prothrombin complex (Bloom 1978, 1981). Large doses of factor VIII concentrate may bring about cessation of bleeding even without producing a measurable increase of procoagulant activity, presumably due to early activity before neutralisation with antibody. Large doses of factor VIII, as well as being costly, have an increased risk of producing haemolysis and transmitting hepatitis B, and in some patients with rapid immunological response an anamnestic rise of inhibitor level will occur. For those who are poor immunological responders and in whom the initial inhibitor level is relatively low, high dose human factor VIII therapy is favoured. Porcine factor VIII, as well as being antigenic, produces thrombocytopenia and is best reserved for emergencies when a once-for-all effect is required.

Another approach to the management of patients with inhibitors is the attempt to by-pass factor VIII in the coagulation cascade by the use of activated clotting factors. In the preparation of vitamin K-dependent factors for use in factor IX deficiency, activation during the fractionating process rendered the product thrombogenic, and although their content included factor II, VII, IX and X, preparations thereafter were known as 'activated factor IX'. These were deliberately produced in the activated form so that they possessed factor VIII inhibitor by-passing activity (Feiba) and their activity is measured in Feiba units. Such products have been shown to be effective when compared with placebo in clinical trials of the treatment of patients with haemophilia A, although in vitro evidence in their plasma is not striking; there is some shortening of the kaolin-cephalin clotting time, prothrombin time, non-activated partial thromboplastin time and, most consistently, the whole-blood clotting time. Prothrombin complex concentrates (as they are more accurately known) are available as Feiba and Autoplex. They carry a small risk of transmitting hepatitis B, and a theoretical risk of disseminated intravascular coagulation in view of the reported rise of fibrinopeptide A and occasional reduction of fibrinogen.

Bloom (1981) considers that treatment is most successful if circulating levels of factor VIII are demonstrable, and recommends human factor VIII concentrate at dosages of 50 units/kg for common bleeding episodes in patients with inhibitors, irrespective of the titre, although he reserves a place for activated PCC in brisk immunological responders. A high antibody titre may call for plasmapheresis in addition to administration of concentrates (Wensley et al 1980).

Haemophilia B (factor IX deficiency)

Haemophilia B, originally known as Christmas disease, resembles haemophilia A closely both clinically and genetically. Heterozygous female carriers of the sex-linked recessive gene may occasionally exhibit a mild clinical haemorrhagic tendency.

As with factor VIII deficiency, it is evident that there is phenotypic and genetic variability of haemophilia B and this has been studied in a series of 92 patients from 71 kindreds by Kasper and his colleagues (1977). In addition to the separation of factor IX procoagulant activity from factor IX-related antigen, some patients with haemophilia B also exhibit a prolonged accelerated clotting time with bovine thromboplastin. Of 12 patients with mild haemophilia B characterised by procoagulant levels between 4 and 22%, none had a prolonged bovine thromboplastin time and antigen levels above 25%; seven had a greatly prolonged activity. The remaining 80, whose activity was below 4%, were designated 'severe' or 'moderately severe'. Of these, 48 had a normal bovine thromboplastin time and no measurable excess of antigen over procoagulant activity; eight had a normal bovine thromboplastin time and antigen levels above 25% seven had a greatly prolonged bovine thromboplastin time and normal levels of antigen; and 17 had a mildly prolonged thromboplastin time and antigen levels above 25%. Thus, about one-third of all the subjects had evidence of an abnormal factor IX molecule. The success of detecting carriers by relating antigen levels to procoagulant activity was confined to those kindreds where the affected male subjects demonstrated an excess of antigen over activity.

IRON DEFICIENCY AND OVERLOAD

The total body content of iron is approximately 72 mmol (4 g), the greater part (about 70%) being found in haemoglobin as an integral constituent of the haem molecule. Other forms of haem iron are contained in myoglobin and many tissue enzymes, thus contributing both to oxygen carriage and to tissue respiration. Non-haem iron is to be found in the iron stores in the form of ferritin and haemosiderin and is also involved in iron transport, bound to the iron-carrying protein, transferrin.

The basal requirement for iron is 0.5–1 mg daily, necessary to replenish loss from skin, hair, nails, faeces and urine, and an additional increment of a similar amount represents the demands of growth, menstruation and pregnancy. As there is no mechanism for active excretion, iron balance is governed by regulation of intestinal absorption of ingested iron. The average iron content of the European diet is 14 mg daily and the normal intestinal absorption is approximately 10% of the intake, although it is capable of increasing to 50% in the presence of iron deficiency. Iron in the intestinal epithelial cell is either delivered to the circulating transferrin by serosal transfer or sequestered in the cell as ferritin, depending on the iron status of the body as reflected in the intracellular iron pool. This mechanism and other aspects of iron metabolism were reviewed in the previous edition.

Iron stores

The amount of iron present in the body stores varies greatly, representing the balance between intake and loss. In the normally nourished male, storage iron may measure 18–36 mmol (1–2 g) while in females the level is usually considerably less, especially in those of fertile age where demands of menstruation and pregnancy as well as a lower dietary intake have their effect upon iron status. Storage iron consists of ferritin and haemosiderin which are chemically related substances. Ferritin is water-soluble and consists of a protein shell of apoferritin in which are deposited micelles of iron in the ferric form, either as hydroxide or phosphate; the iron content of ferritin is approximately 20%. The stimulus for the synthesis of apoferritin is excess of iron delivered to the intracellular pool, exemplified by the regulatory mechanism for iron absorption in the intestinal epithelium. Haemosiderin is water-insoluble and is visible microscopically in tissue sections and bone marrow smears where it can be stained by the Prussian blue reaction. It appears to consist of aggregates of ferritin molecules and has a higher iron content of about 30%. The normal proportion of ferritin and haemosiderin is 65:35 but as the level of storage iron increases there is a relatively greater increase of haemosiderin, as occurs characteristically in conditions of iron overload, and where the higher iron content of haemosiderin allows more economical storage. Chemical and immunological studies have shown that ferritin derived from different tissues and ferritin present in plasma exhibit heterogeneity and represent the existence of several isoferritins. These differ according to the relative proportions of H or L subunits depending on the sialic acid content of carbohydrate residues (Worwood 1980, Jacobs 1982).

Iron stores are essentially located in two tissues, namely the liver parenchyma and the cells of the reticuloendothelial system. The total hepatic content of non-haem iron is between 2.2 and 8.1 mmol (120–450 mg) and that of the bone marrow storage pool, a little less (5.16 mmol in males and 1.77 mmol in females). The content of the spleen is about 10% of that of the liver. Skeletal muscle, apart from myoglobin, contains non-haem iron in its reticuloendothelial cells, and although the concentration is low, the total muscle mass allows such iron to make up 30% of stores. Storage iron therefore is divided in roughly equal proportions between liver, skeletal muscle and bone marrow.

Liver parenchymal cells derive their iron from plasma transferrin transported from the gut, and this is shown to excess in idiopathic haemochromatosis where absorption is poorly regulated. The reticuloendothelial cells remove iron from the haemoglobin of destroyed red cells and are thus the chief recipients in haemolytic anaemia and transfusional haemosiderosis. Ferritin is found predominantly in parenchymal cells while haemosiderin is mostly located in reticuloendothelial cells, including Kupffer cells. While iron can be mobilised from both ferritin and haemosiderin, that most recently laid down, namely ferritin, is more readily available. In addition, iron from haemoglobin breakdown is largely recycled for further haemoglobin synthesis. There is thus little mixing in the functional use of iron from storage sites (Torrance & Bothwell 1980, Jacobs 1982).

The estimation of storage iron is now best accomplished by the measurement of serum ferritin with which it is in equilibrium. Such levels have been shown to compare well with those derived from controlled phlebotomy (Jacob et al 1980). The normal range of serum ferritin is 20–300 μg/l. While low levels are invariably found in iron deficiency anaemia, it is rarely necessary to perform this test when the characteristic haematological findings are accompanied by a low serum iron and high iron binding capacity, indicating low saturation of transferrin. It is valuable confirmatory evidence of iron overload where levels of 25 000 μg per litre have been recorded. It is also useful in the investigation of 'anaemia of chronic disease' where a low serum iron is usually accompanied by a low transferrin and where serum ferritin is frequently increased. Such circumstances exist in rheumatoid arthritis, malignant disease and chronic infection. However, serum ferritin may be increased in any event during infections and is known to be raised also in a number of malignant conditions including Hodgkin's disease and leukaemia (Cook 1980, Jacobs 1982).

Iron deficiency

When negative iron balance occurs because of failure of intake to compensate for loss or increased requirement, there follows a process which ultimately results in the appearance of hypochromic, microcytic anaemia. There is first a mobilisation of storage iron and an increased absorption of dietary iron which maintains haemoglobin synthesis and tissue enzyme activity. During this stage there is a progressive fall of serum ferritin and disappearance of stainable iron from the bone marrow. Further depletion results in a fall of serum iron levels and an overall rise of transferrin indicating desaturation which, when it reaches 16%, produces defective erythropoiesis and hypochromic anaemia. Even at this stage, compensatory mechanisms delay the onset of symptoms; diminished affinity of haemoglobin for oxygen allows normal oxygen delivery to the tissues until the level falls below 10g/dl.

Tissue changes such as koilonychia, glossitis, angular stomatitis and a post-cricoid web are consequences of long-standing iron deficiency and with the diminishing likelihood of its escaping detection, they are becoming increasingly rare. However, early tissue depletion will cause symptoms due to impaired enzyme action independent of the haemoglobin level (Dallman et al 1978). The tissue iron compounds involved are the haem products which include myoglobin and haem enzymes, the non-haem enzymes and a third group which, although not actually iron-containing, require its presence as a co-factor. The first group contains cytochromes, catalase and peroxidase; myoglobin is necessary for oxygen storage and utilisation in muscle, while the cytochromes provide oxidative energy within cells and aid in protein synthesis and in detoxication. The second group aids the uptake of iron by mitochondria and includes iron–sulphur proteins and metalloflavoproteins such as NADH dehydrogenase, succinic dehydrogenase and xanthine oxidase. The third group includes aconitase and tryptophan pyrrolase. Depletion of such enzyme activity does not parallel the degree of anaemia or iron deficiency but depends also on cellular activity and rapidity of turnover. Dallman et al (1978) quote evidence suggesting impaired function of striated muscle, nervous tissue, white blood cells and the gastrointestinal tract in the presence of iron deficiency. Experimental animals exhibit dysfunction of striated muscle which is not corrected by transfusion and therefore not caused exclusively by haemoglobin lack; this responds to iron administration and correlates with the rise of mitochondrial enzymes. In the brain, the effect of iron deficiency on enzymatic degradation of catecholamines and serotonin may account for apparent behavioural changes, although comparative observations are difficult to assess (Leibel et al 1979). While there may be theoretical justification in regarding iron deficiency as protective against infection, clinical experience would favour the reverse impression. Unsaturated transferrin is said to deprive micro-organisms of iron obtained from the host environment by the production of siderochromes and this ability diminishes with transferrin saturation. On the other hand, there is evidence of diminished neutrophil and lymphocyte function in iron deficiency, which is more likely to influence susceptibility to infection.

Iron overload

When excessive iron occurs in storage sites, particularly liver, the term *haemochromatosis* is used to describe predominant overloading of parenchymal cells with associated tissue damage, while *haemosiderosis* is applied to overloading of reticuloendothelial cells. In the liver there is frequently considerable overlap of the two. Primary idiopathic haemochromatosis is an inherited disorder affecting iron absorption, while secondary haemochromatosis occurs with alcoholic cirrhosis and with excessive iron ingestion over a long period. Haemosiderosis occurs most commonly as a result of multiple blood transfusions and becomes clinically apparent when the total amount exceeds 100 units. This is much more likely to occur when the original anaemia is associated with ineffective erythropoiesis and increased absorption of iron, as in thalassaemia, or an abnormality of iron utilisation as in sideroblastic anaemia.

Primary idiopathic haemochromatosis

This is an inherited condition characterised by increased iron deposition, predominantly in parenchymal cells of the liver, accompanied by cirrhosis and frequently with involvement also of pancreas, myocardium, pituitary and adrenal glands. Because of the failure of the normal control of iron absorption by the intestinal epithelial cells, iron is taken up irrespective of body requirements. Iron load gradually accumulates until the recognisable clinical syndrome presents, usually in middle age, when the iron stores frequently exceed 20g. The severity of the condition is influenced also by sex, blood loss and alcohol consumption; it is 10 times more common in males than females, in whom menstruation and a lower dietary intake delay the clinical onset. Hepatic cirrhosis and skin pigmentation are virtually constant findings and hypogonadism, arthropathy and diabetes are common. Although the myocardium is frequently involved histologically, heart failure is uncommon (Crosby 1977, Bomford 1979).

The biochemical findings are essentially a raised serum iron with a high degree of saturation of transferrin which persists even after depletion of iron stores by venesection. Serum ferritin is markedly raised, being a sensitive index of storage iron. When the investigations are performed at the time of overload, iron absorption is usually normal, but venesection results in a marked increase well before iron stores are reduced to normal limits. When reaccumulation of storage iron occurs, absorption again declines so that equilibrium may be achieved at a high storage level.

While the nature of the defect appears to lie in the failure of intestinal regulation of iron absorption, there also seems to be a relative inability of reticuloendothelial cells to retain iron, thus delivering more iron to parenchymal cells via circulating transferrin. A common tissue defect therefore might possibly involve impaired sequestration of ferritin by intestinal and reticuloendothelial cells, resulting in relatively unchecked absorption by serosal transfer and increased delivery to circulating transferrin (Bomford 1979, Jacobs 1982).

Genetic studies have shown an increased frequency of HLA-A3 and HLA-B14 antigens in patients with idiopathic haemochromatosis, and the gene is closely linked with the histocompatibility loci on the sixth chromosome. It is possible that homozygous inheritance results in severe iron overload with the whole galaxy of complications, while the heterozygous state produces a milder condition of which the clinical manifestation depends on other environmental factors such as alcohol consumption (Jacobs 1982). Alternatively, there may be two genes on the sixth chromosome which together produce the full picture of haemochromatosis, but which separately account for an individual defect (Bomford 1979). Thus, one gene may promote accumulation of iron stores and account for high storage iron with relatively normal plasma levels, while the other influences iron absorption and results in relatively high plasma as compared with storage iron.

Early diagnosis of haemochromatosis may thus be possible by investigating families with an affected member, and treatment may limit the extent of tissue damage caused by unrestricted accumulation of iron. Bassett et al (1979) studied 18 unrelated families with affected members and concluded that the most reliable diagnostic indices were serum iron, transferrin saturation and serum ferritin levels. HLA typing was of some value in detecting affected siblings but not offspring. Siblings with identical HLA patterns to those of the probands should be regarded as being at risk and meriting regular observation.

Treatment by regular phlebotomy results in a markedly improved prognosis. There is a 64% survival at 5 years in treated subjects compared with 15% in untreated. There is improved liver function, better diabetic control and fewer cardiac complications, but with longer survival there is an increase of malignancy which is not confined to the incidence of primary hepatoma (Crosby 1977).

MEGALOBLASTIC ANAEMIA

Megaloblastic change in the early red cell series of the bone marrow results from impaired nuclear synthesis of DNA. This is caused by a deficiency of one or more of its immediate precursors, of which the purine derivatives are deoxyribose adenine triphosphate (dATP) and deoxyribose guanine triphosphate (dGTP), and the pyrimidine derivatives are deoxyribose thymine triphosphate (dTTP) and deoxyribose cytosine triphosphate (dCTP). Impaired synthesis of DNA results in defective formation and fragmentation of the strands of the replication fork and this presumably accounts for the characteristic change in the appearance of the nuclear chromatin of the megaloblast.

Folate deficiency (directly) and vitamin B_{12} deficiency (indirectly) produce these changes by inhibiting the formation of dTTP. The conversion of deoxyuridylate to thymidylate (dTMP) depends upon the co-enzyme 5, 10, methylenetetrahydrofolate, and during this reaction the tetrahydrofolate of the co-enzyme is reduced to dihydrofolate. Its reconversion to the active tetrahydrofolate state requires the enzymatic action of dihydrofolate reductase. Drugs which inhibit dihydrofolate reductase activity will block this reconversion and prevent the formation of THF co-enzyme, thus impairing the synthesis of thymidylate. This is exemplified by methotrexate and pyrimethamine, and theoretically by trimethoprin and triamterine. Hydroxyurea, by contrast, inhibits ribonucleotide reductase and thus inhibits production of dATP and dCTP (Hoffbrand 1980, Hoffbrand & Wickremasinghe 1982).

The role of vitamin B_{12}

Lack of vitamin B_{12} results in megaloblastic anaemia and neuropathy (subacute combined degeneration of the spinal cord).

Although first isolated as cyanocobalamin, this particular compound is present in the body only in traces. The three naturally occurring analogues are hydroxocobalamin, adenosylcobalamin and methylcobalamin. The basic structure of the molecule is essentially a corrin ring and a nucleotide; individual cobalamins are distinguished by the radical attached to the central cobalt atom of the corrin ring — hydroxyl, adenosyl or methyl. Methylcobalamin accounts for 70% of the vitamin in circulating plasma, while adenosyl and hydroxocobalamin predominate in the liver and other organs. The cobalamins act as co-enzymes for two important chemical reactions: these are the conversion of homocysteine to methionine (methionine synthetase reaction) and the conversion of methylmalonic acid to succinic acid (methylmalonyl mutase reaction). Methylcobalamin, being a transmethylator, is responsible for the methionine synthetase reaction, accepting methyl radicals from methyltetrahydrofolate and transferring them to homocysteine in the formation of methionine. A deficiency of methylcobalamin will result in an accumulation of methyltetrahydrofolate and an inability to form the active tetrahydrofolate co-enzyme necessary for thymidylate synthesis. This 'methylfolate trap' hypothesis is thus invoked to explain the megaloblastic anaemia induced by vitamin B_{12} deficiency.

However, this does not explain all phenomena of impaired folate utilisation in the presence of vitamin B_{12} deficiency, where uptake of folates without the methyl radical can also be shown to be deficient. Chanarin and colleagues (1980, 1981) have studied the interrelationships of folate and cobalamin in the production of megaloblastic anaemia by using experimental animals made B_{12}-deficient by exposure to nitrous oxide (N_2O). Cobalamin is capable of cleaving N_2O and is oxidised in the process, and as it is a co-factor of methionine synthetase, N_2O is a specific inhibitor of the conversion of homocysteine to methionine. These animals thus serve as models for 'biochemical PA'. The authors conclude that the failure of methionine synthesis itself, rather than the trapping of methyltetrahydrofolate, is responsible for the deficiency of thymidylate and thus of DNA. Methionine is a source of formate for the formation of formyltetrahydrofolates and it is from these that the folate co-enzyme is produced. Methionine, by its derivative S-adenosyl methionine, is also necessary for RNA synthesis in nervous tissue. Prolonged exposure to N_2O caused a neuropathy in experimental animals that could be prevented by administration of methionine. A similar neuropathy could be induced in animals by cycloleneine, an inhibitor of S-adenosyl methionine. There is therefore a possible explanation, on this hypothesis, for the neuropathy of vitamin B_{12} deficiency.

The major causes of megaloblastic anaemia due to vitamin B_{12} deficiency are well known. Gastric conditions resulting in loss of intrinsic factor include Addisonian pernicious anaemia and total or partial gastrectomy. Intestinal malabsorption can result from the stagnant loop syndrome, coeliac disease, small bowel resection and infestation with a fish tapeworm. Rare causes of cobalamin deficiency arise as inborn errors of metabolism. Juvenile pernicious anaemia is inherited as an autosomal recessive character and is caused by lack of intrinsic factor in an otherwise normal gastric mucosa with normal acid secretion. Imerslund–Gräsbeck disease is also inherited as an autosomal recessive disorder, resulting in selective malabsorption of vitamin B_{12} and normal intrinsic factor, frequently associated with albuminuria. Abnormalities of the transport proteins are also known to occur and demonstrate the relative part played in the dynamic turnover of vitamin B_{12}. A congenital deficiency of transcobalamin II produces megaloblastic anaemia through the impaired availability of vitamin B_{12} even though the level of the vitamin in the plasma is not significantly reduced. It usually occurs in the first few weeks of life and requires large doses of hydroxocobalamin to induce and maintain remission. Conversely a congenital deficiency of transcobalamin I and III will result in a low plasma B_{12} without any anaemia. Defective synthesis of one or more cobalamin co-enzymes can arise as a congenital defect. Adenosylcobalamin is responsible for the methylmalonyl mutase reaction, and its deficiency results in methylmalonicaciduria without any anaemia or neuropathy. When synthesis of both adenosylcobalamin and methylcobalamin is defective, the clinical picture is of variable severity but at worst consists of megaloblastic anaemia, neuropathy and dementia, methylmalonicaciduria and homocystinuria. Total plasma cobalamin may not be reduced but tissues are grossly depleted of cobalamin co-enzymes and hydroxocobalamin is in relative excess (Matthews & Linnell 1979).

APLASTIC ANAEMIA

The diagnosis of aplastic anaemia depends upon the combination of pancytopenia in peripheral blood and a hypocellular appearance of bone marrow sections obtained by trephine biopsy of the iliac crest.

Normal haemopoiesis

The earliest productive elements in the bone marrow are the pluripotential stem cells. These are capable of maintaining their own numbers and of differentiation into more specialised cells committed to the production of an individual cell line, under the influence of long-range regulators. Of these regulators, erythropoietin has been positively identified and extensively studied.

The existence of pluripotential stem cells and committed progenitor cells and their role in haemopoiesis have been illustrated by in vivo and in vitro techniques. A mouse spleen assay has been developed which employs, for a model, a mouse irradiated to produce haemopoietic ablation. Infusion of a suspension of syngeneic cells from bone marrow, liver or spleen results, after 7 days or more, in the establishment of numerous discrete colonies of haemopoietic cells in the spleen of the recipient. These can each be shown to originate from a common ancestral cell, in that the cells of one colony may all contain an identifying chromosome not present in other colonies; colonies may also contain cells of one or more lines — erythroid, granulocytic or megakaryocytic. Suspensions of cells from such a colony can be injected into another recipient and produce further colonies in the spleen. It is clear therefore that donor cells are capable of producing colonies in which stem cells reproduce themselves and also differentiate into committed cell lines. These are referred to as 'spleen colony-forming units' (CFU-S) and are representative of pluripotential stem cells. Study of committed progenitor cells has depended upon an in vitro technique of marrow culture on soft agar or methyl cellulose. This requires a feeder layer of cells, usually macrophages, necessary to produce 'colony stimulating factor' essential for the growth of marrow cells. By this means, colonies can be grown producing monocytes and granulocytes and the derivative cells are referred to as CFU-Cs. When erythropoietin is used as a stimulator, two types of erythroid colony are produced. Burst-forming units (BFU-E) require a high concentration of erythropoietin and are so named because of the large clusters of erythroid colonies that arise. Other colonies more sensitive to erythropoietin and thus requiring a lower concentration, are referred to as 'CFU-E'. It is also suggested that megakaryocytes (CFU-M) and B and T lymphocytes (CFU-L) have a similar origin from committed progenitor cells under the influence of specific regulators (Alter et al 1978, Schofield 1979, Geary 1979, Meadenovic & Adamson 1982).

The haemopoietic microenvironment

While the committed progenitor cells of the marrow can be shown to be influenced by humoral regulators, pluripotential stem cells (as represented by CFU-S) seem to depend upon the haemopoietic microenvironment for their survival and proliferation. Although stem cells can be found in the circulating blood of experimental animals, it is only in the haemopoietic sites that they proliferate and differentiate; when lethally irradiated animals are infused with donor marrow cells, it is again only in these sites that the graft will survive. In a particular type of congenital hypoplastic anaemia found in mice (Steel anaemia) there is considered to be a defect of the microenvironment, and in these animals an infusion of normal marrow cells does not result in repopulation of the haemopoietic sites. However, successful transplantation of splenic cells can be achieved, as they provide a suitable microenvironment. Irradiation of bone marrow in experimental animals, sufficient to destroy both haemopoietic and stromal tissues, will result in permanent aplastic anaemia, whereas mechanical destruction by curettage results in only temporary marrow failure, and recovery of haemopoiesis is preceded by regeneration of the marrow stroma. This all suggests that the mechanical supportive tissue of the bone marrow also provides the necessary functional stimulus to haemopoietic proliferation. Experimental confirmation of this is found in the in vitro techniques of marrow culture on cellulose acetate. Here a monolayer of cells is necessary to sustain growth of stem cells and thus provide a suitable microenvironment. Such effective cell layers are mononuclear phagocytes, and 'marrow-derived adherent cells' (MDAC) which are predominantly fibroblasts capable of producing collagen. It seems likely therefore that similarly derived cells in vivo are necessary to sustain proliferation and differentiation of pluripotential stem cells (Bentley 1982).

Causes of aplastic anaemia

Haemopoietic failure can arise as a result of a deficiency, both in number and function, of pluripotential stem cells or committed progenitor cells. Failure of the pluripotential compartment is likely to result in pancytopenia, while failure of committed progenitor cells is more likely to affect one or other individual cell line, unless all elements are depressed simultaneously. The most commonly occurring example of a single-line deficiency is pure red cell aplasia, where erythropoiesis is selectively depressed and leucopoiesis and thrombocytopoiesis are largely intact. Other factors possibly involved in aplastic anaemia are the haemopoietic microenvironment and the humoral regulators of cellular proliferation.

Approximately 50% of patients with aplastic anaemia have no demonstrable cause for the condition and are therefore arbitrarily classified as idiopathic. This proportion is likely to diminish as mechanisms become more clearly understood and further marrow depressants are identified. The idiopathic group tends to have a poorer prognosis as it is likely to contain examples of chemically induced aplasia where the agent has not been recognised and withdrawn.

Exposure to irradiation will damage both stem cells and microenvironment and is thus more likely to result in irreversible marrow aplasia. Drugs and other toxic agents may produce either an obligatory or an idiosyncratic response. Thus, cytotoxic drugs used in the treatment of malignant disease will inevitably cause marrow aplasia if administered in sufficiently high dosage over a prolonged period. On the other hand, drugs may affect a susceptible individual either during administration, when withdrawal can be followed by recovery, or some time after initiation, when the outlook is less favourable. Involvement of the committed progenitor compartment of marrow cells may give rise to single-line deficiencies, and sparing of the pluripotential stem cells allows replenishment of committed progenitors on withdrawal of the offending agent. Nevertheless, many drugs which depress committed progenitor cells will ultimately cause damage to pluripotential stem cells also.

Drugs producing pancytopenia make up a formidable list and include antibacterial, antirheumatic, anticonvulsant and antithyroid agents as well as many miscellaneous compounds. Chloramphenicol, for so long the most frequent cause of aplasia, has been declining in prominence in recent years, the risk being about one in 25 000. Phenylbutazone and oxyphenbutazone are a particular hazard to elderly women. The overall mortality from phenylbutazone is 2.2 per 100 000 and from oxyphenbutazone, 3.8 per 100 000, while for men under 65 the overall figure is 1 per 100 000 and for women over 65, 6 per 100 000.

Drugs may produce single cell-line deficiencies, although in the case of agranulocytosis and thrombocytopenia, this is commonly due to destruction of circulating cells and frequently involves an immune mechanism. Chlorpromazine, however, can produce agranulocytosis, particularly in the elderly, by its effect upon committed progenitor cells. Pure red cell aplasia may also be induced by such drugs as gold, azathioprine, sulphonamides, sulphonylureas, phenytoin, chloramphenicol and phenylbutazone (Alter et al 1978).

The part played by virus infections in the aetiology of aplastic anaemia is exemplified by infective hepatitis, where aplasia may develop within 10 weeks of infection. Although the infective illness may be clinically mild, the aplastic anaemia is usually very severe, calling for bone marrow transplantation.

Constitutional aplastic anaemia embraces several examples of rare congenital and sometimes inherited conditions. Fanconi's anaemia is transmitted as an autosomal recessive character and has numerous associated features such as hyperpigmentation, mental retardation, renal abnormalities, hypoplasia of thumbs or radii, strabismus and deafness. Chromosomal abnormalities are demonstrable and the condition may be preleukaemic. Other congenital disorders of bone marrow function are amegakaryocytic thrombocytopenia, dyskeratosis congenita and Shwachman-Diamond syndrome. The latter condition, also transmitted according to an autosomal recessive pattern, is characterised by neutropenia, pancreatic insufficiency and metaphyseal dysostosis; the marrow depression may progress to pancytopenia. The Diamond-Blackfan syndrome is an example of a congenital single cell line deficiency, namely, pure red cell aplasia. There may be chromosomal abnormalities and acute leukaemia may develop (Alter et al 1978, Wasser et al 1978).

It seems likely that autoimmune processes also contribute to the development of bone marrow aplasia (Parkman 1978). The association of pure red cell aplasia with a thymoma in 50% of cases suggests such an aetiology, and antibodies against either erythroid precursors or circulating erythropoietin have been demonstrated in this condition. There is evidence also that cell-mediated immunity may play a part; patients' T lymphocytes have been shown to have a marked inhibitory effect upon CFU-C proliferation in bone marrow culture. Some patients prepared for bone marrow transplantation by the administration of immunosuppressive drugs have undergone spontaneous recovery with autologous repopulation of their bone marrow, and similar responses have been claimed for antilymphocytic globulin (Shahidi 1979).

THE HAEMOGLOBINOPATHIES

The haemoglobinopathies are inherited disorders which are common in the world at large, particularly in areas where malaria is prevalent. Although rare in the United Kingdom, they are increasing in frequency due to immigration from Asia and the Mediterranean countries.

The haemoglobin molecule is tetrameric in structure, being made up of four polypeptide chains each embracing a haem group. There are two alpha and two non-alpha chains, the latter determining the distinctive type of haemoglobin, the prevalence of which depends upon the stage of embryonic development. During fetal life alpha and gamma chains predominate, producing haemoglobin F ($\alpha_2\gamma_2$), while after birth gamma chains are replaced by beta and to a much less extent by delta, so that adult haemoglobin is made up of 97% Hb A ($\alpha_2\ \beta_2$), 2.5% Hb A_2 ($\alpha_2\ \delta_2$) and approximately 0.5% Hb F ($\alpha_2\ \gamma_2$).

The synthesis of each globin chain is under the control of a separate group of genes and their site is now identifiable by techniques of chromosome mapping (Weatherall 1982). There are four genes controlling alpha chain synthesis, two on each chromosome 16. The genes controlling non-alpha chains are all located on chromosome 11 where gamma genes are also duplicated, but delta and beta genes are single.

The haemoglobinopathies can be classified into qualitative and quantitative disorders. The former are the structural haemoglobin variants, where the polypeptide chains are themselves abnormal and the latter are the thalassaemias, where chain synthesis is defective or lacking (Lehman & Huntsman 1974, Stamatoyannopoulos & Nute 1974, Higgs 1981). A third category combines features of both, when qualitatively variant globin chains are synthesised at a reduced rate; and finally a group of disorders exists where haemoglobin F persists beyond the neonatal period and these are known collectively as hereditary persistence of fetal haemoglobin (HPFH).

Structural haemoglobin variants

These arise as the result of changes in any of the globin chains, in the form of either amino acid substitution, deletion or insertion. There are over 300 known variants, many of which have no clinicopathological significance. They are inherited according to a simple Mendelian pattern and can exist in both the heterozygous and homozygous form. When a clinical abnormality exists, it occurs either as a haemolytic anaemia due to haemoglobin insolubility, or as a disorder of oxygen transport. Sickle-cell disease is the commonest example of the former, but haemolysis can also occur with the unstable haemoglobins and can be drug-induced. Abnormalities of oxygen transport include permanent methaemoglobinaemia and congenital polycythaemia associated with increased oxygen affinity.

Sickle-cell disease

In this condition haemoglobin S results from a substitution of valine for glutamic acid in the sixth position of the beta globin chain. It occurs overwhelmingly in Negroes although it is also seen in India, the Middle East and the Mediterranean. The disorder may exist in the heterozygous state as the sickle-cell trait, as the homozygous sickle-cell anaemia, and in combination with other structural haemoglobin variants.

In situations of low oxygen tension, Hb S becomes rapidly insoluble resulting in distortion of the red cells and sludging of blood in peripheral capillaries. This in turn causes further stagnation and deoxygenation. This effect may be modified by the presence of another haemoglobin in the red cell as in sickle-cell trait or in heterozygous combination with haemoglobin D or E. Conversely, haemoglobin C when present will enhance this effect and produce a more severe haemolytic anaemia in those with such a dual inheritance.

The clinical features of homozygous sickle-cell disease are essentially caused by the haemolytic anaemia and by intermittent vascular occlusion resulting in sickle-cell crises. In the infant, growth and development are normal for the first few months owing to the persisting haemoglobin F, but mild abdominal colic may occur and such children are prone to septicaemia and sudden unexplained death. Splenomegaly is apparent by 6 months in many, but auto-splenectomy occurs progressively so that splenomegaly is undetectable by 6–8 years and by adult life the spleen is reduced to a small remnant. Bone infarction is confined to carpal and tarsal bones in the early years, producing the hand-foot syndrome of children, but in adolescence infarction of long bones is increasingly frequent. The peak of hospital admission is in the first decade when the manifestations are acute, often infective, and frequently leave no permanent residue unless there has been cerebral infarction. In adult life, in contrast, life-threatening complications are chronic and organ-related, chronic renal disease being such an example. Other clinical features described are leg ulcers, priapism and a pulmonary disorder that is caused either by infarction or pneumococcal infection (Powars 1975).

Being a low-affinity haemoglobin, Hb S will deliver more oxygen than haemoglobin A, and the disability of a low haemoglobin level is consequently less in a patient with sickle-cell disease. Acute aplastic crises occur as a complication of the haemolytic anaemia, and are often precipitated by infection. Haemolytic crises with splenic sequestration occur in the early years before the onset of autosplenectomy. The haematological values demonstrate a chronic anaemia with reticulocytosis and irreversible sickle cells and target cells in the blood film.

The existence of the sickle-cell trait is usually symptomless unless the subject is exposed to situations of low oxygen tension. The well-known hazard is a general anaesthetic when the complication of a sickle-cell crisis may occur. It is essential, therefore, to check every Negroid patient for the sickle trait, before embarking on any procedure requiring general anaesthesia.

The sickling test is performed by incubation of a wet blood film with a sealed coverslip at 37°C for 1 hour, when sickling of the cells is noted. It can be aided by the addition of a reducing agent such as sodium dithionite. The presence of haemoglobin S is confirmed by haemoglobin electrophoresis.

The thalassaemias

In the thalassaemias there is deficient production of one or more of the globin chains, resulting in poor cellular haemoglobinisation and increased haemolysis. They can be classified into α, β, $\delta\beta$, δ and $\gamma\delta\beta$ thalassaemias according to which chain is deficient, and should probably also include some examples of hereditary persistence of fetal haemoglobin — HPFH (Bank 1978, Weatherall 1982).

β thalassaemia

This is a heterogeneous condition depending upon whether β chains are totally absent ($\beta°$) or reduced in number ($\beta+$). The clinical classification into thalassaemia major, intermedia and minor is based more upon the severity of the anaemia and its complications than on strict genetic determination. The geographical distribution of the gene is predominantly around the Mediterranean coast and in Asia, particularly China and India. While it can occur in Anglo-Saxons, the vast majority of patients in the United Kingdom are of immigrant stock. Modell (1977) in a study of 300 cases of thalassaemia major in Britain found 60% to be of Cypriot origin, 30% Indian and less than 10% Italian or Chinese.

The heterozygous state rarely produces symptoms and any anaemia is usually very mild and well tolerated. It may be discovered fortuitously on routine blood examination, or on screening of relatives of a known case. There is a hypochromic, microcytic picture with a low MCH and MCV and with target cells and basophilic stippling shown on the freshly made film. Osmotic fragility of the red cells is reduced and there is a demonstrable increase of Hb A_2 and more variably of Hb F. Occasionally the gene may be 'silent' without measurable increase of these haemoglobins and diagnostic confirmation then depends upon estimation of globin chain synthesis.

In the homozygous state, the absence ($\beta°$) or marked reduction ($\beta+$) of β chains and the consequent unbalanced excess of α chains results in marked instability of the haemoglobin in red cell precursors. There is thus marked intramedullary haemolysis and ineffective erythropoiesis with the development of profound anaemia. Some of the free α chains combine with available γ chains to produce Hb F which is present in some of the cells that survive to reach the circulation. However, as this is a high-affinity haemoglobin it contributes to a relative tissue anoxia and this is a further stimulus to erythropoietin production. There is a vast expansion of erythropoietic marrow resulting in skeletal deformities, a tendency to fractures and a characteristic 'hair on end' appearance of the skull radiograph. In addition there is marked extramedullary erythropoiesis with gross hepatosplenomegaly. There is delayed growth and development and a hypermetabolic state with weight loss. Although the homozygous infant is not necessarily anaemic at birth, there is clear evidence of the condition after the first year, and usually death before 5 years in the untreated.

The treatment of thalassaemia major consists of blood transfusion to maintain haemoglobin, splenectomy to prevent hypersplenism and chelation therapy to minimise iron overload (Pearson & O'Brien 1975). Modell (1977) found that 93% of homozygotes were transfusion-dependent in that they were otherwise unable to maintain a haemoglobin level greater than 7 g/dl. The remaining 7% did not require blood transfusion and fitted the clinical category of thalassaemia intermedia. Blood transfusion was calculated to maintain the haemoglobin at a mean level of 11.5 g/dl. In splenectomised subjects where the element of hypersplenism was eliminated, this amounted to an annual requirement of 150–300 ml/kg. An increased requirement over expectation indicated hypersplenism and where this exceeded 50%, splenectomy was called for. Thereafter patients were maintained on prophylactic penicillin in view of the susceptibility to infection. Patients treated according to a high transfusion schedule ('hyper transfusion') benefited from a reduction of all the complications of bone marrow expansion, including cardiomegaly, hepatosplenomegaly, stunted growth, facial deformity and pathological fractures, and there was also reduction of the expanded blood volume and of the excessive gastrointestinal absorption of iron. They were superficially indistinguishable from normal children up to age 13, but there was a gradual retardation of growth and development starting some years before this, due to accumulating iron overload. Where this is untreated, death is likely at 16–24 years of age.

The accumulation of iron can be reduced by chelation therapy, the agent in current use being desferrioxamine. Most transfusion programmes lead to the deposition of 15–25 mg of iron in the tissues per day and chelation therapy must eliminate a similar amount to restore normal iron balance. The recommended dose of desferrioxamine is 25 mg/kg daily by intramuscular injection and, if this is started at the age of 3 years, iron balance can be achieved by the age of 6 years. In effect, the amount usually given is 500 mg daily intramuscularly and 2 g intravenously with every unit of blood. As desferrioxamine has a short half-life and is known to be much more effective when given by slow intravenous infusion, it may be possible in the future to devise a means of slow continuous administration (e.g. subcutaneously) by infusion pump (Graziano & Cerami 1977). Desferrioxamine therapy may be potentiated by the simultaneous administration of ascorbic acid by mouth in a dose of 200 mg daily.

Claims have been made for even higher transfusion programmes aimed at keeping the haematocrit above 35% ('supertransfusion') and for using blood with a high content of young red cells (neocytes). These are collected in a continuous flow separator from the zone just lateral to the buffy coat (Propper et al 1980).

α thalassaemia

As stated earlier, the genes controlling α chain synthesis are duplicated, with two on each chromosome 16 and thus four functioning genes. When non-functioning genes are inherited there are four possible combinations depending upon their number. Where there is only one non-functioning gene, the individual is only mildly affected, with a slight reduction of MCH and MCV. These findings are proportionately greater where two non-functioning α genes occur in the heterozygous state. When only one functioning α gene exists there is a marked surplus of β chains which results in the formation of Hb H (β4) and the development of a severe haemolytic anaemia (Hb H disease). The last possible combination is the total absence of functioning α genes which results in the production of Hb Barts (γ4) and is incompatible with postnatal survival owing to the development of hydrops fetalis (Bank 1978, Higgs 1981). There is evidence that in α thalassaemia also there is considerable heterogeneity at the molecular level (Weatherall 1982).

REFERENCES

Disorders of the haemostatic mechanism

Abildgaard C F, Suzuki Z, Harrison J, Jefcoat K, Zimmerman T S 1980 Serial studies in von Willebrand's disease: variability versus variants. Blood 56: 712–716

Bloom A L 1978 Clotting factor concentrates for resistant haemophilia. British Journal of Haematology 40: 21–27

Bloom A L 1981 Factor VIII inhibitors revisited. British Journal of Haematology 43: 319–324

Cuttner J 1980 Thrombotic thrombocytopenic purpura: a 10-year experience. Blood 56: 302–310

Holahan J R, White G C 1981 Heterogeneity of membrane surface proteins in Glanzmann's thrombasthenia. Blood 57: 174–181

Kaden B R, Rosse W F, Hauch T W 1979 Immune thrombocytopenia in lymphoproliferative diseases. Blood 53: 545–551

Karpatkin S 1980 Review. Autoimmune thrombocytopenic purpura. Blood 56: 329–343

Kasper C K, Osterud B, Minami J Y 1977 Haemophilia B: characterisation of genetic variants and detection of carriers. Blood 50: 351–366

Koutts J, Howard M A, Firkin B G 1979 Factor VIII physiology and pathology in man. Progress in Haematology XI: 115–145

Lee H, Nurden A T, Thomaidis A, Caen J P 1981 Relationship between fibrinogen binding and the platelet glycoprotein deficiencies in Glanzmann's thrombasthenia type I and type II. British Journal of Haematology 48: 47–57

McDonald T P 1981 Assay and site of production of thrombopoietin. British Journal of Haematology 49: 493–500

Malmsten C 1979 Prostaglandins, thromboxanes and platelets. British Journal of Haematology 41: 453–458

Marcus A J 1979 The role of prostaglandins in platelet function. Progress in Haematology XI: 147–171

Miescher P A, Graf J 1980 Drug-induced thrombocytopenia. Clinics in Haematology 9: 505–520

Miller C H, Graham J B, Goldin L R, Elston R C 1979 Genetics of classical von Willebrand's disease. I. Phenotypic variations with families. II. Optimal assignment of the heterozygous genotype. Blood 54: 117–145

Mitchell J R A 1981 Anticoagulants, aspirin and anturan in transient cerebral ischaemic attacks. In: Tunbridge M (ed) Advanced medicine. Royal College of Physicians and Pitman Medical, London, p 276–286

Packham M A, Mustard J F 1977 Clinical pharmacology of platelets. Blood 50: 555–573

Pegels J G, Bruynes E C E, Engelfriet C P, von dem Borne A E G K 1981 Post transfusional purpura: a serological and immunochemical study. British Journal of Haematology 49: 521–530

Sixma J J 1980 The prethrombotic state. British Journal of Haematology 46: 515–522

Stuart M J 1975 Inherited defects of platelet function. Seminars in Haematology 12: 233–253
Tavassoli M 1980 Megakaryocyte–platelet axis and the process of platelet formation and release. Blood 55: 537–543
Wensley R T, Stevens R F, Burn A M, Delamore I W 1980 Plasma exchange and human factor VIII concentrates in managing haemophilia A with factor VIII inhibitors. British Medical Journal 281: 1388–1389

Iron deficiency and overload

Bassett M L, Halliday J W, Powell L W, Doran T, Bashir H 1979 Early detection of idiopathic haemochromatosis: relative value of serum ferritin and HLA typing. Lancet 2: 4–7
Bomford A 1979 Haemochromatosis. Journal of the Royal Society of Medicine 72: 311–314
Cook J D 1980 Iron methodology: An overview. Methods in Haematology 1: 1–14
Crosby W H 1977 Haemochromatosis: the unsolved problems. Seminars in Haematology 14: 135–143
Dallman P R, Beutler E, Finch C A 1978 Effects of iron deficiency exclusive of anaemia. British Journal of Haematology 40: 179–184
Jacob R A, Sanstead H A, Klevay L M, Johnson L K 1980 Utility of serum ferritin as a measure of iron deficiency in normal males undergoing repetitive phlebotomy. Blood 56: 786–791
Jacobs A 1982 Disorders of iron metabolism. In: Hoffbrand A V (ed) Recent advances in haematology 3. Churchill Livingstone, Edinburgh, p 1–24
Leibel R, Greenfield D, Pollitt E 1979 Biochemical and behavioural aspects of sideropenia. British Journal of Haematology 41: 145–150
Torrance J D, Bothwell T H 1980 Tissue iron stores. Methods in Haematology 1: 90–115
Worwood M 1980 Serum ferritin. Methods in Haematology 1: 59–89

Megaloblastic anaemia

Hoffbrand A V 1980 Megaloblastic anaemia. In: Hoffbrand A V, Lewis S M (eds) Postgraduate haematology. Heinemann, London, p 72–111
Hoffbrand A V, Wickremasinghe R G 1982 Megaloblastic anaemia. In: Hoffbrand A V (ed) Recent advances in haematology 3. Churchill Livingstone, Edinburgh, p 25–44
Chanarin I, Deacon R, Lumb M, Perry J 1980 Vitamin B_{12} regulates folate metabolism by the supply of formate. Lancet 2: 505–508
Chanarin I, Deacon R, Perry J, Lumb M 1981 How vitamin B_{12} acts. British Journal of Haematology 47: 487–491
Matthews D M, Linnell J C 1979 Vitamin B_{12}: an area of darkness. British Medical Journal 2: 533–535

Aplastic anaemia

Alter B P, Potter N U, Li F P 1978 Classification and aetiology of the aplastic anaemias. Clinics in Haematology 7: 431–465
Bentley S A 1982 Bone marrow connective tissue and the haemopoietic microenvironment. British Journal of Haematology 50: 1–6
Geary C G 1979 The pathogenesis of aplastic anaemia. British Journal of Hospital Medicine 24: 392–402
Meadenovic J, Adamson J W 1982 Erythroid colony growth in culture: analysis of erythroid differentiation and studies in human disease states. In: Hoffbrand A V (ed) Recent advances in haematology 3. Churchill Livingstone, Edinburgh, p 95–108
Parkman R 1978 The immunology of marrow failure. Clinics in Haematology 7: 475–486
Schofield R 1979 The pluripotential stem cell. Clinics in Haematology 8: 221–237
Shahidi N T 1979 Aplastic anaemia: aetiological and therapeutic dilemmas. British Journal of Haematology 43: 163–166
Wasser J S, Yolken R, Miller D R, Diamond L 1978 Congenital hypoplastic anaemia (Diamond-Blackfan syndrome) terminating in acute myelogenous leukaemia. Blood 51: 991–995

Haemoglobinopathies

Bank A 1978 Critical review. Thalassaemia syndrome. Blood 51: 369–384
Graziano J H, Cerami A 1977 Chelation therapy for the treatment of thalassaemia. Seminars in Haematology 14: 127–134
Higgs D R 1981 The haemoglobinopathies. Hospital Update 7: 1267–1278
Lehman H, Huntsman R G 1974 An introduction to the structure and function of haemoglobin. Clinics in Haematology 3: 217–223
Modell C B 1977 Total management of thalassaemia major. Archives of Disease in Childhood 52: 489–500

Pearson H A, O'Brien R T 1975 The management of thalassaemia major. Seminars in Haematology 12: 255–265

Powars D R 1975 Natural history of sickle cell disease. The first 10 years. Seminars in Haematology 12: 267–285

Propper R D, Button L N, Nathan D G 1980 New approaches to the transfusion management of thalassaemia. Blood 55: 55–60

Stamatoyannopoulos G, Nute P E 1974 Genetic control of haemoglobin. Clinics in Haematology 3: 251–287

Weatherall D J 1982 The molecular genetics of haemoglobin — the thalassaemias. In: Hoffbrand A V (ed) Recent advances in haematology 3. Churchill Livingstone, Edinburgh, p 45–68

8

Developments in medical oncology

C. J. Williams and J. M. A. Whitehouse

INTRODUCTION

There are few areas of medicine today which have not attracted the word 'specialisation'. Improved understanding of the pathology, biochemistry and other complex factors which influence disease, and the consequence of improved pharmacological manipulation, have combined with modern technology to change patterns of disease management so that it would be almost unrecognisable to the physician of the 1940s. Despite the emphasis which some have given to technology, the danger of depersonalising medicine is now well appreciated and the contributions to be made by sophisticated technology can be more clearly identified to serve a specific function within the framework of medicine as a whole. This represents a retrenchment of attitudes from several years ago when it appeared that technology might dominate.

Although specialisation has threatened the practice of the 'generalist' by removing whole areas such as gastroenterology, cardiology, endocrinology and respiratory medicine, there is little doubt that the concentration of expertise which resulted has led to improved management policies. Specialisation inevitably leads to greater critical appraisal so that unnecessary or irrelevant medical practices are abandoned. Cancer has long suffered, not so much from lack of specialisation but from the clinician's sense of desperation in an apparently intractable situation. Since most cancers ultimately disseminate, even after presenting as apparently localised disease, local therapies used in isolation have only limited usefulness. Surgery and radiotherapy used judiciously are, however, invaluable in their proper roles. No longer is surgery regarded as useful only in the curative situation: it has a vital role in reducing tumour volume to a minimum (this in itself may require major surgical reconstruction) and in defining disease extent precisely. Radiotherapy, too, has a curative role in the management of certain localised tumours, exchanging temporary morbidity for long-term preservation of function. It was the patients in whom local therapy failed or was unsuitable whose disease progression and subsequent distress led to a commonly held and, sadly, still frequently found view of the hopelessness of cancer.

The discovery of agents with anticancer activity in the early 1940s had far-reaching effects extending well beyond their immediate anticancer activity. The germ for this change came from the possibility that chemotherapy might offer a realistic management for the majority of cancers for which no therapy was available. At first, responses were confined to rare conditions and resulted in prolongation of survival only. When newer drugs were used in combination and with greater effect, some cures were identified. Optimism overreached therapeutic realism for a time but gradually a new speciality of internal medicine has arisen and 'Medical Oncology', as it is now known, became the latest and newest speciality. In the USA and many countries of Europe, Medical Oncology has become well established, whereas in the UK separate medical oncology units have been set up mainly in academic centres. This delay in making the speciality available has meant that the ideal relationship between radiotherapist, surgeon and medical oncologist exists in only a few major centres. However, within those centres the emphasis on critical evaluation of therapy is paramount. The concentrated experience of supporting services such as pathology, haematology and radiology means that each has a vast personal experience to draw upon — diagnostic errors are minimised, fundamental variations in natural history of disease subtypes are recognised and management made more relevant to the individual patient. Most treatment is arranged within the framework of the clinical trial so that valuable clinical practice is retained and improved and those practices of dubious benefit evaluated and, where appropriate, made obsolete.

Much of the management of the conditions described in this chapter is no longer appropriate for the non-specialist clinician, for neither he nor his clinical team can devote their attention or resources to ensure the optimum outcome of management: nevertheless it is essential that family doctor and generalist alike are aware of the very real progress which has taken place in the treatment of these conditions and the means by which this is achieved. Their close collaboration is essential to achieve the maximum therapeutic benefit and each has a vital part to play in the complex contribution to patient support essential for the achievement of this aim.

This chapter deals with areas of the medical management of cancer where developments are most apparent.

METHODS OF SELECTING ANTICANCER DRUGS FOR CLINICAL USE

At present, anticancer drugs for use alone or in combination are selected according to empirical rules. The selection of drugs by rational means has long been a goal of chemotherapists and the development by Hamburger and Salmon of an assay that can be used to grow human tumour cells in short-term culture may be a first step towards this goal.

The technique used by Hamburger and Salmon was first reported in 1978 (Salmon 1980) and since then these workers have gone on to characterise the cells which form colonies and to correlate the sensitivity patterns of drugs in vivo and in vitro. A suspension of single cells is plated out into 0.3% agar with nutrients in a Petri dish with a lower feeder layer of 0.5% agar containing further nutrients and growth stimulants. The 0.3% agar is of a sloppy consistency which allows the cells to grow but prevents their movement. A single clonogenic cell therefore forms a local colony. The sloppy agar also inhibits the growth of fibroblasts which would normally overgrow the specimen. Colonies form in 1–2 weeks and may be counted with an inverted phase microscope. Drug sensitivity is tested by exposing cells to varying low doses of the drug to be tested for about an hour. After washing, the cells are plated out and the number of colonies formed is compared with the colonies formed by control cells not exposed to the drug. Criteria for in vitro sensitivity for individual drugs have been derived and are based on an initial set of patients who were studied in vitro and within clinical trials.

Types of tumours that form colonies in the clonogenic assay

Since the first reports of Hamburger and Salmon, over 2500 tumour specimens have been plated in the assay. The wide spectrum of different tumours that have been grown in the system is shown in Table 8.1. Cells from various sources can be used to

Table 8.1 Human tumour types which have formed colonies in agar after culturing directly from biopsies. (More than 1500 biopsy samples tested included primary tumour and metastases)

Carcinomas	Sarcomas and other neoplasms
Adrenal	Chronic lymphocytic leukaemia
Bladder	Diffuse lymphomas
Breast	Ewing's tumour
Colon	Fibrosarcoma
Kidney	Giant-cell tumour
Liver	Glioblastoma
Lung (small-cell, adenocarcinoma,	Hodgkin's disease
large-cell, squamous-cell)	Islet-cell tumour
Ovary	Liposarcoma
Pancreas	Macroglobulinaemia
Prostate	Malignant schwannoma
Stomach	Melanoma (melanotic & amelanotic)
Thyroid	Mesothelioma
Upper airways (head and neck)	Multiple myeloma
Uterus (corpus and cervix)	Nephroblastoma (Wilm's tumour)
Unknown primary (squamous)	Neuroblastoma
Head and neck	Nodular lymphomas
	Osteogenic sarcoma
	Rhabdomyosarcoma
	Testicular teratoma
	Testicular seminoma

grow tumours and, as shown in Table 8.2, cells derived from ascites and cavity washings produce greater plating efficiencies and this probably reflects the difficulty of maintaining cell viability when making single-cell suspensions from solid lumps of

Table 8.2 Growth of tumour stem-cell colonies categorised by source of specimen (from Salmon et al 1982)

Source of specimen	Percentage of tumours which formed colonies
1. Malignant effusions (ascites, pleural, pericardial)	80–90
2. Solid tumours (primaries and metastases)	50–60
3. Marrow (e.g. neuroblastoma, myeloma, oat cell)	80–90
4. Cavity washings (bladder, peritoneum, bronchus)	80–90

tumour. Although Salmon's group use mechanical dissociation, several other groups are trying enzymatic methods of cell disaggregation; this area of the assay needs improvement.

Studies showing that the colonies are composed of malignant cells

It is important to find out whether the colonies grown in the assay are composed of tumour cells identical to those growing in the patient's tumour. The following techniques have been used to test this:

1. Light microscopy with or without cytochemistry has confirmed that the nature of the cells is grossly the same as in the primary tumour.
2. Electron microscopy has confirmed the transitional nature of bladder carcinomas growing in the assay, and desmosomes and neurosecretory granules have been identified in neuroblastoma colonies.
3. The results of chromosome-analysis studies are consistent with the malignant nature of the colonies, and characteristic cytogenetic abnormalities have been identified in several tumours.
4. A large number of tumour markers have been shown to be secreted by cells in the colonies growing in the assay. These markers are the same as those secreted by the tumour in the patient and have included somatostatin, melanogens, catecholamines, human chorionic gonadotrophin, α-fetal protein, parathormone and idiotypic immunoglobulin.
5. Cells from colonies grown in the assay have been injected as xenografts into nude mice. These cells form tumours identical to the primary human tumour.

Correlation of drug sensitivity patterns

It is beyond the scope of this chapter to detail the procedure for testing drug sensitivity beyond that previously outlined. Two major groups (that of Salmon in Tucson and of Von Hoff in San Antonio) have reported the widest experience correlating the in vitro results compared with in vivo sensitivity of drugs. The data from both groups are summarised in Table 8.3. It can be seen from this that the correlation for resistance in vitro and in vivo is 97% although the correlation for in vitro and in vivo sensitivity is less good at 60%. These findings are highly significant ($P < 10^{-9}$) and have been obtained in two separate laboratories.

Table 8.3 Composite update of correlations of in vitro — in vivo sensitivity to anticancer drugs (Salmon et al 1982)

Investigative Group	No. of Patients	No. of Clinical Trials for Correlations	Tumour sensitive both in vitro & in vivo	Tumour sensitive in vitro & resistant in vivo	Tumour resistant in vitro & sensitive in vivo	Tumour resistant both in vitro & in vivo
Tucson	96	193	34	20	5	134
San Antonio	101	146	15	6	2	123
Total	197	339	49 (60% true positive)	26	7	257 (97% true negative)

With the Chi square test the association of in vitro and in vivo results was highly significant ($P < 10^{-9}$).

Problems with the human tumour stem-cell assay

One of the major problems is in obtaining a single-cell suspension without undue damage to the cells. Studies of different methods are continuing and there is some evidence that different disaggregation techniques will be required for different tumour types. Even when large numbers of viable cells are available it is not always possible to ensure that enough colonies will be grown to perform drug sensitivity studies. Further efforts are being made to improve the plating efficiency. At present the assay is time-consuming and is not suitable for routine clinical use. Results are available at about 10–14 d but the assay may be made simple and faster by the introduction of automated colony counters which will allow results to be available within as little as 4 d.

Although much emphasis has been placed on the potential role of this type of assay in selecting drugs for clinical use, the assay is a model that can be used in basic biology, the study of drug resistance, screening for new drugs and as a diagnostic tool for detecting minor tumour infiltration. The assay remains experimental and must be extensively assessed and improved before it can become a clinical tool.

CIS-DIAMMINEDICHLOROPLATINUM (DDP)

The discovery of this drug is a story of serendipity. Rosenberg in 1965 found that the replication of *E. coli* was inhibited when he passed an electric current between platinum electrodes in a path of the bacteria. He found that the inhibition was caused not by the electric current but by several platinum compounds that were formed. The development of cis platinum has been extensively reported in the Proceedings of a Conference in Atlanta in 1979 (Prestayko et al 1980).

DDP is the first of a new class of anticancer drugs, the heavy metals; its structure and those of its early analogues are shown in Figure 8.1. Its mode of action appears to be similar to that of the alkylating agents, and studies have shown that it selectively inhibits the synthesis of DNA but not of RNA.

The drug is given intravenously, either by bolus or infusion, and pharmacokinetic studies have shown that the 'free' active drug has a terminal half-life of about 30 min. The drug is rapidly bound to plasma and tissue proteins. The terminal half-life of

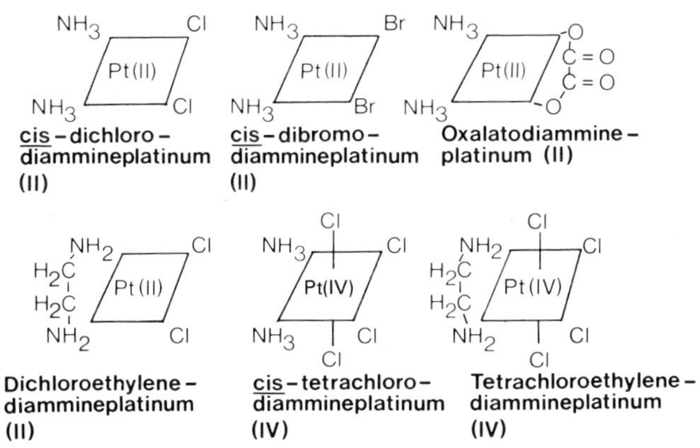

Fig. 8.1 Structure of cis-diamminedichloroplatinum

'total' platinum (free and bound) is about 48 h and tissue-bound platinum can be detected for several months.

The initial dose-limiting toxicity of DDP was acute and chronic renal failure. This problem has largely been overcome by the administration of large volumes of intravenous fluids before, and for some hours after, the DDP is given. Some groups also use diuretics although this does not appear to be necessary if hydration is adequate. Using this simple technique, renal toxicity is rarely troublesome and repeated injections of platinum can be given.

Anticancer activity

Testicular teratomas

DDP is probably the most active single agent in testicular cancer (see p. 185–189) and is an integral part of all current regimens. When used as a single agent in a mixed group of treated and untreated patients, an objective response rate of 60% (20% CR) has been reported. However, most remissions were temporary and the drug is now used in combination.

Ovarian carcinoma

DDP has about a 30% objective remission rate in previously treated patients and has been included in combinations with other drugs. Several combinations, especially those with Adriamycin (doxorubicin) and cyclophosphamide have produced high complete remission rates. It remains to be seen whether these will translate into improved survival; randomised studies are under way.

Head and neck carcinoma

Several groups have reported encouraging single-agent response rates (30%) for DDP. It has been used recently in combinations, particularly with bleomycin and methotrexate, although there is no good evidence of improved survival.

Bladder cancer

Studies showing an objective response rate of up to 30% encouraged studies of combinations with Adriamycin (doxorubicin) but these have shown no better results than with Adriamycin alone. Further studies of DDP-containing combinations continue.

Miscellaneous tumours

Responses have been shown in a variety of other tumours including lung cancer, lymphomas, gynaecological malignancies, osteogenic sarcomas, and thyroid cancers. It appears to be inactive in leukaemias and colonic cancer.

Toxicity

The major toxic effects are renal toxicity, nausea and vomiting, myelosuppression, ototoxicity, anaphylactic reactions, neurotoxicity and transient hypomagnesaemia.

The nephrotoxicity is dose-related but is avoided by scrupulous attention to hydration so that a brisk diuresis is induced for some hours after the drug has been given.

Nausea and vomiting are clinically the major problem in the day-to-day use of the drug. Most antiemetics fail to prevent this side effect. Clinical ototoxicity consisting of tinnitus and hearing loss (4000–8000 Hz) occurs in less than 10% of patients.

Myelosuppression is not severe with DDP although both neutropenia and thrombocytopenia do occur. Anaemia is commonly seen and transfusion is often required if multiple courses of DDP are given.

Anaphylactic reactions have been reported infrequently and were controlled with antihistamines, corticosteroids or adrenaline. Neurotoxicity is uncommon and consists of a predominantly sensory peripheral neuropathy; seizures have also been seen. Chemical hypomagnesaemia is common (up to 50% of patients) although clinical evidence of the disturbance is uncommon: it is probably attributable to DDP-induced tubular damage causing loss of tubular reabsorption. This effect is usually transient but magnesium replacement therapy is required in symptomatic patients.

Platinum is the first of a new group of antitumour agents and is highly active in a variety of tumour types. It is also a toxic drug and further evaluation is needed before its role in the treatment of many common tumours can be defined.

VP16-213

The other active new drug introduced during the past 5 years is a member of the podophyllotoxin group. Stahelin modified portions of the podophyllotoxin ring system to produce less toxic compounds suitable for clinical use. One compound (Fig. 8.2), 4[1]-demethyl-epipodophyllotoxin-9-(4, 6-0 ethylidene-D glucopyranoside) has been shown to be clinically active and is now commercially available in Britain (VP16-213 or etoposide). The proceedings of the first international

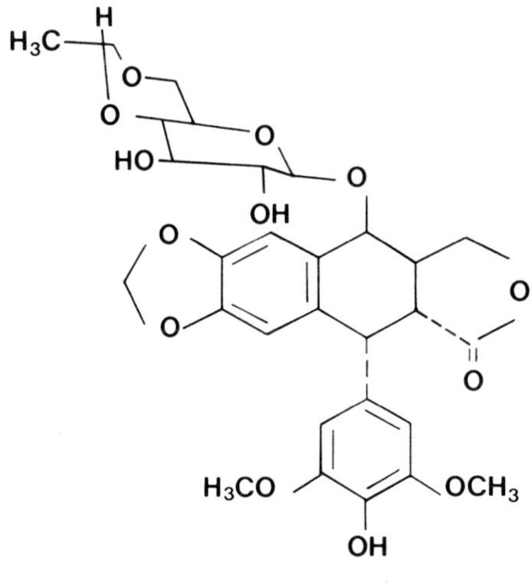

Etoposide (VP-16-213)

Fig. 8.2 Structure of VP16-213

symposium on the podophyllotoxins has recently been published in *Cancer Chemotherapy and Pharmacology*.

Alteration of the parent compound has resulted in a different mode of action. VP16-213 arrests cells in late S or G_2 phases of the cell cycle and produces single-strand breaks in DNA. It does not produce metaphasic arrest, as does the parent compound podophyllotoxin. It may be given either intravenously or orally. When given intravenously it should be given as an infusion over at least 30 min because hypotension can result from rapid administration. Bioavailability studies suggest that only about 50% of the drug is absorbed, compared with i.v. administration. Although no clinical studies have adequately explored dose scheduling, most workers agree that the drug is better given over several days and most give it over 3–5d.

Clinical activity

VP16-213 has been shown to be highly active in small-cell lung cancer and is also active in the lymphomas, Hodgkin's disease, teratomas, the acute leukaemias and choriocarcinoma. It has shown no significant activity in breast, ovarian or GI tract carcinoma or in melanoma and sarcomas.

Toxicity

The major dose-limiting toxicity is myelosuppression. Neutropenia occurs with a nadir around day 8–10 and thrombocytopenia is usually about 2–3d later. Counts have usually recovered by about day 20.

Gastrointestinal toxicity, mainly nausea, occurs in about 25% of patients. Alopecia, less severe than with Adriamycin or cyclophosphamide, occurs in about one-third of patients. Hypersensitivity has been reported.

VP16-213 is the first of a new class of anticancer agents to enter clinical use. Its main indication is in lung cancer although it is active in a wide variety of other tumour types. It is schedule-dependent and is best administered over 3–5d. Toxicity is predictable and reversible.

ACUTE MYELOGENOUS LEUKAEMIA

Introduction

Although rare, acute myelogenous leukaemia (AML) continues to excite interest as a therapeutic problem. The rapidity of disease progression in untreated patients and the life-threatening consequences of the leukaemic process are, in combination, a formidable challenge to modern medical expertise. However, its sensitivity to some of the new anticancer drugs offers the potential for an improved prognosis.

Little is known of the aetiology of leukaemias in man although, in some animals, viruses capable of inducing leukaemia have been identified. Exposure to irradiation and to benzene are known to be associated with an increased risk of acute leukaemia. Long-term administration of alkylating agents in such conditions as carcinoma of the ovary, and the use of both chemotherapy and radiotherapy in the same patient, are now also recognised as being associated with an increased risk of second malignancy.

AML may result from the neoplastic transformation of a single cell which then produces a daughter population and subsequently a clone of malignant cells or, alternatively, it may represent a defect of maturation so that normal and abnormal granulopoiesis are inextricably interrelated. From the point of view of therapy the former theory is more attractive, for while the elimination of a clone of abnormal cells is conceivable with available therapies, restoration of normal maturation would be likely to require an entirely different approach to management.

Classification

The term 'acute myelogenous leukaemia' implies origin from a myeloid stem cell and is used broadly to include all those acute leukaemias of presumed bone marrow origin. Over the past few years it has been possible to subclassify the acute myelogenous leukaemias by combining conventional morphology with an increasing number of objective laboratory tests. The classification currently in use is summarised in Table 8.4.

Cytogenetic studies have revealed abnormal karyotypes in a significant proportion of patients with AML (Trujillo et al 1974). These have been found to be due to changes in the number of chromosomes, to chromosome breakage, or to specific structural chromosome changes. Both hyper- and hypo-diploidy are found. Banding techniques have improved the precision of cytogenetic analysis, but so far no consistent changes have been identified. These techniques have also thrown some light on the evolution of the neoplastic process and, indeed, some evidence of involvement of red cell precursors in AML has been shown (Blackstock & Garson 1974). It would be a considerable asset, both for diagnosis and for monitoring during therapy, if a definitive marker could be demonstrated on the cell surface of the leukaemic cells but no specific AML antigen has been identified.

Table 8.4 Classification of acute myelogenous leukaemia

Acute myelogenous leukaemia (AML)
Myeloblastic
Myelomonocytic
Promyelocytic
Erythroleukaemia
Hypoplastic
Monoblastic

Clinical features and diagnosis

There is no classic history which is diagnostic of AML. However, many patients complain of a 'flu'-like illness 4–6 weeks previously with persisting ill-health and the subsequent development of anaemia, thrombocytopenia or infection. Despite the fact that many patients are granulocytopenic at the time of diagnosis, infection is a fairly unusual presenting feature. Commonly, the patient is anaemic and a careful search will reveal evidence of purpura, particularly in the lower limbs, in the axilla and on the trunk. Retinal haemorrhages may be present in those patients who are profoundly thrombocytopenic.

Lymphadenopathy and splenomegaly, both fairly common in acute lymphoblastic leukaemia, are found infrequently in patients with AML. Gum hypertrophy is a feature of acute monocytic and acute myelomonocytic leukaemia and is found only where teeth remain. Acute promyelocytic leukaemia is a rare variant of AML and almost invariably is associated with disseminated intravascular coagulation to a greater or lesser extent.

Although there may be a high clinical suspicion of AML (a diagnosis which is made more likely by the presence of large numbers of circulating blast cells), the diagnosis can be established only following bone marrow examination. Routine investigation should include the following:

1. Full blood count including differential white count, platelet count and examination of film
2. ESR
3. Blood urea and electrolytes
4. Serum calcium
5. Serum immunoglobulin and serum protein electrophoresis
6. Liver function tests
7. Serum B_{12} and B_{12}-binding protein
8. Serum folate and red cell folate
9. Serum urate
10. Chest radiograph both PA and lateral (to show anterior mediastinum)
11. Bone marrow aspirate and trephine including iron stains
12. Blood group.

Other investigations which may be indicated include tests for haemolysis, cytogenetic studies (for Philadelphia chromosome to exclude chronic granulocytic leukaemia), leucocyte alkaline phosphatase, surface marker characteristics of cell population, lymph node biopsy for histology and imprint for cytology.

Management

The management of the acute leukaemias has now become so complex that patients are tending to be referred to centres with particular experience of the intensive treatment and support of such patients. Within these centres, patients have their progress carefully monitored. Flow charts are used so that peripheral blood and other selected characteristics can be graphically displayed. These facilitate treatment supervision, allow an immediate appreciation of the development of significant side effects and are particularly useful in the follow-up of patients receiving intensive chemotherapy.

There are two major phases of therapy. The first relates to the induction of complete remission, that is complete eradication of all disease detectable by any available method, and the second phase is concerned with the maintenance of this status, that is the perpetuation of an apparent disease-free state. During remission induction, many forms of supportive care may be needed and are of critical importance. Considerable attention is now being paid to the stress experienced by the patient with acute leukaemia, and the particular problems that this creates for the family.

Remission induction

General care. While the initial investigations are being processed, a careful assessment of the patient's clinical state can be carried out. Since a major consequence of antileukaemic therapy is bone marrow suppression, any anaemia, thrombocytopenia or granulocytopenia at the time of presentation is likely to be made worse by therapy. General measures to be taken before chemotherapy are summarised in Table 8.5. Infection in the granulocytopenic patient (less than 500 granulocytes/mm^3) should be investigated promptly and treatment with intravenous gentamycin plus carbenicillin (or a cephalosporin) started immediately.

Table 8.5 Supportive care that may be required before chemotherapy is given in acute leukaemia

1. Anaemia — transfusion
2. Control infection
3. Treat haemorrhagic tendency appropriately
4. Exclude renal failure
5. Prevent hyperuricaemia — allopurinol
6. Exclude other metabolic changes:
   Hypokalaemia
   Hyperkalaemia
   Hyperphosphaturia
   and correct if present

A significant haemorrhagic tendency will nearly always be due to thrombocytopenia although a coagulation screen may indicate an element of disseminated intravascular coagulation (DIC). The former should be treated by regular transfusions. The management of DIC is controversial, but heparin infusions have been used. The risk of DIC developing in acute promyelocytic leukaemia is highest 3–4 d following the start of chemotherapy. Renal dysfunction may result from leukaemic infiltration, but renal functional impairment may also be produced by the breakdown products of leukaemic cells, and this may result in acute or chronic renal failure. In the event of hyperuricaemia at the time of presentation, chemotherapy must be delayed until the hyperuricaemia is controlled. However, since effective therapy carries the risk of causing or accentuating hyperuricaemia, allopurinol 300 mg daily should be given throughout the period of intensive chemotherapy.

In those patients with high peripheral blast counts there is a risk of hyperkalemia, so that careful monitoring throughout the early part of a chemotherapy course and appropriate corrective management are essential. During induction therapy, platelet transfusions should be given when thrombocytopenia is associated with a clinical haemorrhagic tendency, for example the development of haemorrhages, microscopic haematuria, or new purpura. Prophylactic platelet transfusion makes excessive demands on the supply of platelets with no obvious advantage. The requirement may be exacerbated, however, in septicaemic patients. Platelet transfusions are usually given every 24–48 h.

Prevention of infection is the ultimate aim in patients with acute leukaemia. Although a significant proportion of patients have no evidence of infection at presentation, the prolonged period of neutropenia during remission induction chemotherapy means that if no precautions are taken, infection is almost certain to occur, and will be the immediate cause of death in a significant number of patients. The major risk is of endogenous infection, and this is reflected in the difficulty of demonstrating a clear advantage in nursing the patient in isolation units. Prophylactic antibiotics and gut sterilisation have been shown to decrease the frequency of severe infections, without an obvious improvement in remission rates or survival.

The policy of treating febrile episodes in neutropenic patients has a sound basis. It does mean, however, that if the fever is not bacterial in origin, then inappropriate treatment is being given. Other explanations for fever should constantly be sought, and in special centres the patient at risk may be given granulocyte transfusions. Granulocyte transfusions are not of such clearly established benefit as are platelet transfusions, but the serious consequences of infection in the granulocytic patient make all approaches to supportive care worthy of critical evaluation.

Other infections during remission induction may include viral or presumed viral infections, for example, infectious mononucleosis, cytomegalovirus, hepatitis B, and

Table 8.6 Combination chemotherapy for remission induction in acute myelogenous leukaemia

Reference	Agents used	Complete remission (%)
Rosenthal & Moloney 1972	Vincristine Daunorubicin Cytosine arabinoside	55
Whitecar et al 1972	COAP Cyclophosphamide Vincristine Prednisolone Cytosine arabinoside	44
Yates & Holland 1973	Daunorubicin Cytosine arabinoside	44
Crowther et al 1973	Daunorubicin Cytosine arabinoside	54
MRC 1974	5 trials, varying combinations: 6-Mercaptopurine Daunorubicin Prednisolone Cytosine arabinoside 6-Thioguanine L-Asparaginase	34
Curtis et al 1975	CAV Cyclophosphamide Cytosine arabinoside Vincristine	46
Clarkson et al 1975	'L6' Protocol 6-Thioguanine Cytosine arabinoside	56
Preisler et al 1977	Adriamycin (doxorubicin) Cytosine arabinoside	62
Gale & Cline 1977	Daunorubicin Cytosine arabinoside 6-Thioguanine	82
Weinstein et al 1980	Vincristine Adriamycin (doxorubicin) Prednisolone Cytosine arabinoside	70

herpes simplex. Monilial infection is common and while this may involve only the nasopharynx, it can produce severe discomfort. However, extension down the oesophagus is not uncommon and generalised haematological dissemination may occur. *Pneumocystis carinii,* a protozoan, may cause fatal lung infections but can be treated by high-dose co-trimoxazole. Systemic fungal infections require treatment with amphotericin and this drug requires careful supervision. Superficial fungal infections including oesophagitis usually respond to local nystatin mouthwashes and amphotericin lozenges.

Chemotherapy. Some of the more widely used chemotherapy combinations are summarised in Table 8.6, from which it can be seen that complete remission rates have been increasing over the past decade. These combinations may have involved the more effective use of different drugs, but part of the improvement in complete remission rate is undoubtedly a reflection of improved supportive care. Courses of treatment are usually given at 2- to 3-weekly intervals or less, depending on the protocol, and complete remission assessed by bone marrow biopsy before the second or third course of therapy. Treatment is usually better tolerated as the marrow recovers and leukaemic infiltration is reduced. The exact interpretation of complete remission varies between institutions, and is subject to the vagaries of individual haematologists, but in complete remission the patient must by definition be in good general health, free of clinical evidence of disease, the peripheral blood count should be normal and the bone marrow should contain fewer than 5% blast cells. Once complete remission is attained, further additional chemotherapy (consolidation) may be given with the intention of further reducing the leukaemic burden. This practice is based on experimental animal studies which have shown increased curability when consolidation chemotherapy is given.

Remission maintenance

The ideal management of the patient who has achieved complete remission has not yet been identified. Sadly, the aspirations for immunotherapy have never been attained and indeed, any benefit is marginal in the majority of studies; it remains an interesting area for further study. Because the majority of patients with AML ultimately relapse, any maintenance chemotherapy is given, not with a concept of disease eradication, but of disease control. Life for the AML patient achieving complete remission should be made as tolerable as possible. The patient receiving maintenance chemotherapy who ultimately relapses has a 10% chance of achieving a second complete remission, while the patient who has an unmaintained complete remission tends to have a short disease-free interval, and second, third, and even fourth complete remissions can be obtained, but there is no prolongation of survival. However, disease-free intervals well in excess of a year are now being reported with more intensive maintenance regimens.

Only about 5% of patients survive beyond 2 years with conventional chemotherapy. Further intensive treatment given during complete remission may result in an improvement in this figure. In a recent study from the Sidney Farber Cancer Centre (Weinstein et al 1980) 83 patients under the age of 50 were treated intensively for 14 months following CR. Actuarial analysis predicts that almost 50% will remain in CR at 2 years. At the present time the most promising approach in AML has come from bone marrow transplantation where the percentage of long-term survivors exceeds that anticipated in patients receiving conventional chemotherapy only. Patients undergoing bone-marrow transplantation are inevitably selected to some degree and continuing studies are therefore essential to determine the real impact of this procedure.

THE LYMPHOMAS

Interest in the lymphomas stems principally from the encouraging results of modern therapy in Hodgkin's disease and the apparent sensitivity of many lymphomas to both radiotherapy and chemotherapy. It is unfortunate that because of their apparent derivation from cells of lymphoid origin, lymphomas are frequently regarded as one clinical entity. The spectrum of disease they cause ranges, however, from one requiring no initial therapeutic intervention to that which untreated may be rapidly fatal within a few days. Although they are uncommon, it is their very heterogeneity which makes some knowledge of the different lymphomas of particular value to those concerned with diagnosis. Fundamental differences exist between those lymphomas identifiable as Hodgkin's disease because of the presence of Reed-Sternberg cells, and the remainder — called naïvely, the non-Hodgkin's lymphomas. Neither group is common in general clinical practice and for this reason, management by the specialist clinician is to be encouraged.

Classification

Hodgkin's disease

Four subtypes of Hodgkin's disease are recognised: lymphocyte-predominant; nodular sclerosing; mixed cellularity; lymphocyte-depleted.

Attempts to subclassify these further using morphological or immunological techniques have proved to be of little help in making a prognosis. Nodular sclerosing disease is by far the commonest variety, accounting for up to 80% of referrals. Lymphocyte-predominant and lymphocyte-depleted Hodgkin's disease are both uncommon. Despite this subclassification, only lymphocyte-depleted Hodgkin's disease is associated with a poorer prognosis; it also tends to be more widespread at presentation than the other types.

Non-Hodgkin's lymphomas

This group of conditions has been so labelled despite the fact that, in some, the cell of origin may not be the lymphoid cell but macrophage/histiocyte. The most commonly used classification is that devised by Rappaport based on morphological criteria only. This differentiates between a lymph node in which the nodular pattern is lost (diffuse) and one in which the nodular pattern is largely retained (nodular). Table 8.7 reproduces the classification in full. Many now feel that is is appropriate to include chronic lymphocytic leukaemia and the acute lymphoblastic leukaemias within the spectrum of the non-Hodgkin's lymphomas, for many of the lymphomas have bone marrow involvement with a minor degree of haematological overspill. The Rappaport classification has been used to divide patients into two major groups: (1) the indolent lymphomas, which are often stage III or IV at diagnosis but have a long

Table 8.7 Non-Hodgkin's lymphoma: modified Rappaport classification

Architectural patterns
Nodular (N) includes partially nodular
Diffuse (D)
Cell types
Lymphocyte (L)
well differentiated (WD)
intermediate differentiated (ID)
poorly differentiated (PD)
Histiocytic (H)
Mixed lymphocytic-histiocytic (M)
Lymphoblastic (LB)
Undifferentiated (U)
Burkitt's (BUR)

median survival (>5 years); (2) the aggressive lymphomas, which are less widespread at diagnosis but have a shorter median survival.

Immunological techniques which have permitted determination of the surface characteristics of neoplastic cell population have shown that many apparently similar populations of cells have differing characteristics. For this reason, alternative classifications have been proposed on the basis of the immunological characteristics of the neoplastic cells. No classification has so far superseded that of Rappaport in clinical usefulness but an alternative morphological classification has been proposed by Lennert and is commonly used in Europe; this is reproduced in Table 8.8. The majority of clinical trials being published still use the Rappaport classification and until a viable alternative can be found this does, at least, permit some degree of comparison of results between different centres. An NCI study of 1153 patients in four institutions comparing six currently used classifications is to be published shortly and may help to determine a classification which is internationally accepted and which is based on current cytological and immunological studies.

Table 8.8 Non-Hodgkin's lymphoma:

Lennert-Kiel classification
Lymphocytic, chronic lymphocytic leukaemia
Lymphoplasmacytoid
Centrocytic
Centroblastic-centrocytic with and without sclerosis, follicular and follicular and diffuse
Centroblastic-centrocytic diffuse
Centroblastic
Lymphoblastic convoluted cell type
Lymphoblastic other
Immunoblastic

Management

Hodgkin's disease

Treatment of Hodgkin's disease is perhaps the most extensively explored of any malignancy. However, some 40% of those presenting with Hodgkin's disease will have died of this condition within 10 years despite optimum therapy at a major centre. For this reason it is clearly essential to continue to evaluate management critically and, if possible, to identify those patients who require more intensive therapy at the outset. Patients whose disease can be clearly shown to be localised within lymph nodes (stage IA–IIIA) and who receive radiotherapy to the 'mantle' or inverted 'Y' areas, or total nodal irradiation, can expect a survival determined by their pathological stage before therapy. Approximately 90% of those with stage IA disease will be cured, but the local failure rate in stage IIA disease approaches 20%. However, within this latter group those patients with large mediastinal masses have a poorer prognosis, with some centres reporting a relapse rate as high as 50%. Among patients with stage IIIA disease who receive total nodal irradiation, 34% have relapsed by 5 years. Patients at particular risk of relapse are those with bulky mediastinal tumours, extensive splenic involvement, disease at four or more nodal sites or involvement of the lower abdominal nodes (designated stage III_2 by Stein et al (1979)). Attempts to select patients at high risk for relapse have been made because they may benefit from radiotherapy and chemotherapy.

In an attempt to reduce the relapse rate in patients receiving extensive radiotherapy for pathological stage I, II and III disease, adjuvant MOPP was given in a randomised controlled trial starting in 1968 at Stanford (Rosenberg et al 1979). 253 patients were evaluable for analysis. Disappointingly, it was found that while relapse-free survival was improved in patients with IA, IIA, IIIA and IIIB disease, it was not improved in patients with IB and IIB disease. Furthermore, there are only borderline survival advantages in symptom-free patients after 10 years of study. Current Stanford studies use less extensive radiotherapy. The role of adjuvant chemotherapy in those at particular risk of relapse following radiotherapy is not yet substantially supported by available clinical data.

Patients receiving MOPP for stage IIIB and IV disease have a temporary but appreciable morbidity. Widening of the interval between courses and the substitution of vinblastine for vincristine led to MVPP with a lessening of the toxicity (Nicholson et al 1970). Substituting chlorambucil for mustine in the MVPP regime followed. Both MVPP and chlorambucil VPP appear to produce overall responses paralleling those of MOPP. Of 73 previously untreated patients who received chlorambucil VPP at the Royal Marsden Hospital (Kaye et al 1979), 67% achieved complete remission. Response rates were higher, as expected, in those previously treated with radiotherapy (90%). Preliminary survival data appear similar to that for MOPP and MVPP, but analysis of the cohort over a period of at least 10 years will be necessary before final conclusions can be reached.

Salvage of patients relapsing following radiotherapy is appreciable, response rates to MOPP or equivalent combinations being around 90%. In those patients who previously received chemotherapy the results are much less encouraging. While most patients who relapse following complete remissions obtained with MOPP will once again respond to MOPP, durable remissions are rarely obtained.

Combining Adriamycin (doxorubicin), bleomycin, imidazole carboxamide and vinblastine (ABVD), Bonadonna and his colleagues reported that this appeared to be active in patients relapsing following MOPP (Santoro & Bonadonna 1979). In a subsequent study MOPP and ABVD have been compared in previously untreated patients, and appear to be equally effective in inducing complete remissions.

However ABDV, while producing some responses among MOPP-relapsing patients (6/27 in a Stanford series), results in durable remissions in only about a quarter of patients treated. Preliminary results of trials using alternating combinations of MOPP and ABVD have been reported but long-term follow-up is awaited (Bonadonna et al 1978).

Interest in combining chemotherapy and radiotherapy is manifest in a number of clinical studies where attempts are being made to improve the overall cure rate. It is very important that the contribution made by combined modality should be evaluated for the risk of second malignancy. Those patients receiving both chemotherapy and radiotherapy for the treatment of Hodgkin's disease have an increased incidence of second tumours. Both acute myelogenous leukaemia and, in long survivors, non-Hodgkin lymphoma, occur at greater than expected frequency among patients who have received combined modality treatment with radiotherapy and MOPP or MVPP (Krikorian et al 1979). In patients receiving ABVD and radiotherapy the risk of second malignancy has been reported to be less (Valagussa et al 1980). Further long-term observation will clarify the situation. All men treated with MOPP or similar regimens containing an alkylating agent and procarbazine are likely to be sterile. Bonadonna has claimed that infertility is very much less common after ABVD treatment. Any treatment including adjuvant chemotherapy in stages IA–IIIA must take these long-term toxicities into account.

Non-Hodgkin lymphoma

For the non-Hodgkin's lymphomas a staging system similar to that for Hodgkin's disease is used but has proved to be of limited use. In Hodgkin's disease, spread appears to be from one contiguous lymph node group to another, and cure of Hodgkin's disease by local radiotherapy is well established. This is not a feature of NHDL. True stage I non-Hodgkin's lymphoma is extremely uncommon and only in those few patients whose disease is shown to be confined to one lymph node group by exhaustive staging including laparotomy, is cure to be expected in some patients treated with radiotherapy. For this reason, and because of the increased morbidity in older patients, staging laparotomy is rarely considered in the non-Hodgkin's lymphomas, but in all other respects the staging investigations should be as thorough as in Hodgkin's disease. Patients with nodular lymphomas and well-differentiated diffuse lymphomas, whose disease is confined to one anatomical lymph node site, may benefit from local radiotherapy. However, the advantages of such therapy are by no means proved. It is apparent that, in some patients with clinical stage II–IV nodular poorly differentiated and well differentiated diffuse lymphoma, who are both asymptomatic and who do not have bulky disease, the disease may remain stable or fluctuate over a period of years.

In studies from Stanford and St Bartholomew's Hospital comparing chlorambucil alone with a cyclophosphamide, vincristine and prednisolone combination (CVP) in patients with indolent lymphomas, the complete remission rate was slightly higher in the CVP group. An additional group in the Stanford trial using total nodal radiotherapy (TNI) together with CVP produced a similar complete remission rate. However, no survival advantage was noted in any of the groups in either trial.

Toxicity was greater in the CVP and TNI group. In the young patients with indolent lymphomas, a median survival of 8–10 years represents a considerable threat. For this reason, several studies have examined the role of intensive chemotherapy and whole-body irradiation in these patients. Whereas the response rate and morbidity have been high, these approaches have not conferred improved survival.

Using the Rappaport classification, two subgroups of the nodular lymphomas have distinguished themselves from NLPD by their different behaviour. In several studies, those patients with mixed nodular histology have had a high complete remission rate and a long disease-free survival (Lister et al 1978a) Histiocytic nodular disease, however, appears to have a more aggressive course than NLPD, and these patients are in many studies singled out for immediate therapy with combinations such as C-MOPP.

The rapid evolution of the diffuse lymphomas (with the exception of well-differentiated cell types) and poor prognosis have led to investigation of many different treatment combinations. Interpretation of data from different centres is complicated by difficult interpretation of classifications, grouping together of different subgroups and the use of a variety of treatment regimens. However, complete remission rates rarely exceed 50% and median survivals are under 2 years. Of particular interest within the group are those which are included in some series of 'large-cell lymphomas'. Most of the cases identified as large-cell lymphomas are reported as 'histiocytic diffuse' but a small proportion are also identifiable as 'diffuse undifferentiated' in the Rappaport classification. These together make up approximately 25% of all non-Hodgkin lymphomas, and 40% of the diffuse lymphomas (DHL 31%, DUL 9%).

While clinical staging implies a progressive increase in number of patients in each successive stage from I–IV, pathological staging (staging laparotomy plus or minus whole-body scanning) reveals that the majority of cases are stage IV (>50%); that the number of stage II cases (<20%) often exceeds those that are stage III (<20%) and that rather less than 10% prove to have stage I disease.

Five-year survival for stage I and II disease treated primarily with radiotherapy approaches 45%. Most series report a significant difference in survival between pathological stage I and II disease. Stage I and IE may be cured using radiotherapy alone in approximately 75% of cases, while 30–40% of stage II and IIE disease are cured using a combination of surgery and radiotherapy alone. Recent reports of a small number of cases having stage I or II diffuse histiocytic lymphoma treated with either chemotherapy and radiotherapy or chemotherapy alone (Miller & Jones 1979) show no significant survival advantage for either approach. In view of the high risk of relapse in stage II disease treated by radiotherapy, first-line chemotherapy for this group merits further clinical trials.

Stage III and IV diffuse histiocytic lymphomas should always receive combination chemotherapy. The role of radiotherapy in these patients is not established. Several careful studies from major centres have identified complete response rates around 50% or more (C-MOPP, BACOP, CHOP, HOP, OPAL, COMLA): median survivals exceed 3 years and approximately half of the patients achieving complete remission may prove to be cured. Survival rates of partial remitters and of non-responders do not differ significantly. Poor prognostic factors include stage IV disease, bone marrow involvement, CNS involvement, gastrointestinal involvement, and a tumour mass exceeding 10 cm in diameter. Constitutional 'B' symptoms have also been reported to be associated with a poorer prognosis than is found in those patients without such symptoms. The difference in outlook between stage III and stage IV disease is now emphasised in several studies. In addition, a high incidence of CNS involvement appears to be a feature of those with bone marrow involvement (Lister et al 1978b). No studies have suggested any advantage for maintenance chemotherapy.

Key features which have been identified for further study are: chemotherapy alone in stage I and II disease; the use of more effective combinations to improve complete remission rates in stage III disease; more effective chemotherapy for stage IV disease, and the role of central nervous system prophylaxis. Finally, correlation of newer classifications, either cytologically or immunologically based, with response to therapy and disease characteristics, is required. A preliminary report from the NCI indicates that large cleaved-cell lymphomas have a good prognosis (Strauchen et al 1978). This is in contrast to another study which reports large non-cleaved cells as a majority group within the complete responders. Further detailed clinical trials are thus essential.

Central nervous system involvement

Involvement of the central nervous system is extremely rare in Hodgkin's disease, but is a recognised complication of the non-Hodgkin lymphoma. Young et al (1979a) reported that, of 445 patients with non-Hodgkin lymphoma, 38 (8.5%) developed this complication. This risk is highest in lymphoblastic and Burkitt lymphoma. The use of craniospinal prophylactic irradiation with or without intrathecal methotrexate was introduced on the basis of benefit observed in childhood acute lymphoblastic leukaemia. The advantage in patients with non-Hodgkin lymphoma is less easy to define. Young et al (1979b) have suggested that only 1.5% of patients with nodular lymphomas and 5% of those with diffuse lymphomas might benefit from prophylaxis. Anecdotal reports imply a reduced risk of central nervous system involvement in diffuse histiocytic lymphoma when treated with regimens containing either high-dose methotrexate or cytosine arabinoside.

Because radiotherapy given prophylactically to the CNS may compromise the ability to give adequate chemotherapy, it may be more appropriate to reserve cranial prophylaxis for the recognised high-risk groups. Alternative systemic regimes which may confer some degree of CNS protection are under investigation.

OVARIAN CARCINOMA

Despite the use of radiation therapy and cytotoxic chemotherapy there has been no improvement in the median survival of this disease in the past 30 years. It is increasing in incidence and its advanced state at diagnosis in 60% of patients means that it is the commonest fatal gynaecological malignancy.

There have been several changes in the therapy of this disease that may result in the improved survival of patients and this section will concentrate on these changes.

Radiotherapy

In a series of papers Dembo, Bush and their co-workers (1979) have reported on their randomised trials of extensive radiotherapy in stage I, II and asymptomatic III* ovarian cancer.

One hundred and ninety patients were randomly allocated according to the scheme shown in Figure 8.3. Patients with stage I or II underwent a three-way random allocation to groups in which pelvic radiotherapy (PEL) was compared with pelvic radiotherapy/chlorambucil (P + CB) or both pelvic + abdominal radiotherapy (P + AB). Patients with asymptomatic stage III disease were randomly allocated to groups receiving pelvic radiotherapy/chlorambucil or pelvic + abdominal radiotherapy only.

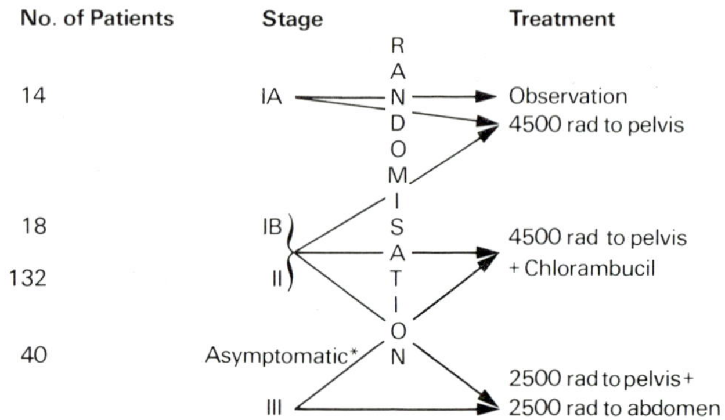

* Absence of pelvic or abdominal symptoms 4-6 weeks after operation.

Fig. 8.3 Randomisation scheme in the study reported by Bush et al (1979)

An interim analysis suggested that pelvic irradiation alone was inferior to the other two therapies; accrual to this group was therefore stopped after 43 patients had been entered. For the remaining 147 patients the trend for survival favours P + AB over P + CB (60% vs 45% surviving at 5 years) but is not significant ($P = 0.13$). However, if the group of patients who did not have a complete bilateral salpingo-oophorectomy and total abdominal hysterectomy (BSOH) is excluded, then a significant difference between P + CB and P + AB is seen. The 5-year survival rate for those completing BSOH (65.7%) is significantly better than for those not undergoing BSOH (23.7%) and this difference ($P < 0.005$) is independent of stage.

For those patients with incomplete BSOH there was no difference in the 5-year survival for each of the three treatments. In contrast, the survival of BSOH-completed patients is markedly influenced by the postoperative therapy. At 5 years, the actuarial survival rate of those patients is 81% for P + AB and only 51% for P + CB ($P = 0.02$). The 5-year survival of P + CB is no better than that for PEL and

---

*In this series asymptomatic is defined as the absence of abdominal or pelvic symptoms attributable to residual carcinoma or of ascites 4–6 weeks postoperatively.

the apparent superiority of P and CB, seen in an interim analysis, appears to represent a 10-month delay in time to relapse.

An analysis of the treatment failures in BSOH-completed patients shows that the failure rate in the pelvis was similar for all three treatments. However, when this pelvis was free of disease at relapse, only patients receiving P + AB had long-term control of upper abdominal disease. The addition of AB to pelvic irradiation controls occult abdominal disease in about 25% more BSOH patients than do the other two therapies. It is this significant ($P < 0.01$) reduction in isolated abdominal relapse that accounts for the improved survival rate for P + AB patients.

The trials described by Bush and Dembo underline the importance of the underestimation of the extent of disease in early-stage patients and the need to control abdominal disease as well as the pelvic tumour. It appears that pelvic and abdominal radiotherapy are capable of controlling residual disease provided that the tumour bulk is small.

Young and co-workers at the NCI (1978) have reported on a combination of drugs (Hexa-CAF) which appears to be superior to conventional alkylating agents in advanced disease (FIGO III and IV). All the alkylating agents are active in this disease, with an overall objective response rate of about 50%. Unfortunately most of these responses are incomplete and relatively short-lasting. The study by Young et al using a combination of hexamethylmelamine, cyclophosphamide, methotrexate and 5-fluorouracil has shown a significantly improved overall survival rate (75% vs 54%, $P < 0.05$) for the combination when compared with melphalan alone in a randomised study of 80 patients. The complete remission rate (surgically documented) was also better in the Hexa-CAF group (33% vs 16%), and the median survival (29 months vs 17 months, $P < 0.02$) favoured the combination group. Patients with minimal residual disease had a significantly higher response rate than those with extensive residual disease and the advantage in Hexa-CAF patients was best seen in those with tumours of histological grades 2 and 3. This study is the first to show that a drug combination is more effective than a single alkylating agent, but it must be remembered that the complete pathological remission rate for Hexa-CAF is only 33% and most of the patients have died of their disease.

Platinum-based combinations (Williams et al 1982) have been reported to give high response rates in advanced disease and are now being tested in randomised trials. It seems likely that combination chemotherapy will be used in advanced disease, but this treatment must be used with caution in view of the increased toxicity and lack of randomised trials defining the most active regimens and the best ways to use them.

TERATOMAS

Despite their apparent rarity testicular teratomas are the most common malignant tumour in young adult men (15–39 years). Their incidence is increasing in Western countries, although no clear causal factor apart from maldescent of the testis has been identified. Although the great majority of teratomas are testicular in origin, the tumour may also arise in the mediastinum, abdomen and ovary. Detailed reviews of this subject can be found in the proceedings of the Boerhaare course in 1980.

The major changes and improvements in the management of this disease have concerned better staging, the introduction of routine tumour markers and more active antineoplastic chemotherapy. Various staging systems have been used in the past and new classifications are being introduced. The main aim of these classifications is to subdivide patients by disease bulk as well as by site, large volume abdominal disease thus representing a worse prognostic factor than minimal lung disease. Table 8.9 outlines a recently reported classification which attempts to rationalise the staging and consequent treatment in testicular teratomas.

Table 8.9 Staging classification for testicular teratoma (Royal Marsden)

Royal Marsden Stage	Description
I	Lymphogram/CT scan negative, no evidence of metastases including AFP and β HCG
II	Lymphogram/CT scan positive, metastases confined to abdominal nodes, 3 subgroups recognised.
	A. Maximum diameter of metastases < 2 cm B. Maximum diameter of metastases 2–5 cm C. Maximum diameter of metastases > 5 cm
III	Involvement of supra- and infra-diaphragmatic lymph nodes. No extra lymphatic metastases. Abdominal status: A, B, C as for stage II.
IV	Extra-lymphatic metastases. Suffixes as follows: 0—lymphogram/CT scan negative; A,B,C as for stage II
	Lung status — $L_1 < 3$ metastases $L_2 < 2$ cm maximum diameter L_3 multiple > 2 cm diameter.
	Liver status — H + = Liver involvement

In addition to improved staging systems which reflect our better understanding of the natural history of the disease, the introduction of accurate and reproducible assays for β HCG and AFP have improved our ability to detect and follow disease. Either β HCG or AFP may be detected in teratomas and over 90% of patients with metastatic disease have one or both of these markers raised. In pure seminomas AFP levels are never increased although a few patients have slight increases in β HCG levels. The potential uses of these markers are outlined in Table 8.10. False-positive AFP and β HCG levels occur occasionally but can usually be excluded. Modest rises in β HCG may occur if testicular endocrine function is suppressed but this can be corrected with injections of depot testosterone.

Treatment of stage I and minimal stage II disease

Results of local therapy in these patients are good and most modern series quote 2-year disease-free survivals in excess of 85%. Relapse usually occurs within the first year and very rarely after 2 years. In the UK, local treatment (after an initial inguinal orchidectomy) is usually radiotherapy. This should be reserved for retroperitoneal disease of diameter less than 2 cm, treatment being given to the para-aortic lymph nodes and to the iliac lymph nodes on the side of the tumour. In the USA, further surgery is usually performed after orchidectomy. This comprises a total

Table 8.10 Potential uses of AFP and β HCG in the testicular teratomas

Diagnosis	1. Aid in the differential diagnosis of a scrotal mass if levels are elevated. Negative values do not obviate surgical exploration
	2. Elevated AFP does not occur in pure seminoma and an elevated βHCG may indicate poor prognosis in a seminoma
Staging	Persistently raised levels of βHCG and AFP after orchidectomy indicates metastatic disease. Normal markers should *not* prevent staging
During or after treatment	1. Serial measurements are invaluable for assessing the adequacy of local treatment in stage I or II disease. Persistently raised markers indicate extralymphatic disease
	2. Serial measurements are very helpful in assessing tumour response to chemotherapy. A graph of fall in β HCG and AFP should be compared with the expected fall calculated from the known half-life of the markers
	3. Normal markers (when previously raised) in the face of a persistent mass may indicate that the lesion has evolved into a benign teratoma. Surgical excision of such masses should normally be undertaken
	4. In patients in apparent complete remission rising markers are often the first sign of recurrent tumour

retroperitoneal lymphadenectomy; the surgery is major and includes dissection of retroperitoneal tissue from behind the great vessels below the renal arteries, ligation of the inferior mesenteric artery, and ligation of the lumbar arteries below the renal pedicles. Mortality and postoperative morbidity is low, reflecting the age of the patients, but the risk of retrograde ejaculation and subsequent sterility is high. Modifications of surgical approach based on histopathological studies of the spread of testicular teratoma suggest that a more limited unilateral approach may be appropriate, reducing the risk of retrograde ejaculation.

Some studies of adjuvant chemotherapy after surgical or radiotherapeutic treatment of early-stage patients have begun. There is little indication that such treatment is currently needed, as with careful follow-up the small proportion who do relapse ($<15\%$) should be curable with modern combination chemotherapy. With present staging techniques and treatment the survival rate of these patients should approach 100%.

Treatment of advanced stage II and minimal stage III and IV

In the USA, patients with advanced stage II (without disease above the diaphragm) undergo laparotomy and an attempt to excise all tumour. This surgery is usually followed by combination chemotherapy. In Britain, patients with this type of disease receive combination chemotherapy because radiotherapy is of much less use in patients with bulky retroperitoneal disease (>2 cm in diameter). For patients with minimal disease above the diaphragm the initial treatment, in the USA and Europe, is combination chemotherapy. Combination chemotherapy has improved greatly during the past 20 years, starting with the combinations of Li in the early 1960s and the development of highly active combinations by Samuels and Einhorn in the 1970s. Results obtained by Einhorn, the Memorial Sloan-Kettering group and the Charing Cross group suggest that intensive chemotherapy regimens including cis diamminedichloroplatinum are capable of producing complete clearance of all detectable disease (including markers) in about 60–70% of cases.

After chemotherapy, a proportion of patients have detectable disease. Excision of such masses shows that about one-third are mature teratoma, one-third are fibrous tissue and one-third are malignant teratoma. In Einhorn's series, results of further chemotherapy in those patients found to have persisting malignant teratoma have not been encouraging, although others have claimed good responses in these patients.

The platinum, vinblastine and bleomycin regime of Einhorn remains particularly toxic, despite the reduction in the initial dose of vinblastine. The multidrug regimens used by several other groups are claimed to be less toxic although no results are available from controlled trials comparing the toxicity and antitumour effects of current regimens. With current chemotherapy, between 45–55% of patients are alive and disease-free after 2 years. Most relapses occur in the group with very advanced bulky disease.

Treatment of bulky stage IV disease

Those patients with bulky disease and liver disease have a lower initial response rate and overall survival. Although most patients initially respond to the current drug regimens, complete remissions are less frequent and early relapse is common. Chemotherapy is the mainstay of treatment and new and more active regimens are needed. Despite poorer results in these patients, combination chemotherapy must be given because a proportion (40%) do well on current regimens.

Areas of change

The major subjects of debate regarding the testicular teratomas are:

1. Whether further treatment (beyond orchidectomy) is required for a patient with a stage I tumour which has been carefully staged.
2. Whether adjuvant chemotherapy should be given to patients with minimal spread of disease following potentially curative surgery or radiotherapy. Some groups in the USA are using adjuvant chemotherapy in these patients, whereas others are waiting till relapse occurs (in probably less than 15% of the patients) and then treating with intensive chemotherapy. It will not be possible to use controlled trials to test these two philosophies as the number of patients relapsing is small and in a rare disease there will be too few patients to run studies.
3. The role of surgery and, in Europe, radiotherapy, after intensive chemotherapy remains unsettled. Most centres recommend surgery for persistent masses after chemotherapy, provided that there is no evidence of active disease. The key to possible benefits from this surgery lies in the results obtained in the one-third of

patients shown to have active tumour. Good results, with further chemotherapy, in these patients will be an incentive to pursue this type of surgery.

4. The need to reduce the toxicity of current intensive drug regimens. This is particularly important in those with minimal metastatic disease and for those trials using intensive adjuvant chemotherapy.

5. The need for more effective drug regimens for patients with very advanced disease.

Mediastinal teratomas are rare and no large series are available. The principles of management are similar to those for the testicular teratomas but early results suggest that mediastinal teratomas are less easily eradicated. Teratomas of the ovary are also less common than those of the testis and several recent studies using regimes developed for testicular tumours have shown response rates and survival data similar to those reported in testicular tumour.

SMALL-CELL BRONCHOGENIC CARCINOMA (SCBS)

The histological cell type, extent of tumour dissemination and performance status are the most important prognostic features in patients with lung cancer. Small-cell lung cancer (see Table 8.11 for WHO classification) accounts for about a quarter of the cases of carcinoma of the bronchus diagnosed each year.

Table 8.11 WHO classification of bronchogenic carcinoma

Stage	Description
I	Epidermoid (squamous)
II	Small-cell anaplastic
	1. Fusiform
	2. Polygonal
	3. Lymphocyte-like
	4. Others
III	Adenocarcinoma
IV	Large-cell carcinoma

During the past decade, the importance of a correct histological diagnosis has become more obvious as it has been shown that the natural history and response to therapy of this type of lung cancer differs markedly from those of the other types. Although small-cell carcinoma of the lung has been divided into several subtypes, there is no evidence that there is any biological or therapeutic rationale for this.

Although the extent of disease in lung cancer is usually defined according to the TNM system this has not been found to be useful in SCBC. Instead, a crude system of limited or extensive disease is used. Limited disease is defined as disease confined to one hemithorax, with or without mediastinal adenopathy and with or without ipsilateral supraclavicular nodes. Extensive disease is any tumour beyond these limits.

The prognosis of untreated SCBC is very poor; in a VA Lung Study Group trial of supportive care only, the survival in 118 patients with limited or extensive disease was 3.1 and 1.4 months respectively. In most patients surgery has not been beneficial, because of the rapid and extensive spread of the tumour. In an autopsy study of patients dying (of non-tumour related causes) within 30 d of an apparently 'curative' resection of SCBC, 70% of patients had distant metastases and a similar percentage had recurrent local tumour. Most surgical series have reported very low 5-year survival rates and routine resection of SCBC has been abandoned. However, in patients presenting with solitary peripheral lesions (SCBC is usually central in origin) resection is capable of achieving a 30% 5-year survival rate. Such patients should probably receive chemotherapy after surgery. These patients are few and far between and, with good staging, few patients technically are resectable by current surgical criteria. Detailed references to all aspects of SCBC are included at the end of the chapter.

Staging

Staging of this tumour has an important bearing on the selection of therapy and is helpful in indicating the investigations necessary to confirm a complete remission. CT scans of the thorax have been very useful in assessing the extent of local tumour in the thorax. Fibreoptic bronchoscopy is used by some centres and is useful in the reassessment of tumour response. Up to 60% of patients with SCBC have hepatic involvement at autopsy. One study has shown that abnormal SGOT, bilirubin and alkaline phosphatase levels indicate liver metastases. If only one or two of these tests is abnormal the accuracy of predicting liver involvement is reduced. Ultrasonic liver scans are more useful than isotope liver scans, which have been disappointing. CT scans of the liver are still being evaluated and experimental techniques such as

Table 8.12 Staging procedures for SCBC (modified from Ihde, Hansen et al 1980)

	Routine	Special clinical indication
Intrathoracic		
CXR	*	
CT scan	* (if available)	
Thoracocentesis and cytology		*
Fibreoptic bronchoscopy		*
Mediastinoscopy/thoracoscopy		*
Extrathoracic		
Hepatic		
Biochemical liver function tests	*	
CT scan	* (if available)	
Ultrasound	*	
Peritoneoscopy with biopsy		*
Bone		
Peripheral blood examination	*	
Bone marrow aspirate/biopsy	*	
Isotope bone scans	*	
Skeletal X-rays		*
CNS		
CT scan	* (if available)	
LP with cytology		*
Myelogram		*
Other sites		
CT scan of the abdomen	* (if available)	

peritoneoscopy with liver biopsy have been useful but are too cumbersome for routine staging.

Bone marrow involvement has occurred in about 20% of patients in recent series, and a bone marrow aspirate and biopsy are recommended. Bone disease is best assessed by an isotope scan and a skeletal survey is not necessary. Up to 10% of patients present with CNS involvement, but these can be detected by a careful history and physical examination. There is little evidence that routine staging brain scans or lumbar punctures are useful in detecting occult cases although in one study CT scans revealed occult metastases in 7.4% of 81 patients.

Other metastatic sites (pancreas, adrenals, abdominal lymph nodes) are probably best assessed by CT scan if this is available. A suggested schema for staging SCBC is shown in Table 8.12.

Treatment

Radiotherapy in a controlled trial (Medical Research Council) was little better than surgery, even in patients with apparently operable cancer. Although the radiation appeared to control local disease within the irradiation portal, it soon became apparent that failure in the irradiated site was common if the patient survived long enough.

There are few randomised trials of single-agent chemotherapy but those that have been reported show a modest advantage for chemotherapy over no treatment. During the past 10 years there have been numerous studies of combination chemotherapy and the improvement in survival, both for limited and extensive disease, is largely due to the development of more active drug therapy. The results of therapy with various single agents is shown in Table 8.13.

Table 8.13 Single agent chemotherapy in SCBC (adapted from Broder 1977 and Ihde & Bunn 1982)

A. Drugs with established activity (objective responses in > 15% of minimum of 40 patients: active in two studies of 10 or more patients)

Drug	No. of patients	Objective responses %
VP16-213	201	44
Nitrogen mustard	55	44
Vincristine	43	42
Cyclophosphamide	636	38
Adriamycin (doxorubicin)	53	30
Methotrexate	73	30
Hexamethylmelamine	69	30

B. Drugs with probable activity (objective responses in > 15% but not meeting above conditions)

Drug	No. of patients	Objective responses %
Ifosfamide	14	85
Procarbazine	19	47
Methyl CCNU	19	26
Dibromodulcitol	17	24
BCNU	15	20
CCNU	76	14

Although no formal studies have tested the impact of increasing the number of drugs in chemotherapy combinations for SCBC, the evidence available suggests that optimum combinations contain three or four drugs. Studies testing intensive regimens against low-dose regimens indicate that drugs should preferably be given at high dose, although such trials can be used only as a rough guideline because the results are valid only for the combinations being tested. A recent trial of very intensive therapy showed no benefit, but increased toxicity, when compared with the same drugs given in a conventional high dose. Despite this, by taking three or four of the active drugs in Table 8.14 and using them at maximally tolerated doses, it has been possible to obtain complete remissions in SCBC and to improve survival. However, most patients eventually relapse and, for this reason, several groups have tested the addition of alternate courses of non-cross-resistant drug regimens. This has shown some benefit but it has been small; it remains to be proved that this approach is useful. Table 8.14 shows the results in compiled chemotherapy series between 1975–1980. About half the patients with limited disease achieve complete remission, whereas less than one-third of patients with extensive disease become clinically free of disease. The median survival in many current series is in excess of 1 year for patients with limited disease and about 10 months for those with extensive disease. More important, some patients are now surviving for more than 2 years and remain free of disease. Weiss (1980) has collected a substantial number of patients who have survived for more than 2 years in complete remission and although most trials do not report data in this way, 2-year disease-free survival is probably the best indicator of superior therapies.

The role, intensity and duration of maintenance therapy are uncertain. Many investigators give prolonged (2-year) maintenance therapy, often using modest drug doses to avoid toxicity. Such low-dose maintenance is theoretically suspect because high drug doses may be needed to eradicate a small tumour burden. In addition, some studies not using maintenance have produced survival equivalent to that in similar studies that differ only in the duration of therapy. Table 8.15 shows the results of treatment with vincristine, Adriamycin (doxorubicin) and cyclophosphamide and radiotherapy. The only difference between the three studies was the duration of the treatment.

Chemotherapy was originally introduced as an adjuvant to radiotherapy but trials are now testing whether radiotherapy improves the results of chemotherapy alone. There is little evidence that radiotherapy improves the results achieved with drug therapy in extensive disease. In limited disease some of the best results have been in trials using both radiotherapy and chemotherapy early in the course of treatment (Table 8.14). Excellent results have also been reported with chemotherapy alone, and randomised trials testing the role of radiotherapy are under way. Most trials have used relatively low doses of radiation (3000 rad in 10 fractions over 14d) and new studies of more intensive radiotherapy are also being conducted. A further area of study is how to time the administration of radiotherapy and chemotherapy to achieve maximal benefit whilst avoiding the toxicity seen in the study of Johnson et al (1978).

Prophylactic brain irradiation has been shown to be effective in preventing CNS relapse; however, it is best reserved for patients who obtain a complete remission. Such radiotherapy will be shown to contribute to improved survival only if a substantial proportion of patients achieve 2-year disease-free survival.

Although there have been great improvements in the treatment of SCBC in the

Table 8.14 Effectiveness of combination chemotherapy in SCBC (after Ihde & Bunn 1982)

	Limited disease				Extensive disease				
No. of trials	No. of patients	Mean CR(%)	Mean med. surv.	% Mean 2-yr disease-free surv.	No. of trials	No. of patients	Mean CR(%)	Mean med. surv.	% Mean 2-yr disease-free surv.
3 drugs									
3	88	44	8.5	6	11	364	27	7.0	1
4 drugs									
2	84	27	10.0	0	9	286	27	8.5	1
5 + drugs (usually sequential combinations)									
3	74	59	11.5	9	4	147	34	9.0	7

Table 8.15 Results of varying duration of therapy in limited SCBC

Authors	Duration of therapy (months)	No. of patients	Med. survival (months)	% 2-year disease-free surv.
Johnson et al 1978	3–4	36	18.5	28
Greco et al 1979	14	32	17	25
Einhorn et al 1978	24	19	17	26

past decade, the rate of progress has slowed during the past 3 years. New drugs and approaches are needed. Further studies of sequential non-cross-resistant drug regimes are being conducted. Drugs may also be selected according to the results obtained from assays in vitro (p. 166) although the validity of this approach has not yet been confirmed. Another area of interest is the use of very high doses of drugs, with or without whole-body radiotherapy, and autologous bone marrow transplantation. Anecdotal reports of success with this approach encourage formal trials. Further trials of radical radiotherapy and intensive chemotherapy in localised disease continue. When considering the use of these expensive and toxic treatments, it is worth remembering that the majority of SCBCs are directly related to cigarette smoking.

REFERENCES

Methods of selecting anticancer drugs for clinical use

Salmon S E (ed) 1980 Cloning of human tumour stem cells. Alan Liss, New York

Salmon S E, Von Hoff D D, Williams C J 1982 In vitro evaluation of anti-cancer drugs with the human tumour stem cell assay. Williams C J, Whitehouse J M A (eds). In: Recent advances in clinical oncology 1. Churchill Livingstone, Edinburgh

Cis-diamminedichloroplatinum (DDP)

Prestayko A W, Crooke S T, Carter S K 1980 Cisplatin: current status and new developments. Academic Press, New York

VP16-213

Proceedings of the First International Symposium on the Epipodophyllotoxins. Southampton 1981 Cancer Chemotherapy and Pharmacology Vol 7, 1982

Acute myelogenous leukaemia

Blackstock A M, Garson O M 1974 Direct evidence for involvement of erythroid cells in acute myeloblastic leukaemia. Lancet 2: 1178–1179

Clarkson B D, Dowling M D, Gee T S, Cunningham I B, Burchenal J H 1975 Treatment of acute leukaemia in adults. Cancer 36 (supplement 2): 775–795

Crowther D, Powles R L, Bateman C J T, Beard M E J, Gauci C L, Wrigley P F M et al 1973 Management of adult acute myelogenous leukaemia. British Medical Journal 1: 131

Curtis J E, Cowan D H, Bergsagel D E, Hasselback R, McCulloch E A 1975 Acute leukaemia in adults: assessment of remission induction with combination chemotherapy by clinical and cell culture criteria. Canadian Medical Association Journal 113: 289–294

Gale R P, Cline M J 1977 High remission induction rate in acute myeloid leukaemia. Lancet 1: 497–499

MRC Council Report 1974 Treatment of acute myeloid leukaemia with daunorubicin, cytosine arabinoside, mercaptopurine, L-asparaginase, prednisolone and thioguanine. Results of treatment with five multiple drug schedules. British Journal of Haematology 27: 373–389

Preisler H D, Bjornsson S, Henderson E 1977 Protected environment unit in the treatment of acute leukaemia. Seminars in Oncolology 2: 369–377

Rosenthal D S, Moloney W C 1972 The treatment of acute granulocytic leukaemia in adults. New England Journal Medicine 286: 1176–1182

Trujillo J M, Cork A, Hart J S, George S L, Freireich E J 1974 Clinical implications of aneuploid cytogenetic profiles in adult acute leukaemia. Cancer 33: 824–834

Weinstein H J, Mayer R J, Rosenthal D S, Camitta B M, Coral F S, Nathan D G et al 1980 Treatment of acute myelogenous leukaemia in children and adults. New England Journal of Medicine 303: 473–478

Whitecar J P, Bodey G P, Freireich E J, McCredie K B, Hart J S 1972 Cyclophosphamide (NSC-26271), vincristine (NSC-67574), cytosine arabinoside, (NSC-63878) and prednisolone (NSC-10023) (COAP) combination chemotherapy in acute leukaemia in adults. Cancer Chemotherapy Reports 56: 543–550

Yates J W, Holland J F 1973 A controlled study of isolation and endogenous microbial suppression in acute myelocytic leukaemia patients. Cancer 32: 1490–1498

Lymphomas

Bonadonna G, Fossati V, De Lena M 1978 MOPP vs MOPP plus ABVD in stage IV Hodgkin's disease. Proceedings of the American Association for Cancer Research 19: 363

Kaye S B, Juttner C A, Smith I E et al 1979 British Journal of Cancer 39: 168

Krikorian J G, Burke J S, Rosenberg S A, Kaplan H S 1979 Occurrence of non-Hodgkin's lymphoma after therapy for Hodgkin's disease. New England Journal of Medicine 300: 452–458

Lister T A, Cullen M H, Beard M E J, Brearley R L, Whitehouse J M A, Wrigley P F M et al 1978a Comparison of combined and single-agent chemotherapy in non-Hodgkin's lymphoma of favourable histological type. British Medical Journal 1: 533–537

Lister T A, Cullen M H, Brearley R B, Beard M E J, Stansfeld A G, Whitehouse J M A et al 1978b Combination chemotherapy for advanced non-Hodgkin's lymphoma of unfavourable histology. Cancer Chemotherapy and Pharmacology 1: 107–112

Miller T P, Jones S E 1979 Chemotherapy of localised histiocytic lymphoma. Lancet 1: 358–360

Nicholson W M et al 1970 Combination chemotherapy in generalized Hodgkin's disease. British Medical Journal 3: 7–10

Rosenberg S A, Kaplan H S, Brown B W 1979 In: Jones S E Salmon S E (eds) Adjuvant therapy of cancer II. Grune and Stratton, New York, p 109

Santoro A, Bonadonna G 1979 Prolonged disease-free survival in MOPP-resistant Hodgkin's disease after treatment with adriamycin, bleomycin, vinblastine and dacarbazine (ABVD). Cancer Chemotherapy and Pharmacology 2: 101–105

Stein R S, Golomb H M, Ultman J E, Wiernik P H, Diggs C, Hellman S et al 1979 Anatomic substages of stage III Hodgkin's disease (HD): a collaborative study. Proceedings of the American Association for Cancer Research 20: C-614, 438

Strauchen J A, Young R C, De Vita V T, Anderson T, Fantone J C, Berard C W 1978 Clinical relevance of the histopathological subclassification of diffuse 'histiocytic' lymphoma. New England Journal of Medicine 299: 1182–1387

Valagussa P, Santoro A, Kenda R, Fossati Bellani F, Franchi F, Banfi A et al 1980 Second malignancies in Hodgkin's disease: a complication of certain forms of treatment. British Medical Journal 1: 216–219

Young R C, Howser D M, Anderson T, Jaffe E, De Vita V T 1979a CNS infiltration: a complication of diffuse lymphomas in CNS complications of malignant disease. In: Whitehouse J M A, Kay H E M (eds). Macmillan, London, Ch 11, pp 121–130

Young R C, Howser D M, Anderson A et al 1979b CNS complications of non-Hodgkins lympyhoma: a potential role for prophylactic therapy. American Journal of Medicine 66: 435

Ovarian carcinoma

Dembo A J, Bush R S, Beale F A, Bean H A, Pringle J F, Sturgeon J et al 1979 Ovarian carcinoma: improved survival following abdomino-pelvic irradiation in patients with a completed pelvic operation. American Journal of Obstetrics and Gynecology 134: 793-800

Williams C J, Mead G M, Arnold A, Green J, Buchanan R, Whitehouse J M A 1982 Chemotherapy of advanced ovarian carcinoma: initial experience using a platinum-based combination. Cancer 49: 1778- 1783

Young R C, Chabner B A, Hubbard S P, Fisher R I, Bender A A, Anderson T et al 1978 Advanced ovarian adenocarcinoma: a prospective clinical trial of melphalan (L-PAM) versus combination chemotherapy. New England Journal of Medicine 299: 1261–1266

Teratomas

Van Oosterom A T, Muggia F M, Cleton F J (eds) 1980 Therapeutic progress in ovarian cancer, testicular cancer and the sarcomas. Leiden University Press, The Hague

Small-cell bronchogenic carcinoma

Arnold A M, Williams C J 1979 Small cell lung cancer: a curable disease? British Journal of Diseases of the Chest 73: 327–347

Bunn P A 1977 Advances in small cell bronchogenic carcinoma. Cancer Treatment Reports 61: 333–342

Einhorn L H, Bond W H, Hornbank N, Beng-Tek J 1978 Long-term results in combined-modality treatment of small cell carcinoma of the lung. Seminars in Oncology 5: 309–313

Greco F A, Richardson R L, Snell J D, Stroup S L, Oldham R K 1979 Small cell lung cancer: complete remission and improved survival. American Journal of Medicine 66: 625–630

Johnson R E, Brereton H D, Kent C H 1978 Total therapy for small cell carcinoma of the lung. Annals of Thoracic Surgery 25: 510–515

Weiss R B 1980 Small cell carcinoma of the lung. Journal of the American Society of Haematology 56: 575–584

9

Renal disease

R. Wilkinson

URINARY TRACT INFECTION

This subject was thoroughly reviewed in the last edition of this book and only subsequent developments will be described here.

Treatment of asymptomatic urinary tract infection

In *non-pregnant women and girls without renal scarring* and without vesicoureteric reflux, treatment of asymptomatic infections is not necessary. Renal function and renal growth are not affected by withholding treatment, and symptomatic infections are not prevented by giving treatment (Cardiff-Oxford Bacteriuria Study Group 1978). Indeed, Asscher has suggested that all that may be achieved by treatment is the replacement of an asymptomatic by a symptomatic infection. Furthermore, as the infection has cleared spontaneously in about one-third of women when reviewed at 1 year (Asscher et al 1969) and 50% of those initially cured by treatment are again infected at 1 year, little is achieved by the treatment.

In *pregnancy,* the value of treatment of asymptomatic bacteriuria is, of course, well established (Kass 1960) and has been shown to reduce the risk of acute pyelonephritis.

With regard to *older women,* about 10% of those aged 60 years have asymptomatic bacteriuria. The usual approach to this is, as in younger women, to withold treatment although a single attempt at clearing the infection is often made. This approach may have to be changed in the light of the observation that survival is significantly reduced in the elderly bacteriuric patient (Dontas et al 1981), although it was not possible to be certain from this study whether the urinary infection was the cause of death or simply a consequence of the debility that contributed to earlier death. Clearly, controlled trials of treatment of asymptomatic bacteriuria in the elderly are required to resolve this issue.

Urinary infection in patients with renal scarring

In *children with vesicoureteric reflux,* sterilisation of the urine with continuous low-dose nitrofurantoin or trimethoprim–sulphamethoxazole allows normal renal growth in the majority of cases. Furthermore, there is spontaneous resolution of the reflux in most cases (Edwards et al 1977). Thus, there is universal agreement that even asymptomatic infections should be treated in this group of patients.

In *adults with scarred kidneys* the causative vesicoureteric reflux has usually resolved, and progressive scarring of the kidneys and deterioration of renal function is usually very slow (Gower 1976). However, frequent and persistent urinary infection is associated with poorer prognosis and it is normally considered to be advisable to treat even asymptomatic infections arising in these patients, in the hope of preventing progression of the renal damage.

This distinction between the recommended management of asymptomatic infections in patients with and without renal scarring gives a purpose to the investigation of patients with urinary tract infection.

Investigation of patients with urinary infection

Adults without renal scars at the outset will not develop scarring as a result of infection unless a calculus or obstruction develops; their symptoms may be treated by their family doctor, as necessary: Those patients with renal scarring, however, require hospital follow-up with regular screening for asymptomatic infection, culture before and after a course of treatment, and monitoring of renal function and blood pressure because approximately 70% of such patients will eventually develop hypertension.

If the need for detecting renal scars is accepted, how can this can be achieved with reasonable economy and minimal unnecessary irradiation? If an intravenous urogram (IVU) were to be performed in all adult women with asymptomatic urinary infection, approximately 18% would show abnormalities (Sussman et al 1969). To improve this yield the suggestions made in the last edition remain reasonable i.e. an IVU should be performed in a woman with any of the following:

1. A history of urinary infection or persistent enuresis in childhood
2. Proteinuria between infections
3. Raised plasma urea or creatinine levels
4. Relapse after an adequate course of antibacterial therapy
5. Three definite episodes of urinary tract infection in adult life.

Even a negative IVU is of practical value in that it enables one to decide to manage the patient outside the sphere of a hospital clinic.

THE TREATMENT OF GLOMERULONEPHRITIS

Glomerulonephritis occurring without evidence of systemic disease is still a condition for which there is no satisfactory treatment.

Membranous nephropathy

There have been reports of apparent temporal relationships between remission and steroid treatment in patients with membranous glomerulonephritis. A recent study has shown a reduction in the number of patients progressing to renal failure over a 3-year period following a 2-month course of prednisone 2 mg/kg (maximum 120 mg) on alternate days (Collaborative Study 1979). However, 25% of patients with this condition remit spontaneously and it is therefore clearly necessary to repeat the Collaborative Study protocol in an unselected, previously untreated group of patients with idiopathic membranous nephritis; such a study has been started under the auspices of the British Medical Research Council. Until clear evidence of benefit from steroid or immunosuppressive drugs becomes available, such treatment should be reserved for the unusual patient with severe nephrotic syndrome in whom the combination of diuretics, sodium restriction and high-protein diet does not adequately control oedema, or for patients in whom renal function is deteriorating. If high doses of steroid are given they should be stopped after 2 months if there is no evidence of improvement.

Rapidly progressive 'crescentic' nephritis

Most interest recently has been directed towards the treatment of rapidly progressive, 'crescentic', nephritis which, when untreated, commonly leads to irreversible renal failure. Previous treatments consisted of various combinations of steroids, immunosuppressives, anticoagulants and antiplatelet agents. The technique of plasmapheresis in combination with prednisone and cyclophosphamide has been applied with success to the treatment of patients with rapidly progressive glomerulonephritis attributable to circulating anti-glomerular basement membrane antibodies (GBM) which includes most cases of Goodpasture's syndrome, (Lockwood et al 1976, Kincaid Smith & d'Apice 1978). Although the efficacy of the technique has not been demonstrated by controlled trial in this condition (and because of the clear benefits observed will probably never be subjected to this test), it is now in general use for the treatment of anti-GBM nephritis. This has led to its use, again in an uncontrolled way and again with apparent success, in the treatment of crescentic glomerulonephritis associated with immune-complex deposition in the glomeruli and without anti-GBM antibody (Lockwood et al 1977, Harmer et al 1979). However, plasmapheresis is not without risk: vascular access with its attendant risks is necessary for the procedure; arrhythmias may occur during the exchange, and bleeding complications afterwards, because of depletion of clotting factors. Although recently reported studies of plasmapheresis in immune-complex nephritis (Ahmad et al 1981, Russ & d'Apice 1981) have shown overall benefit, they have included patients with systemic disease (systemic lupus, polyarteritis, Wegener's granulomatosis), and it is not clear whether patients with disease limited to the kidney have obtained similar benefit. Our present policy is to limit this treatment to patients who have rapidly deteriorating renal function and who, on renal biopsy, have more than 70% of glomeruli with crescents. The wider application of this treatment is really justified only as part of a controlled trial. However, the practical difficulties of such a trial are immense. Because of the rarity of the condition, a multicentre, and probably even a multinational, study would be required, with all the attendant problems. We may therefore expect a trend towards the use of plasmapheresis combined with immunosuppression in more and more mild cases of crescentic nephropathy, despite the paucity of firm evidence of its beneficial effects.

Wegener's granulomatosis

This may lead to renal failure, with crescents histologically indistinguishable from the changes seen in patients with rapidly progressive glomerulonephritis without extrarenal disease. However, Wegener's granulomatosis responds well to immunosuppressive drugs without plasmapheresis (Fauci et al 1978).

Polyarteritis nodosa

Polyarteritis nodosa also may be responsible for crescentic nephropathy. Although the response to steroid and immunosuppressive drugs is not as consistent in this condition as that seen in Wegener's granulomatosis, dramatic responses to treatment with cyclophosphamide and steroids have been reported (Fauci et al 1979).

Systemic lupus erythematosis (SLE)

SLE can be shown by renal biopsy to involve the kidney to some extent in more than 95% of cases (Mahajan et al 1977). There is clinical evidence of renal disease in approximately 50% of cases at presentation and, on follow-up, about 75% develop proteinuria or deterioration of renal function.

Diagnosis of renal lupus

The only histological feature which is almost pathognomic of SLE is the haematoxylin body and this, in our experience, is so rarely seen that it can almost be discounted. The diagnosis is therefore made from the finding of anti-double-strand DNA antibody in serum, or less specifically by the presence of antinuclear antibody in serum, or with less sensitivity and specificity by a positive LE cell test in blood (positive in only 65% of patients with SLE). The renal histological changes are not specific for SLE: however, if immunofluorescent or peroxidase staining techniques demonstrate the presence of unexpected numbers of immunoglobulins and complement components, this should make one consider the diagnosis of SLE, as should the finding of a lowered serum complement (Williams 1981).

There are several histological types of renal lupus which differ in their course, and in their need for and response to treatment, as described below.

The mesangial type accounts for approximately 15% of cases. There is immunoglobulin and complement deposition in the mesangium, associated with little or no change on light microscopy, and little or no abnormality in the urine. No treatment is required.

The focal proliferative type also accounts for about 15% of cases. There is more widespread deposition of immunoglobulins and complement, affecting the capillary wall as well as the mesangium, and leading to endothelial as well as mesangial proliferation with resultant proteinuria and haematuria in most cases. Treatment would be indicated only for the unusual patient in whom deterioration of renal function or troublesome nephrotic syndrome developed.

The membranous pattern of renal involvement is also seen in approximately 15% of patients. There is subepithelial immunoglobulin and complement deposition, as seen in other forms of membranous nephritis. Light microscopy shows that there is diffuse thickening of the basement membrane. All patients have proteinuria and the majority develop the nephrotic syndrome. Treatment of the membranous form is ineffective and should be withheld.

Diffuse proliferative glomerulonephritis is seen in about 50% of cases of lupus nephritis and the other forms may progress to this. There are diffuse mesangial, sub-endothelial and subepithelial deposits of IgG, IgM, C3, C4 and sometimes IgA, leading to the characteristic light-microscopic picture of diffuse proliferative changes with wire loops and, in severe cases, necrotising lesions and epithelial crescents. Proteinuria and haematuria is almost universal in these patients: some develop nephrotic syndrome and some, progressive renal failure. Unfortunately, it is not possible to predict, even from the severity of the histological changes, which patients will progress to renal insufficiency (Cameron et al 1979), although the presence of subendothelial deposits appears to signify a poor prognosis (Hecht et al 1976). Serological tests are an equally unreliable means of identifying those patients with active disease who will progress (Williams 1981).

Steroids

Steroid drugs have been shown to be of value in proliferative lupus nephritis (Baldwin et al 1977, Donadio et al 1978). However, even with steroid treatment, the 5-year survival in patients with this type of lesion was only about 25% in those treated before 1970 (Pollak et al 1973) and is still only 40–60% in patients treated more recently (Donadio et al 1978, Cameron et al 1979, Decker 1979).

Cytotoxic agents

Because of the poor results of treatment with steroids used alone, combinations of prednisolone and azathioprine or cyclophosphamide have been used. Unfortunately, the addition of the cytotoxic agents probably does not affect the long-term outcome (Donadio et al 1981) despite earlier encouraging reports. In view of this, the improvement in survival since 1970 may be attributable merely to the acquisition of greater skill in the use of steroids. Whether or not azathioprine improves the prognosis when added to prednisolone therapy, it is of value in that it enables the dose level of steroids to be reduced, with a concomitant reduction in side effects, while itself causing few problems if used with care. Cyclophosphamide, however, is not suitable as a steroid-sparing agent because its prolonged use is associated with serious side effects including gonadal damage, haemorrhagic cystitis, and bladder and other cancers. Nevertheless, cyclophosphamide may be more effective than azathioprine and probably has a role when it is given as a short course (up to 8 weeks) with prednisolone in patients with rapidly progressive disease.

Methylprednisolone pulse therapy

In severe cases with rapidly deteriorating renal function, increasing serum creatinine, or signs of activity of SLE in other systems, in conjunction with proliferative glomerulonephritis, treatment with methylprednisolone (1 g doses infused over 30 min on 3 consecutive days) followed by oral prednisolone with or without cyclophosphamide, has been reported in uncontrolled studies to be beneficial (Ponticelli et al 1981).

Plasmapheresis. Plasmapheresis has also been used, with promising results, in patients with severe proliferative lupus nephritis (Russ & d'Apice 1981).

Treatment decisions

It is easy to decide to treat the patient with deteriorating function or nephrotic syndrome. However, even patients with diffuse proliferative lupus nephritis may have stable renal function and little proteinuria, and these patients do not require specific therapy. Early warning of activity of disease may be given by falling serum complement and rising anti-double-strand DNA antibody titre, but unfortunately these measures may be misleading and should be taken as an indication for closer surveillance rather than for action, treatment being introduced only when proteinuria increases or renal function begins to decline.

It can also be difficult to decide when to reduce or to stop treatment. The serological tests can be helpful, and repeat renal biopsy may also be of value.

The management of SLE remains difficult, therefore, but there has been an improvement in the overall 5-year survival rate for patients with SLE, from 70% before 1968 to 93% in 1977 (Cameron 1977).

DIABETES AND THE KIDNEY

The death rate in diabetics in middle age is two to six times greater than that of the general population, mainly because of an increase in cardiovascular and renal disease (Marks & Krall 1971). Uraemia causes about one-third of deaths (Deckert et al 1978). However, renal disease does not occur inevitably in diabetics and many long-surviving diabetics are free of nephropathy. The reason for this is not clear but several factors have been identified.

Structural changes in the kidney in diabetes

Enlargement

The kidneys are found to be enlarged in the early stages of diabetes (Mogensen & Andersen 1975). This is accompanied by an increase in glomerular size with a consequent increase in the total volume of basement-membrane material and an increase in glomerular filtration rate of about 25%, which persists until diabetic nephropathy develops and renal function deteriorates, although it can be normalised by insulin treatment.

Diabetic glomerulosclerosis

The development of diabetic renal disease is based on microangiopathy. The basement membrane (BM) is of normal thickness at the onset of juvenile diabetes (Østerby 1975); 2 years later there has been an increase in thickness of about 15% and this thickening progresses over the years. At the same time there is enlargement of the mesangium. Ultimately, after a mean of about 20 years in those juvenile-onset diabeties in those who are to develop renal disease, capillary closure becomes extensive and renal function begins to decline. The precise biochemical abnormality leading to the thickening of the basement membrane is not known, but it has been shown that in animals it can be prevented by diabetic control (Rasch 1979). However, once established it is not reversed, even when the diabetes is cured by islet-cell transplantation (Maurer et al, in press).

Proteinuria in diabetes

In the very early stages of diabetes an increase in urinary albumin excretion can be detected, which is above that in normal subjects (usually less than 1.5 mg/dl) although it is not as high as the threshold for detection by 'Albustix' (10–15 mg/dl) (Viberti & Pickup 1981). Even those patients with normal albumin excretion under resting conditions showed an abnormal increase following exercise. Strict control of diabetes corrects both resting and exercise proteinuria in these early cases. One attractive suggestion put forward to explain proteinuria in diabetes is that changes in glycosylation in the glycoproteins of the capillary wall may alter their permeability. Unfortunately, in long-standing diabetics with heavier proteinuria, careful control achieved with continuous subcutaneous insulin infusion continued over 6 months did not result in any reduction in proteinuria.

Prospects for prevention of diabetic renal disease

Metabolic control

The observations on proteinuria, together with the ability to prevent but not reverse basement-membrane thickening, suggest that there may be a point in the natural history of diabetic glomerulosclerosis at which the changes become irreversible, and that only meticulous control of diabetes from its onset can be effective in preventing renal disease.

Hypertension

Hypertension appears to accelerate the decline in renal function in diabetics, whereas control of hypertension delays progression of the nephropathy (Mogensen 1981). Careful control of hypertension should, therefore, be an integral part of the activity of a diabetic clinic.

Cigarette smoking

Cigarette smoking increases the likelihood of diabetic nephropathy (Christiansen & Nerup 1978) and should be strongly discouraged from the earliest stage of the disease.

As the mean time to renal failure in juvenile-onset diabetes is 20 years, and because many patients never develop significant renal disease, the practical difficulties in establishing that the above recommendations will be effective in preventing renal disease, even if they can be achieved, are obviously tremendous.

Treatment of end-stage renal failure in diabetics

Over the past 5–10 years, dialysis and transplantation have been offered to an increasing number of diabetics, in whom such treatment was not previously considered justifiable because of their multi system disease and because of the practical difficulties of delivering this treatment. In Europe at present approximately 2% of patients receiving treatment for end-stage renal failure are diabetics, whereas in one survey (Ahlmén 1975) diabetics constituted 14% of patients presenting with end-stage renal disease, so that they are still less likely than the non-diabetic to be offered treatment.

Difficulties in dialysis of diabetics

Vascular access, whether by arteriovenous shunt or the much more usual Cimino arteriovenous fistula, is made difficult by arterial atheroma in diabetics; however, with increasing experience this is not a major obstacle.

Diabetic control is made difficult by the glucose load which is delivered on dialysis days, usually requiring some adjustment of insulin dosage on that day. Continuous ambulatory peritoneal dialysis (CAPD) avoids this problem as the glucose load is the same on every day and insulin can, if necessary, be given with the dialysate intraperitoneally. However, many patients still prefer to use the subcutaneous route to avoid the risk of peritoneal infection which accompanies the injection of insulin into the dialysate bag.

Blindness afflicts many diabetics by the time that they require dialysis. This makes self-dialysis impossible, whether by home haemodialysis or CAPD, unless they have a willing and able spouse. The alternatives — hospital haemodialysis and hospital peritoneal dialysis — are often oversubscribed and more time-consuming for the patient. The anticoagulation accompanying haemodialysis does not cause problems of bleeding in the eye, as was originally feared (Ritz et al 1981).

Atheroma is present in the majority of diabetics by the time that they reach end-stage renal failure, resulting in an increased incidence of myocardial infarction, strokes and peripheral vascular disease, often leading to amputation. In addition they suffer the other diabetic complications including peripheral sensory and motor neuropathy, autonomic neuropathy and a reduced resistance to infection. The net effect of all of these conditions is to reduce the 2-year survival on dialysis from around 80% in non-diabetics to 55% in diabetics; these figures, of course, vary with the age of the patients admitted to the dialysis programme.

Transplantation in diabetes

Technical problems in transplanting the kidneys of diabetic patients are not insuperable because, if severe atheroma of the iliac vessels is present, endarterectomy can be performed at the time of transplant.

The major problem which may occur after the kidney has been transplanted, concerns atheroma. The 3-year survival in patients with impairment of vision and symptoms or signs of ischaemic heart disease at the time of cadaver transplant has been reported to be as low as 10% (Joint Scandinavian Report 1978). Peripheral vascular disease is still a major problem at this stage, as well as during the dialysis phase of treatment: two of our patients have required amputation of fingers as well as of lower limbs.

Increased susceptibility to infection has not presented a major problem in our patients.

Control of diabetes has not presented problems following transplant, despite the high dose level of steroid drugs. However, in the hope of reducing diabetic complications, simultaneous pancreatic and renal transplantation has been tried and may become a practical form of treatment.

Timing of transplantation. Early transplantation has been recommended in diabetics to avoid the rapid deterioration in vision which often occurs in the months running up to the start of dialysis treatment and during the first months of dialysis. Unfortunately, this has rarely been achieved in practice because of the chronic shortage of kidneys for transplantation. It seems likely that it is not, in fact, necessary if hypertension is avoided by suitable antihypertensive and diuretic therapy in the predialysis phase of treatment, combined with fairly early recourse to regular dialysis.

RENAL BONE DISEASE

Osteomalacia

In the 4 years between this and the last edition the problem of the most troublesome type of renal bone disease — osteomalacia developing in patients after the start of dialysis — has been solved. Although this condition was histologically indistinguishable from the osteomalacia seen in about 20% of patients at the beginning of dialysis (Ellis et al 1977), it was clearly different in that it was not associated with increases in total serum alkaline phosphatase or bone alkaline phosphatase isoenzymes and, most important, it did not respond to 1-α-OH-cholecalciferol, or indeed any other therapy and was a major cause of morbidity in some dialysis centres. The condition was first studied in Newcastle upon Tyne, England, where it was a major problem and this earned it the title 'Newcastle bone disease', although an identical condition was subsequently recognised in other centres. The condition was clearly not an inevitable consequence of dialysis or of prolonged survival with partly controlled uraemia for, in some dialysis centres, no patients were affected. The disease disappeared when water was deionised. Epidemiological studies revealed an association between the aluminium content of the water used in making the dialysate and the incidence of bone disease. The role of aluminium was confirmed when a correlation was observed between the aluminium content of bone and the severity of osteomalacia, and when the disease was reproduced in animals by the administration of aluminium chloride. The source of aluminium in the water supply is aluminium sulphate which is added by the water authorities to remove colour from surface water (Kerr 1981).

Osteitis fibrosa

Approximately 80% of patients show histological evidence of osteitis fibrosa at the beginning of dialysis. The condition can often be detected very early in the course of chronic renal failure by an increase in the levels of serum parathyroid hormone (PTH) and alkaline phosphatase when serum creatinine is as low as 200 μmol/l. At this stage the condition should be treated to prevent hyperplasia of the parathyroid glands, because once the glands have become hyperplastic they may remain so, even when the primary stimulus to their overactivity has been removed by a successful transplant. Treatment consists of control of hyperphosphataemia, if present, by the administration of aluminium hydroxide taken with meals; the patient is given advice about a low-phosphate diet. Unfortunately, both of these measures may be unpopular with the patient as aluminium hydroxide often causes nausea and a low-phosphate diet is unpalatable. Hypocalcaemia, best monitored by measuring serum ionised calcium, is treated by the administration of calcium carbonate (which also tends to reduce phosphate absorption) and by the careful use of 1-α-OH-cholecalciferol, avoiding hypercalcaemia. There is some anxiety that vitamin D therapy may accelerate the decline in renal function and, also, that it may precipitate metastatic calcification. In the later predialysis phase of treatment, during dialysis, and following transplant, subtotal parathyroidectomy is not uncommonly required in patients with persistently increased serum PTH levels who do not respond to the above measures without developing hypercalcaemia or, in the case of those patients who have received transplants, who have persistent hypercalcaemia. Ideally, parathyroidectomy should be performed before metastatic calcification develops, because this is only very slowly, and perhaps incompletely, reversible following surgery.

parathyroidectomy should be performed before metastatic calcification develops, because this is only very slowly, and perhaps incompletely, reversible following surgery.

DIALYSIS ENCEPHALOPATHY

At the time of the last edition, dialysis dementia was a leading cause of death in some units; its aetiology was uncertain, although Alfrey et al (1976) had suggested the possibility of aluminium toxicity. It now seems certain that aluminium in the water supply is the cause of encephalopathy. There is a close association between dialysis osteomalacia and dementia in most areas (Platts et al 1977, Parkinson et al 1979) related to high aluminium levels in the water supply. Furthermore, in Eindhoven, dialysis dementia developed in a group of patients who underwent dialysis using water which had accidentally been contaminated with aluminium from a water heater, but dementia was not seen in another group using the same water supply but without this contamination (Flendrig et al 1976).

CONTINUOUS AMBULATORY PERITONEAL DIALYSIS

Intermittent peritoneal dialysis (IPD) has been used in the treatment of end-stage renal failure for many years. Until recently it usually meant 48 h in hospital for the patient to receive hourly 2-litre exchanges of fluid delivered by a stiff cannula which was inserted under local anaesthetic at the beginning of the procedure and removed following it. Not surprisingly, this form of dialysis was disliked by the majority of patients and staff, so much so that it was used as a form of 'trial by ordeal' by some units in order to select those patients with sufficient moral fibre to warrant long-term haemodialysis.

The discomfort of repeated cannula insertions was overcome with the advent of the soft silastic permanent peritoneal catheter, developed by Palmer and modified by Tenckhoff. However, peritoneal dialysis for chronic renal failure became popular only when, with the introduction of the technique of continuous ambulatory peritoneal dialysis (CAPD) by Popovich et al (1976) and its promotion by Oreopoulos et al (1978), it became possible to avoid the prolonged treatment periods of IPD. In CAPD, 2 litres of a commercial dialysate fluid (sodium 132 mmol/l, chloride 102 mmol/l, calcium 1.75 mmol/l, magnesium 0.75 mmol/l, lactate 35 mmol/l and glucose 13.6 g/l or 38.6 g/l) contained in a soft plastic bag are run into the peritoneal cavity. The empty bag remains connected to the peritoneal catheter, is rolled up and held under a light waistband. After dwelling overnight, or for 4–6 hours during the day, the fluid is drained back into the empty bag; this is discarded, a new bag connected and fresh dialysate run into the abdomen. The exchange can be completed in 30 min.

The biochemical control achieved by CAPD is, in general, better than that on intermittent peritoneal dialysis or haemodialysis (Chan et al 1981) and anaemia is less severe, possibly because of the more efficient removal of 'middle molecules' resulting from the long equilibration periods. These substances, of molecular weight mainly between 800 and 1500, may suppress red-cell production (Scizalla et al 1980). In addition, although hypertriglyceridaemia is common, as it is in all forms of dialysis treatment, HDL-cholesterol is higher in CAPD than in haemodialysis patients, so that the incidence of vascular disease, which is a major cause of morbidity and mortality in patients with end-stage renal disease, may be reduced. In order to limit hypertriglyceridaemia and avoid obesity, patients are usually advised to limit fluid intake to avoid the necessity for using hypertonic dialysate which, of course, delivers a high glucose load to the patient while removing fluid from him. However, despite this constraint, fluid restriction does not usually have to be as strict as it is in patients on haemodialysis.

There are other advantages to CAPD from the physician's point of view. Vascular access is always difficult in children and in diabetic patients and, of course, is unnecessary with CAPD. Haemodialysis imposes a considerable haemodynamic stress, which may be dangerous in the small child and in the elderly; this, too, is avoided by CAPD. Diabetic control is often difficult with the wide fluctuations in glucose load which occur when dialysis is intermittent, but it is facilitated by CAPD. Furthermore, training for home treatment is quicker and easier and, overall, costs a little less than the alternative modes of dialysis.

CAPD has attractions for the patient in calling for less dietary restriction of sodium, potassium and water intake, giving a greater sense of well-being (possibly because of the improved haematocrit) and involving a simpler regime of treatment which does not call for machines and which allows the patient to travel.

What, then, are the problems? Unfortunately, peritonitis remains a major problem and may lead to prolonged hospitalisation and even death in some patients. There are about two episodes of peritonitis per patient year (Chan et al 1981). This is the commonest cause of treatment failure and may limit the long-term application of this technique. Our policy in Newcastle is to use CAPD as the first option in patients with a common tissue type who are likely to be offered a renal transplant within 2 or 3 years, but to recommend home haemodialysis for patients with less-common tissue types, who are likely to have to wait longer for transplantation.

RENAL TRANSPLANTATION

Since 1978, when renal transplantation was reviewed in the last edition, there has been, as predicted, a steady improvement in transplantation techniques without any 'major breakthrough'.

Blood transfusion

In 1978, a prospective trial of blood transfusion before transplantation was anticipated. This trial is now unlikely to take place, because it is generally felt that the retrospective data are so convincing that to withhold transfusion would be unethical. Indeed, on the basis of retrospective analysis of our results, in 1978 we introduced a policy of deliberate transfusion before cadaver transplantation, together with greater emphasis on HLA-B locus matching. We have noted a significant improvement in graft survival which is coincidental with these changes (unpublished work).

The mechanism by which transfusion enhances graft survival remains the subject of controversy (Editorial, Lancet 1981) although some conclusions are emerging. In a study in which patients who had not previously been transfused, or who had received less than three units of blood, were followed, with or without transfusion, through the transplantation procedure, Opelz et al (1981) have helped to clarify several points. Most important is the observation that transfusions probably do *not* exert their effect by excluding strong immune-responders from transplantation. If their non-transfused are assumed to be comparable with their transfused patients, (a not completely valid assumption because the patients were not randomly allocated to transfusion or non-transfusion groups) then less than 30% would be strong responders on the basis of the development of cytotoxic antibodies. However 77% of grafts were unsuccessful in the non-transfused group whereas in those patients who had received the most blood, graft survival was 90% at 1 year. Some factor other than selecting out of non-responders must be responsible for the much improved outcome in transfused patients. A plasma factor may be associated with the α_2-macroglobulin fraction (Proud 1980). There is, in addition, evidence for an increase in suppressor T cell activity following blood transfusion (Smith et al 1981). The other points clarified by Opelz were that graft survival progressively improved with the number of units transfused, and that transfusion at the time of surgery is not of value, although he cites the evidence for the conflicting view.

Tissue typing

There is now good evidence that matching for HLA-B locus antigens results in a significant improvement in cadaver graft survival in patients who have been transfused, and that matching for HLA-A antigens has little effect in these patients (Uldall et al 1977, Brynger & Gelin 1980). Neither HLA-A nor HLA-B antigen matching appears to influence cadaver graft survival in non-transfused patients. These observations are likely to lead to a change in the present policy for the distribution of cadaver kidneys by UK Transplant, away from equal rating of -A and -B antigen matches to a weighting in favour of HLA-B antigen matches.

The mixed lymphocyte reaction test for D-antigen matching takes too long to be of value in cadaver kidney transplantation. However, the D-related or DR-antigen can be identified serologically and it is now possible to DR-type donor and recipient prospectively; cadaver kidney distribution could therefore be based on this. The attraction of changing from the present system of distribution, based on HLA-A and -B antigens, to one based on DR antigens, is that there are far fewer DR antigens so that it should be much easier to match donor and recipient for DR. The attraction of DR matching was even greater when it was thought that matching for only one DR antigen improved graft survival; unfortunately this has now been shown not to be the case (Morris 1980). Further work is continuing on the value of matching for two DR antigens.

Cyclosporin A

The drugs used to achieve immunosuppression in renal transplant recipients have remained essentially unchanged since the introduction of azathioprine in the early 1960s; they comprise azathioprine and prednisone or, more recently, prednisolone. Antilymphocyte globulin (ALG) has been used by some centres for about 15 years but has not gained general acceptance. It is expensive, painful to administer and, probably because of variability in the activity of different preparations, not of clearly confirmed value.

A possible 'major breakthrough' has now emerged in the form of cyclosporin A.

This is a cyclic peptide fungal metabolite which acts mainly on T lymphocytes, suppressing their response in the mixed lymphocyte reaction and to mitogens. There can be no doubt as to its efficacy (Evans 1981): it has often been used as the sole immunosuppressive agent. However, it has not yet been shown to give results which are superior to conventional treatment with azathioprine and prednisolone and its use has been associated with rather alarming side effects. In particular, the Cambridge group noted the development of lymphoma in three of the first 20 patients treated, a rather high rate of death from sepsis, and initial tubular necrosis which could be avoided by adequate hydration. These toxic effects were probably caused mainly by the high dose used: they have diminished following the reduction in initial daily dose from 25 to 17 mg/kg. We therefore must await the long-term results in patients treated with these lower doses of cyclosporin before we can determine its place in clinical transplantation.

Hypertension after transplantation

Approximately 50% of transplant recipients have persistent hypertension. In approximately 10% of these, the hypertension is caused by, or exacerbated by, transplant artery stenosis, while in others it is associated with deterioration of renal function. In patients with good renal function and without renal artery stenosis, we have found a very low incidence of hypertension in patients subjected to bilateral nephrectomy, a correlation between blood pressure levels before and after transplant, a correlation between blood pressure and plasma renin activity and also between blood pressure responses to saralasin infusion and plasma renin activity (McHugh et al 1980). These observations have led us to the conclusion that the host's diseased kidneys are a major factor in post-transplant hypertension. However, we do not recommend bilateral nephrectomy as a routine procedure because it carries a considerable risk of morbidity and even of occasional death, and because, in most cases, the hypertension can be controlled satisfactorily with drugs.

In patients with transplant renal artery stenosis, the approach is again usually medical. Surgical correction is difficult because of fibrosis around the artery, and attempts at repair have often led to graft loss. In patients with severe resistant hypertension, the technique of balloon dilatation (see below) has been applied with some success.

New investigative techniques in renal transplantation

The management of transplant recipients has been facilitated by the widespread availability of the gamma camera and ultrasonography.

The gamma camera

The gamma camera is used to provide a series of images of the transplanted kidney and bladder following the intravenous injection of ^{99}Tc-labelled DTPA. From these images an assessment of renal perfusion can be made. At its crudest, this allows the non-invasive diagnosis of renal artery occlusion. With serial studies and computer analysis of the scans it may be possible to diagnose the onset of rejection in the presence of pre-existing tubular necrosis — a diagnosis which is at present very difficult to make without renal biopsy. Another very major contribution from these scans is in the diagnosis of obstruction to outflow from the kidney. This is achieved by comparing the radioactive counts over the renal pelvis with those over the bladder. The gamma camera is of particular importance in making this diagnosis in the early days following transplantation, when renal function is usually too poor to allow sufficient concentration for an intravenous urogram (IVU), and dilatation of the renal collecting system and ureter are insufficient to allow diagnosis by ultrasonography.

Renal ultrasound
Ultrasound examination is of particular value in the diagnosis of outflow obstruction of late onset, and of lymphocoele which can give rise to ureteric obstruction by stretching the ureter and displacing the bladder. It has become a routine investigation as a means of excluding outflow obstruction in patients with established graft function who develop deterioration of renal function. It is also possible to diagnose acute rejection using ultrasound, because the papillae become swollen: however, as yet we have not had sufficient confidence in the technique to rely on this sign.

RENOVASCULAR HYPERTENSION

Definition

Stenosis of the renal arteries may occur in essential hypertensives as the result of atheroma and is not necessarily the cause of the associated hypertension. Renovascular hypertension is therefore defined as hypertension which is cured or improved by the correction of renal artery stenosis. This distinguishes it from renal vascular disease in a patient with essential hypertension.

Prevalence

The prevalence of renovascular hypertension in a hypertensive population is not known. Estimates range from 0.2% up to 10% (Gifford 1969, McNeil et al 1975, Berglund et al 1976, Tucker & Labarthe 1977). It is, however, of little real value to derive an overall figure for prevalence when in practice we are faced with the decision of whether to investigate a patient of a particular age with a particular level of blood pressure. Thus, it has been reported that as many as 31% of patients with malignant hypertension have renal artery stenosis (Davis et al 1979), although much lower proportions have also been reported: Russell et al (1980) found that only 7% of patients with malignant hypertension had renal artery stenosis. On the other hand, the figure is very much lower when patients with mild hypertension are included. Similarly, there is a higher prevalence of renovascular hypertension among elderly hypertensives than in the middle-aged.

As it is possible to pick out groups of patients in which the yield of investigation is likely to be much higher than for the whole 'hypertensive' population (however that may be defined), we should not be inhibited from all investigation of hypertension by the discouraging figures from cost-benefit analyses (McNeil et al 1975). However, to keep the yield of investigation in perspective, in Newcastle we refer only six to eight patients a year for renal artery surgery or dilatation, despite being a regional centre serving a population of 3 million.

Pathology

Renal artery stenosis is usually due to fibromuscular dysplasia in the younger, usually female, patient and to atheroma in the older, usually male, patient. Although there have been reports that the results of surgical treatment do not differ between the two pathological types (Mackay et al 1981), other have reported higher cure rates in fibromuscular dysplasia (Dean 1981); the results of percutaneous transluminal balloon angioplasty also seem to be better in those patients with fibromuscular dysplasia (Grim et al 1981). In any analysis of results, therefore, the two categories are best analysed separately; it would be a pity if poor results in a 60-year-old atherosclerotic were allowed to discourage intervention in a young woman with fibromuscular dysplasia who might later face the prospect of pregnancy.

Clinical features

There are no clinical features which reliably separate renovascular from essential hypertension (Simon et al 1972). However, there are some clinical features which are more common in renovascular hypertension, for example severe hypertension (see above), the presence of an epigastric bruit (six to eight times more common) and the rapid development of severe hypertension in a patient known to have been normotensive. These features, although by no means diagnostic, should make one suspect renovascular hypertension.

Investigations necessary in all hypertensives

As hypertension may be the presenting feature of renal disease or of an endocrine condition which deserves diagnosis in its own right, regardless of considerations of blood pressure control, all patients under the age of 65 years with diastolic pressure persistently in excess of 100 mmHg should have the following simple investigations. Urinalysis (Labstix®) and microscopy will give a clue to glomerulonephritis and may be abnormal in chronic pyelonephritis; estimation of plasma creatinine, urea and electrolytes will exclude chronic renal insufficiency and hypokalaemic primary aldosteronism; measurement of serum calcium will exclude primary hyperparathyroidism which may account for 0.3% of hypertensives (Berglund et al 1976). Chest radiography and electrocardiography, although desirable as baselines for future changes, are not essential either in diagnosis or in management.

Selection of patients for intravenous urogram and isotope renogram

If no abnormality is found by this simple screening procedure, then before embarking on further investigation one next has to decide whether the patient would be recommended for surgical rather than medical treatment, assuming that a correctable cause had been found. Application of this simple rule immediately excludes some groups of patients:

1. Patients with diastolic pressure less than 110 mmH g, although some would put the level lower than this (for example Dean 1981); in certain circumstances, such as the case of a young woman planning pregnancy, most would agree that investigation is indicated at much lower levels.
2. Older patients, over 45 years, unless drug treatment is difficult for medical or social reasons e.g. employment threatened by the need to take drugs.

3. Patients with evidence of vascular disease in other organs, which would make surgery both more hazardous and less likely to cure the hypertension.

4. Patients who say at the outset that, whatever the findings, they would not wish to have surgery unless medical treatment failed.

5. Patients whose physician would prefer to treat medically initially, whatever the outcome of investigations.

Thus, investigation is concentrated on the more severe hypertensive, in the younger age group, who is without evidence of vascular disease elsewhere and who would accept surgery if offered it. These patients should be given IVU and isotope renogram.

The rapid-sequence IVU

This is positive in 78% of patients with renovascular hypertension and falsely positive in 11% of patients with essential hypertension (Bookstein et al 1972). In addition to identifying renal vascular disease, it is also of value in bringing to light other possible causes of hypertension which, although usually not surgically remediable, do influence the management of the patient; in particular, chronic pyelonephritis, obstructive uropathy and polycystic disease may be diagnosed. Such abnormalities may be detected in about 4% of hypertensives; however, in one hospital-based study the yield of abnormalities on IVU was 12% (Atkinson & Kellett 1974).

The isotope renogram

This gives information similar to that given by the IVU on the likelihood of renovascular disease and has similar sensitivity — positive in 76% of cases of renovascular hypertension. It is cheaper than the IVU and the dose of irradiation is less, but it is more commonly falsely positive in patients without renovascular hypertension; furthermore, it does not give the information provided by the IVU on the morbid anatomy of the kidney. Its role, in my view, is therefore as an adjunct to the IVU to reduce the likelihood of false-negative tests.

Selection of patients for arteriography

1. Patients with diagnostic changes on the IVU
2. Patients with diagnostic changes on the isotope renogram, in whom the IVU is compatible with the diagnosis and excludes parenchymatous renal disease
3. Patients with suggestive changes in both IVU and renogram, or in one of these if there is an abdominal bruit.

In addition, it is reasonable to subject patients with none of these features to arteriography if there are strong clinical indications, to be certain that renal artery stenosis is not being missed. This would include, for example, the young patient with very severe hypertension, patients in whom medical treatment has failed and patients whose employment would be jeopardised by taking drugs. The extreme application of this view is seen in some American centres where all patients with diastolic pressures in excess of 105 mmHg and who do not have significant complicating risk factors are screened with arteriography (Dean 1981).

It must be emphasised that only broad guidelines can be given and the final decision is best made by a physician with experience in managing hypertension of this type.

The assessment of the functional significance of renal artery stenosis

The renal vein renin ratio

This ratio is currently regarded as the best test for assessment of the functional significance of renal artery stenosis, although other tests have their advocates (see below). Both renal veins are cannulated via the femoral veins to allow simultaneous collection of renal vein blood from the two sides. Because renin has a half-life of about 30 min, which tends to diminish differences between the sides due to recirculation, sampling is usually performed during active secretion of renin stimulated by sodium depletion, tilting or vasodilator-induced hypotension. Unfortunately, even this test cannot provide a clear answer on whether or not surgery should be recommended. Most groups report similar findings to those of the Glasgow group (Mackay et al 1981) who found that surgery was successful in all patients having a renal vein renin ratio greater than 2. However, more than half of the patients who responded to surgery had ratios less than this. If the ratio for selection for surgery was set at 1.5:1, then approximately one-third of operations would fail to cure the hypertension and about one-third who would have benefited from surgery would still be denied operation. Again, therefore, no dogmatic advice can be given on whether renal artery stenosis which has been demonstrated angiographically should be corrected.

The final decision must be based on the whole clinical picture and is best made by a team of physician, surgeon and radiologist, with special experience in dealing with the problem. The Glasgow group have analysed the basis of their management decisions in patients with renal artery stenosis (Mackay et al 1981). They noted that, if any test or feature is used alone or in combination as an indication for surgery, it will reduce the chance of an unsuccessful operation but at the expense of reducing the total number of successful operations. They found that best results were associated with youth, unilateral disease, absence of vascular disease elsewhere, good renal function and high renal vein renin ratio, but concluded that every case should be considered individually.

Other tests of functional significance of renal artery stenosis

Divided renal function studies require bilateral ureteric catheterisation which may be traumatic. In addition, ureteric urine collection is often incomplete, thus invalidating the test. Finally, even when the test is technically satisfactory in experienced hands, it does not discriminate between those who will and those who will not respond to surgery (Mackay et al 1981). This test should not, therefore, be used in the investigation of hypertension.

Peripheral vein plasma renin activity (PRA) is not of value in predicting response to surgery. It is normal in 40% of patients with renovascular hypertension and increased in 15–20% of essential hypertensives.

The infusion of an angiotensin antagonist, usually saralasin (1-sarcosine-8-alanine angiotensin II, an analogue and competitive antagonist of angiotensin II) suffers from the same limitations as the measurement of peripheral venous PRA in that it also lowers the blood pressure in high renin essential hypertensives and therefore does not predict response to surgery. It has been suggested that, because PRA is hyperresponsive to saralasin infusion in renovascular hypertension, measurement of PRA after saralasin infusion might result in fewer misclassifications than arise when blood pressure response is used (Maxwell et al 1978). Whether or not this is confirmed, the test remains laborious in that the saralasin should be given as an infusion over 30 min, with close medical supervision during and following this procedure; it is unlikely to find a place in routine use.

Correction of renal artery stenosis

Surgery

The choice of surgical procedure will depend on the angiographic appearance and the surgeon's preference. Possible techniques include endarterectomy, sleeve resection, direct re-anastomosis of the renal artery to the aorta, interposition of a vein graft and autotransplantation of the kidney to the iliac fossa.

Results of surgery. Although some staggeringly good results, with cure or improvement in 96% of patients, have been reported (Dean 1981), the results reported by the Glasgow group (Mackay et al 1981) are more typical with 50% cured, 34% improved and 15% not benefited. These results are similar to those of the Co-operative Study of Renovascular Hypertension (Foster et al 1975).

Percutaneous transluminal balloon angioplasty

The use of this technique to correct atheromatous stenosis in the renal artery was first reported in 1978 by Gruntzig et al, and in 1979 for correction of stenosis due to fibromuscular dysplasia (Millan et al 1979).

The renal artery is cannulated percutaneously from the femoral or axillary artery; a guide wire is inserted through the catheter and the tip lodged in a segmental renal artery. The dilating catheter, incorporating a thick-walled balloon of the required maximum inflated diameter, is then introduced along the guide wire through the stenosis. The balloon is then filled on several occasions under pressure using contrast medium so that the effect on the stenosis can be monitored. The patient is treated with an antiplatelet agent (aspirin or dipyridamole) for 1 week before the procedure and for 1 year afterwards.

Results of balloon dilatation. Because the technique has been introduced so recently the long-term results are not known. Initial reports have been favourable (Geyskes et al 1979, Yune et al 1980). However, a note of caution in applying the technique to patients with atheromatous stenosis has been sounded by the report of Grim and his colleagues (1981), that 11 of 16 patients with atheromatous stenosis had developed re-stenosis at 1 year (as opposed to only one of six patients with fibromuscular dysplasia) and that two patients with single functioning kidneys developed renal failure following the procedure; in one of these, the presence of cholesterol emboli was demonstrated in the kidney.

THE MEDICAL TREATMENT OF RENAL HYPERTENSION

Medical vs surgical treatment

Some of the problems involved in identifying the small percentage of hypertensive patients suitable for surgical treatment have been outlined and this has led to the suggestion that the search for such patients is not worth the expense. No controlled trial comparing medical and surgical management of renovascular hypertension has been reported, although such a trial is currently in progress (Dean 1981). A comparison of medical and surgical treatment conducted at the Mayo Clinic came out in favour of surgery (Hunt et al 1974), but this is balanced by a report that superior control of blood pressure was obtained by medical means (Zech & Pozet 1979).

Whatever the outcome of comparative trials, there will be some patients who will require medical treatment because they are unsuitable for, or unwilling to undergo, surgery.

The choice of drug

Because it seems likely that the renin angiotensin system has a major role in the pathogenesis of renovascular hypertension, it has been suggested that drugs which interfere with renin release (particularly the β-adrenergic blockers) or with the production of angiotensin II (captopril, which blocks the conversion of decapeptide angiotensin I to the active octapeptide angiotensin II) are specifically indicated in the treatment of renovascular hypertension. However, it is by no means certain that β-blockers exert their antihypertensive effect through suppression of renin and, although captopril probably acts mainly by blocking angiotensin II production, it also inhibits the enzyme responsible for the breakdown of bradykinin, which may also contribute to the antihypertensive effect. Certainly, both β-blockers and captopril are effective in the treatment of essential as well as of renovascular hypertension.

The principles of drug therapy of renovascular hypertension are therefore similar to those for treating essential hypertension with, at most, a slight change in emphasis towards β-blockers rather than diuretics as initial treatment.

Treatment plan in renovascular hypertension

β-adrenergic blockers

If there are no contraindications, a β-blocker is usually the initial treatment, the dose being adjusted according to blood pressure response and heart rate.

In the unusual patient in whom there is impairment of renal function, a cardioselective drug such as atenolol or metoprolol is normally used, because we have evidence (unpublished work) that these drugs are less likely to cause further reduction in function than are non-selective drugs. However, it should be emphasised that, despite earlier reports that non-selective β-blockers may cause renal failure, in our experience the effect of any of the β-blockers on renal function is slight.

Diuretic

If the β-blocker does not control blood pressure, or cannot be tolerated, then a diuretic is added. A thiazide is usually chosen and to improve patient compliance may be given as a combined tablet with the β-blocker. If serum creatinine is increased above 200 μmol/l, the thiazide will be less effective and a loop diuretic (frusemide or bumetanide) should be used.

Vasodilator

If blood pressure remains uncontrolled a vasodilator is added, usually hydrallazine which acts directly on the vessel wall and affects mainly the arterioles, or prazosin which is an α-adrenergic blocker and affects mainly the venous capacitance vessels. The recently introduced drug indoramin has actions similar to those of prazosin.

If the three-drug combination does not control blood pressure then Kincaid-Smith (1977) has suggested the use of both hydrallazine and prazosin together with β-blocker and diuretic. We have found that this is very effective in some patients.

Some physicians prefer to use the α- and β-adrenergic blocking drug labetalol in place of β-blockers and hydrallazine or prazosin. There are no data to show which approach is best and it is reasonable to use either.

Centrally acting drugs

If the blood pressure remains uncontrolled with the above combination of drugs, my personal preference is to add methyldopa, which is well-tried, has few toxic effects and (in about 50% of patients) no troublesome side effects. Nevertheless, because of its central action, other patients complain of drowsiness, depression and of impotence.

Clonidine is less used now because of the occurrence of rebound hypertension in some patients following its sudden withdrawal.

New potent vasodilators and angiotensin antagonists

If the blood pressure still remains uncontrolled, then the stage has been reached at which the newer, very potent drugs should be introduced.

In men, minoxidil should be tried, beginning with 2.5 mg daily and increasing slowly to 50 mg if required. This is a very potent vasodilator and therefore causes fluid retention: concurrent high doses of a loop diuretic are therefore usually required. The β-blocker should also be administered concurrently to avoid tachycardia. Obviously, the less potent vasodilators hydrallazine and prazosin should be discontinued and methyldopa can be withdrawn gradually.

Why should this very effective drug be used only at this stage, and then restricted to men? It is a relatively new drug, only recently released for general use in the United Kingdom. It has been reported to cause atrial necrosis in dogs but not in man; however, pericarditis associated with its use has been reported in man (Bennett 1977). Nevertheless, this is a rare complication and probably will not preclude its eventual more frequent use. The reason for confining its use to men, except when all else fails in women, is that it causes a generalised increase in hair growth which, although reversible on stopping the drug, is unacceptable to most women.

Oral diazoxide is as potent as minoxidil but causes hyperglycaemia, usually necessitating oral hypoglycaemic drugs, in about 50% of patients; as it also causes hirsutes, minoxidil is usually preferred.

In women, and in those men in whom minoxidil is for any reason not suitable, captopril is the drug of choice at this stage because it does not cause hirsutes. In patients who are already receiving diuretics and in whom plasma renin activity and angiotensin II levels are high, captopril may have a very dramatic effect. Ideally, therefore, the diuretic should be discontinued for 48 h before introducing captopril. In view of the variable response, the paucity of patients in whom it is required, and the severity of their hypertension, it is reasonable to admit patients to hospital for the initial administration of captopril.

The dose of the drug is 12.5 mg 8 hourly between meals (because food interferes with absorption) increasing to 450 mg daily. Concurrent diuretics may not be necessary because aldosterone secretion is reduced; β-blockers are usually continued but hydrallazine and prazosin are discontinued, and methyldopa can usually be withdrawn.

The reason for reserving this drug for those patients who do not respond to conventional therapy is again related to toxic effects. Bone marrow depression has been reported and regular blood counts are mandatory. Proteinuria, amounting to a nephrotic syndrome in a few patients, with immune complexes in the glomerular basement membrane, has also been reported. Abnormalities of taste, skin rashes and fevers are more common but of less importance. The current trend to use lower doses has very much reduced toxic effects.

Treatment of malignant hypertension

Definition

The term malignant hypertension is now applied to hypertension with exudates and haemorrhages in the fundi, without the requirement that papilloedema should be present (WHO Expert Committee 1978).

Management

In order to ensure prompt control of blood pressure, patients with malignant hypertension should be admitted to hospital. If the hypertension is very severe they should be confined to bed but, unless they are in heart failure, suffering from hypertensive encephalopathy or dissecting aneurysm of the aorta, there is general agreement that parenteral therapy should not be given, because of the risk of precipitating cerebral or coronary thrombosis by a too-rapid reduction in blood pressure. The pressure is best reduced gradually, using a combination of methyldopa and diuretic given orally; however, some prefer to begin with β-blocker and diuretic even though the β-blocker may take several days to exert its full effect.

In patients with left ventricular failure, intravenous frusemide is usually adequate to deal with the acute situation. If additional antihypertensive intravenous therapy is indicated, then nitroprusside is of value because of its vasodilatory effect which reduces pre-load on the heart. However the nitroprusside solution has to be made up just before use and requires minute-to-minute monitoring.

Patients with heart failure are not suitable for treatment with a β-blocker, or with labetalol (which would be my choice in patients with encephalopathy or dissecting aneurysm requiring parenteral therapy), nor for hydrallazine or diazoxide which could make the heart failure worse by causing tachycardia. An alternative to nitroprusside in this situation would be the short-acting ganglion-blocker trimethaphan given by intravenous infusion.

Nevertheless, it should be emphasised that parenteral therapy is very rarely needed.

REFERENCES

Urinary tract infection

Asscher A W, Sussman M, Waters W E, Evans J A S, Campbell H, Evans K T et al 1969 Asymptomatic bacteriuria in the non-pregnant woman II. Response to treatment and follow-up. British Medical Journal 1: 804–806

Cardiff-Oxford Bacteriuria Study Group 1978 Sequelae of covert bacteriuria in schoolgirls. Lancet 1: 889–893

Dontas A S, Kasviki-Charvati P, Panayiotis C, Papanayiotou C, Marketos S D 1981 Bacteriuria and survival in old age. New England Journal of Medicine 304: 939–943

Edwards D, Normand I C S Prescod N, Smellie J M 1977 Disappearance of vesicoureteric reflux during long-term prophylaxis of urinary tract infection in children. British Medical Journal 2: 285–288

Gower P E 1976 A prospective study of patients with radiological pyelonephritis, papillary necrosis and obstructive atrophy. Quarterly Journal of Medicine 45: 315–349

Kass E H 1960 Bacteriuria and pyelonephritis of pregnancy. Archives of Internal Medicine 105: 194–198

Sussman M, Asscher A W, Waters W E, Evans J A S, Campbell H, Evans K T et al 1969 Asymptomatic significant bacteriuria in the non-pregnant woman. I. Description of a population. British Medical Journal 1: 799–803

Glomerulonephritis

Ahmad S, Young J, Quadracci L, Pagel M, Scribner B, Striker G 1981 Comparison of immunosuppression and plasma exchange with immunosuppression or no treatment in crescentic glomerulonephritis. Abstract 8th International Congress of Nephrology, Athens. Karger-University Studio, Thessaloniki, p 284

Baldwin D S, Gluck M C, Lowenstein J, Gallo G R 1977 Lupus nephritis: clinical course as related to morphologic forms and their transitions. American Journal of Medicine 62: 12–30

Cameron J S 1977 Diseases of the urinary system. Treatment of glomerulonephritis by drugs. British Medical Journal 1: 1520–1522

Cameron J S, Turner D R, Ogg C S, Williams D G, Lessof M H, Chantler C et al 1979 Systemic lupus with nephritis: a long-term study. Quarterly Journal of Medicine 48: 1–24

Collaborative study 1979 A controlled study of short-term prednisone treatment in adults with membranous nephropathy: Collaborative Study of the Adult Idiopathic Nephrotic Syndrome. New England Journal of Medicine 301: 1301–6

Decker J L 1979 Systemic lupus erythematosis: evolving concepts. Annals of Internal Medicine 91: 587–604

Donadio J V, Holley K E, Ilstrup D M 1981 Adrenocorticoid and cytotoxic drug treatment of lupus nephropathy. Proceedings of the 8th International Congress of Nephrology, Athens. Karger–University Studio, Thessaloniki, p 643–648

Donadio J V Jr, Holley K E, Ferguson R H, Ilstrup D M 1978 Treatment of diffuse proliferative lupus nephritis with prednisone and combined prednisone and cyclophosphamide. New England Journal of Medicine 299: 1151–1155

Fauci A S, Haynes B F, Katz P 1978 The spectrum of vasculitis: clinical, pathologic, immunologic and therapeutic considerations, NIH Conference. Annals of Internal Medicine 89: 660–676

Fauci A S, Katz P, Haynes B F, Wolff S M 1979 Cyclophosphamide therapy of severe systemic necrotising vasculitis. New England Journal of Medicine 301: 235–238

Harmer D, Finn R, Goldsmith H J, Bone J M, Forbes A W 1979 Plasmapheresis in fulminating crescentic nephritis. Lancet 1: 679 (letter)

Hecht B, Siegal N J, Adler M, Kashgarian M, Hayslett J P 1976 Prognostic indices in lupus nephritis. Medicine (Baltimore) 55: 163–187

Kincaid-Smith P, d'Apice A J F 1978 Plasmapheresis in rapidly progressive glomerulonephritis. American Journal of Medicine 65: 564–566

Lockwood C M, Rees A J, Pearson T A, Evans D J, Peters D K, Wilson C B 1976 Immunosuppression and plasma exchange in the treatment of Goodpasture's syndrome. Lancet 1: 711–715

Lockwood C M, Rees A J, Pinching A J, Russell B, Sweny P, Uff J et al 1977 Plasma exchange and immunosuppression in the treatment of fulminating immune complex crescentic nephritis. Lancet 1: 63–67

Mahajan S K, Ordóñez N G, Feitelson P J, Lim V S, Spargo B H, Katz A I 1977 Lupus nephropathy without clinical renal involvement. Medicine (Baltimore) 56: 493–501

Pollak V E, Pirani C L, Dujovne I, Dillard M G 1973 The clinical course of lupus nephritis; relationship to the renal histologic findings. In: Kincaid-Smith P, Mathew T H, Becker E L (eds) Glomerulonephritis: morphology, natural history and treatment. John Wiley and Sons, New York, p 1171

Ponticelli C, Zucchelli P, Banfi G, Cagnoli L, Scalia P 1981 High-dose parenteral methylprednisolone in diffuse proliferative lupus nephritis. Proceedings of the 8th International Congress of Nephrology, Athens. Karger-University Studio, Thessaloniki, p 649–656

Russ G R, d'Apice A J F 1981 Plasma exchange and immunosuppression in crescentic glomerulonephritis. Proceedings of the 8th International Congress of Nephrology, Athens. Karger-University Studio, Thessaloniki, p 667–673

Williams D G 1981 The role of serological measurements in the management of lupus nephritis. Proceedings of the 8th International Congress of Nephrology, Athens. Karger-University Studio, Thessaloniki, p 655–663

Diabetes and the kidney

Ahlmén J 1975 Incidence of chronic renal insufficiency. A study of the incidence and pattern of renal insufficiency in adults during 1966–71 in Gothenberg. Acta Medica Scandinavica 198 (supplement 582): 1–50

Christiansen J S, Nerup 1978 Smoking and diabetic nephropathy. Lancet 1: 605 (letter)

Deckert T, Poulsen J E, Larsen M 1978 Prognosis of diabetics with diabetes onset before the age of 31. 1. Survival, causes of death and complications. Diabetologia 14: 363–370

Joint Scandinavian Report 1978 Renal transplantation in insulin-dependent diabetics. Lancet 2: 915–917

Marks H H, Krall L P 1971 Onset, course, prognosis and mortality in diabetes mellitus. In: Marble A, White P, Bradley R F, Krall L P (eds) Joslin's diabetes mellitus, 11th edn. Lea and Febiger, Philadelphia, p 209–254

Maurer S M, Steffes M W, Brown D M 1982 The kidney in diabetes. American Journal of Medicine (in press) Cited by Viberti & Pickup 1981 (see below)

Mogensen C E 1981 Long-term antihypertensive treatment (over six years) inhibiting the progression of diabetic nephropathy. Acta Endocrinologica 97 (supplement 242): 31–32

Mogensen C E, Andersen M J F 1975 Increased kidney size and glomerular filtration rate in untreated juvenile diabetes: normalisation by insulin treatment. Diabetologia 11: 221–224

Østerby R 1975 Early phases in the development of diabetic glomerulopathy. A quantitative electron microscopic study. Acta Medica Scandinavica 197 (supplement 574): 1–82

Rasch R 1979 Prevention of diabetic glomerulopathy in streptozotocin diabetic rats by insulin treatment. Glomerular basement membrane thickness. Diabetologia 16: 319–324

Ritz E, Bommer J, Andrassy K 1981 Treatment of diabetic patients with end-stage renal failure: some clinical aspects. Proceedings of the 8th International Congress of Nephrology, Athens. Karger-University Studio, Thessaloniki, p 1107–1115

Viberti G C, Pickup J C 1981 Proteinuria, metabolic control and diabetes mellitus. Proceedings of the 8th International Congress of Nephrology, Athens. Karger-University Studio, Thessaloniki, p 1096–1106

Renal bone disease and dialysis encephalopathy

Alfrey A C, Le Gendre G P, Kaehny W D 1976 The dialysis encephalopathy syndrome. Possible aluminium intoxication. New England Journal of Medicine 294: 184–188

Ellis H A, Pierides A M, Feest T G, Ward M K, Kerr D N S 1977 Histopathology of renal osteodystrophy with particular reference to the effects of 1α-hydroxyvitamin D_3 in patients treated by long-term haemodialysis. Clinical Endocrinology 7: (supplement) 31s–38s

Flendrig J A, Kruis H, Das H A 1976 Aluminium intoxication: the cause of dialysis dementia? Proceedings of the European Dialysis and Transplant Association 13: 355–361

Kerr D N S 1981 Renal osteomalacia. Proceedings of the 8th International Congress of Nephrology, Athens. Karger-University Studio, Thessaloniki, p 221–228

Parkinson I S, Ward M K, Feest T G, Fawcett R W P, Kerr D N S 1979 Fracturing dialysis osteodystrophy and dialysis encephalopathy. Lancet 1: 406–409

Platts M M, Goode G C, Hislop J S 1977 Composition of the domestic water supply and the incidence of fractures and encephalopathy in patients on home dialysis. British Medical Journal 2: 657–660

Continuous ambulatory peritoneal dialysis

Chan M K, Chuah P, Raftery M J, Baillod R A, Sweny P, Varghese Z et al 1981 Three years' experience of continuous ambulatory peritoneal dialysis. Lancet 1: 1409–1412

Oreopoulos D G, Robson M, Izatt S, Clayton S, de Veber G A 1978 A simple and safe technique for continuous ambulatory peritoneal dialysis (CAPD). Transactions of the American Society for Artificial Internal Organs 24: 484–489

Popovich R, Moncrief J W, Decherd J F, Bomar J B, Pyle W B 1976 The definition of a novel portable/wearable equilibrium peritoneal dialysis technique (abstract). Transactions of the American Society for Artificial Internal Organs 5: 64

Scizalla P, Sukiyasova T S, Gudim V I, Grobmann P 1980 Influence of uraemic middle molecules and of uraemic serum on the DNA-synthesis in erythroblasts in vivo. Abstracts EDTA, Prague, p 88

Renal transplantation

Brynger H, Gelin L E 1980 Steroids and rejection treatment in the Gothenberg transplant programmes. Proceedings of the European Dialysis and Transplant Association 17: 395–403

Editorial 1981 Blood transfusion and kidney graft survival. Lancet 1: 1242–43

Evans D B 1981 Cyclosporin A in renal transplantation. Proceedings of the 8th International Congress of Nephrology, Athens. Karger-University Studio, Thessaloniki, p 980–981

McHugh M I, Tanboga H, Marcen R, Liano F, Robson V, Wilkinson R 1980 Hypertension following renal transplantation: the role of the host's kidneys. Quarterly Journal of Medicine 49: 395–403

Morris P J 1980 Powerful effect of HLA-DR matching on survival of cadaveric renal allografts. Lancet 2: 282–285

Opelz G, Graver B, Terasaki P I 1981 Induction of high kidney graft survival rate by multiple transfusion. Lancet 1: 1223–1225

Proud G 1980 Blood transfusions and organ transplantation. Annals of the Royal College of Surgeons 62: 271–79

Smith M D, Williams J D, Coles G A, Salaman J R 1981 The effect of blood transfusions on T-suppressor cells in renal dialysis patients. Transplant Proceedings 13: 181–83

Uldall P R, Wilkinson R, Dewar P J, Murray S, Morley A R, Baxby K et al 1977 Factors affecting the outcome of cadaver renal transplantation in Newcastle upon Tyne. Lancet 2: 316–319

Renovascular hypertension

Atkinson A B, Kellett R J 1974 Value of intravenous urography in investigating hypertension. Journal of the Royal College of Physicians of London 8: 175–181

Berglund G, Andersson O, Wilhelmsen L 1976 Prevalence of primary and secondary hypertension: studies in a random population sample. British Medical Journal 2: 554–556

Bookstein J J, Abrams H L, Buenger R E, Lecky J, Franklin S S, Bleifer K H et al 1972 Co-operative study of renovascular hypertension. 2. The role of urography in unilateral renovascular disease. Journal of the American Medical Association 220: 1225–1230

Davis B A, Crook J E, Vestal R E, Oates J A 1979 Prevalence of renovascular hypertension in patients with Grade III or IV hypertensive retinopathy. New England Journal of Medicine 301: 1273–1276

Dean R H 1981 Indications for operative management of renovascular hypertension. Proceedings of the 8th International Congress of Nephrology, Athens. Karger-University Studio, Thessaloniki, p 1146–1152

Foster J H, Maxwell M H, Franklin S S, Bleifer K H, Trippel S H, Julian O C et al 1975 Renovascular occlusive disease: results of operative treatment. Journal of the American Medical Association 231: 1043–1048

Geyskes G C, Puylaert C B A J, Oei H Y, Boomsma J H B 1979 Intraluminal dilatation of renal artery stenosis. Clinical Science 57: 441s–443s

Gifford R W Jr 1969 Evaluation of the hypertensive patient with emphasis on detecting curable causes. Milbank Memorial Fund Quarterly 47 (part 2): 170–186

Grim C E, Luft F C, Yune H Y, Klatte E C, Weinberger M H 1981 Balloon dilation of renal artery stenosis causing hypertension: contrasting cure rates by lesion type. Proceedings of the 8th International Congress of Nephrology, Athens. Karger-University Studio, Thessaloniki, p 1154–1160

Gruntzig A, Kuhlmann U, Vetter W, Lutolf U, Maier B, Siegenthaler W 1978 Treatment of renovascular hypertension with percutaneous transluminal dilatation of a renal artery stenosis. Lancet 1: 801–802
Kincaid-Smith P 1977 Prazosin in the treatment of hypertension. The Medical Journal of Australia: special supplement 1 & 2: 27–29
Mackay A, Boyle P, Brown J J, Cumming A M M, Forrest H, Graham A G et al 1981 Management decisions in patients with renal artery stenosis. Proceedings of the 8th International Congress of Nephrology, Athens. Karger-University Studio, Thessaloniki, p 1132–1138
McNeil B J, Varady P D, Burrows B A, Adelstein S J 1975 Measures of clinical efficacy. Cost-effectiveness calculations in the diagnosis and treatment of hypertensive renovascular disease. New England Journal of Medicine 293: 216–221
Maxwell M H, Varady P, Zawada E T, Burkhalter J F, Waks U, Marks L 1978 Maximal discrimination of renovascular from essential hypertension by the saralasin test. Clinical Science and Molecular Medicine 55: 297s–299s
Millan V G, Mast W E, Madias N E 1979 Non-surgical treatment of severe hypertension due to renal artery internal fibroplasia by percutaneous transluminal angioplasty. New England Journal of Medicine 300: 1371–1373
Russell G I, Bing R F, Thurston H, Swales J D 1980 Renal artery stenosis in malignant hypertension. Lancet 2: 529 (letter)
Simon N, Franklin S A, Bleifer K H, Maxwell M H 1972 Co-operative study of renovascular hypertension: clinical characteristics of renovascular hypertension. Journal of the American Medical Association 220: 1209–1218
Tucker R M, Labarthe D R 1977 Frequency of surgical treatment for hypertension in adults at the Mayo Clinic from 1973 through 1975. Mayo Clinic Proceedings 52: 549–555
Yune H Y, Klatte E C, Grim C E, Weinberger M H 1980 Transluminal balloon dilatation of renal artery stenosis causing hypertension: 18 months' experience. Clinical Science 59: 483s–485s

Medical treatment of renal hypertension

Bennett W M 1977 Pericardial effusions associated with minoxidil. Lancet 2: 1356 (letter)
Dean R H 1981 Indications for operative management of renovascular hypertension. Proceedings of the 8th International Congress of Nephrology, Athens. Karger-University Studio, Thessaloniki, p 1146–1152
Hunt J C, Sheps S G, Harrison E G Jr, Strong C G, Bernatz P E 1974 Renal and renovascular hypertension: a reasoned approach to diagnosis and management. Archives of Internal Medicine 133: 988–999
WHO Expert Committee 1978 Report on arterial hypertension. World Health Organisation, Geneva
Zech P, Pozet N 1979 Renovascular hypertension: a comparison of medical and surgical treatment. La Nouvelle Presse Médicale 8: 495–498

10

Gastroenterology

O. James

TREATMENT OF DUODENAL ULCER

Histamine H_2-receptor antagonists

Effectiveness

Few, if any, other drugs have ever received the critical attention given to cimetidine since 1975. The spotlight has recently turned upon the first 'son of cimetidine' — ranitidine. An analysis of many papers suggests a healing rate of about 75% for acute or chronic duodenal ulcer after 1 month's treatment with 1 g cimetidine daily. This increases to over 95% healing after 3 months (Editorial, Lancet 1981, Pounder 1981). The healing rate for placebo-treated patients in 18 trials involving over 1000 patients was 43% after 1 month, confirming the intermittent nature of duodenal ulcer disease. There appears to be no significant difference between conventional (1 g/day) cimetidine treatment and treatment with ranitidine 150 mg twice daily for 4 weeks (Walt el al 1981). As was the case with other forms of treatment for peptic ulcer, Korman et al (1981) found that if patients continued to smoke while taking cimetidine, no beneficial effect on ulcer healing could be seen after 1 month's treatment. Other studies using H_2 antagonists do not confirm these findings.

Relapse and maintenance

Burland et al (1980) suggested that the relapse rate both of symptom-producing and of asymptomatic duodenal ulcers after stopping a successful 1-month course of treatment was about 8.5% per month. Similarly, 23 out of 27 patients had symptomatic recurrence of duodenal ulcer within a year of successful healing with cimetidine (Martin et al 1981). It is not clear whether this extremely high likelihood of recurrence is worse after cimetidine treatment than might be expected in the natural course of events. Moshal et al (1979) reported that ultrastructural abnormalities of duodenal epithelium remained even after macroscopic healing of a duodenal ulcer with cimetidine and during maintenance treatment. Pounder has recently used these studies on maintenance treatment with cimetidine (usually 400 mg at night indefinitely, after ulcer healing) to suggest a model of medical treatment for duodenal ulcer. It is suggested that, in a pool of duodenal ulcer patients receiving maintenance treatment and full dose at times of relapse of symptoms, only 3% of patients will be in symptomatic relapse at any one time.

Adverse effects

Cimetidine occasionally causes drowsiness or tremor, particularly in the elderly. Breast enlargement, lactation and impotence are extremely rarely seen; all are reversible. It is also of interest that cimetidine is a potent inhibitor of hepatic microsomal mixed-function oxidases (Roberts et al 1981) and this may lead to prolongation of the effects of benzodiazepines and potentiation of the action of warfarin. It is suggested that a similar effect upon liver enzymes does not occur following treatment with ranitidine (Henry et al 1980).

The most important question concerning histamine H_2-receptor antagonists, particularly in long-term use is, do they cause gastric cancer? This possibility was raised by Elder et al (1979) and is based upon: (1) the parallel between the achlorhydria of pernicious anaemia and H_2-receptor antagonist treatment; patients with pernicious anaemia have about three times the usual frequency of gastric cancer in Britain; (2) the possible production of potential carcinogens, notably nitrosamines in gastric juice in the absence of gastric acid. Although Elder described three patients in whom gastric cancer apparently developed after cimetidine treatment, further case reports have been rare, and it is extremely hard to exclude the possibility of gastric cancer prior to treatment in some cases. Muscroft et al (1981) and others have failed to find evidence of potential formation of nitrosamines in the stomach of patients receiving cimetidine. At present it seems reasonable to agree with the *British Medical Journal* that 'taken overall, the clinical evidence linking cimetidine use with liability to gastric cancer is weak' (Editorial, British Medical Journal 1981a). Nevertheless, while doubts remain, the use of maintenance H_2-receptor antagonists indefinitely for duodenal ulcer must be kept under very critical review.

Tripotassium dicitrato bismuthate (TDB)

Effectiveness

Although far fewer studies have been performed using TDB than with histamine H_2-receptor antagonists, results for healing of duodenal ulcer with TDB appear very comparable — approximately 65% after 4 weeks and 88% after 2 months (Vantrappen et al 1980, Martin et al 1981). In assessing these results, only endoscopically confirmed randomised controlled trials have been considered. It is possible that symptoms arising from the duodenal ulcer are relieved a little more quickly with cimetidine than with TDB.

Relapse and maintenance

The well-conducted study by Martin et al (1981) showed that, whereas 23/27 previously healed patients treated with cimetidine had relapsed within 12 months of stopping treatment, only 11/28 TDB-treated patients had experienced a symptomatic relapse which was shown by endoscopy to be due to a further duodenal ulcer; this was a highly significant difference. Martin (1981) has hypothesised that TDB allows more complete healing of the duodenal mucosa than does cimetidine and that this may be the cause for the apparently reduced relapse rate.

Little, if any, evidence is available at present regarding the effect of long-term maintenance TDB treatment. This may partly be due to the fact that, in Britain at least, TDB is available only as a very unpalatable liquid preparation which must be diluted in water.

Adverse effects

Adverse effects during TDB therapy are very rare indeed. Encephalopathy has been reported in association with the use of bismuth antacids, as has arthropathy, but these have seldom if ever been reported in association with the use of TDB (Serfontein & Meckel 1979).

Antacids

The evidence that antacid treatment leads to healing of duodenal ulcers is rather less convincing than that for histamine H_2-receptor antagonists or TDB. The well-conducted study of Peterson et al (1977) suggests that if duodenal ulcer patients are given enough antacid by mouth (in this case 210 ml/day in seven doses plus antacid tablets as needed) then the proportion of ulcers that will heal — 76% after 1 month — is similar in these patients and in those treated with H_2-receptor antagonists or TDB. Lam et al (1979) found that a mixture of antacid plus sulpiride given seven times daily also healed 78% of duodenal ulcers in 1 month. These very large amounts of antacid, taken frequently, may be unacceptable to patients and are quite different from the use of occasional tablets to relieve symptoms.

Relapse and maintenance

Very little is known of the likelihood of relapse after such a heroic antacid course. It is probably similar to that after a course of cimetidine (Centre for Ulcer Research and Education 1980) and smoking probably increases the likelihood of relapse.

Adverse effects

These depend upon the type of antacid or antacids used. Large quantities of aluminimum hydroxide lead to phosphate deficiency, anorexia, muscle weakness and, ultimately, osteomalacia. This is due to increased urinary and faecal excretion of calcium and decreased absorption of fluoride (Spencer & Lender 1979). Magnesium-containing antacids produce diarrhoea. Calcium-containing antacids cannot be used because of the ensuing alkalosis and hypercalcaemia leading to renal damage (Robson & Heading 1978). Antacids may also alter the absorption and excretion of other drugs — notably antibiotics, anticonvulsants and warfarin.

Conclusions

This consideration of the three leading contenders in the field of duodenal ulcer healing has excluded such other agents as carbenoxolone and gefarnate. It is likely that the widespread use of cimetidine has altered the management of duodenal ulcer very radically. The referral rate for elective operations for duodenal ulcer and even the number of emergency operations has fallen in most parts of Britain in the past 5 years (Thompson 1981). There is no evidence at present that patients who come to surgery after failing to respond to cimetidine have a worse surgical outlook than any other patients undergoing a vagotomy procedure (Blackett & Johnston 1981).

What should be recommended as the current management of uncomplicated duodenal ulcer? I would suggest the following:

1. Make an endoscopic diagnosis before starting treatment;
2. The heroic doses and 'impressive list of potential adverse effects' (Editorial, British Medical Journal 1981b) rule out antacid treatment alone as the treatment of choice, but antacid tablets or liquid may be used to relieve symptoms in conjunction with other treatment;
3. A full course, for 1–2 months, of histamine H_2-receptor antagonist — probably in a twice-daily dose — is acceptable to patients and has a high likelihood of healing ulcers and relieving symptoms. Major questions must remain over ulcer recurrence following this treatment and over the desirability of maintenance treatment over a period of years;
4. TDB is less palatable than H_2-receptor antagonists but appears to be equally effective. Relapse is probably less likely after a treatment course of 1–2 months, but maintenance treatment is at present unexplored.

UPPER GASTROINTESTINAL HAEMORRHAGE

Mortality

A superficial appraisal of mortality following admission to hospital for upper gastrointestinal (GI) haemorrhage suggests that little advance has occurred in management over the past 60 years. The reported mortality from GI haemorrhage in the first three decades of this century was 4% in one large series (Conybeare 1934) and 13% in a second (Bulmer 1927); after the advent of blood transfusion, Jones (1947) reported a mortality of 10% in 687 patients with upper GI bleeding. These figures may be compared with 9.7% (Allen & Dykes 1976) and 8.1% (Birnie et al 1981) in the post-endoscopy era.

The statistics may be misleading for a number of reasons. Allen & Dykes have pointed out that in the past decade a greater proportion of patients admitted with upper GI bleeding are over 60 years of age: 48% in their own series versus 2% of the series of Bulmer 60 years earlier. Elderly patients have a higher mortality following any surgical procedure. The proportion of patients with malignancy and those bleeding from oesophageal varices with severe liver disease is also probably higher in the past decade compared with earlier series. Thus, of the overall mortality of 8.1% out of 769 patients admitted to hospital with upper GI bleeding reported by Birnie et al (1981), half died of irremediable malignancy of hepatic failure and a similar proportion of Allen & Dykes' patients also died from malignancy or liver disease, whereas only 20% of the patients in Bulmer's series and 18% of Avery Jones' patients who died were said to have liver disease or cancer. Nevertheless, in 1981 Vellacott et al reported a mortality rate of 10.5% in 1373 patients admitted to hospital with bleeding peptic ulcer. These figures must lead us to ask three questions:

1. What is the place of endoscopy in the management of upper GI haemorrhage?
2. In what circumstances should surgery be carried out?
3. What new effective non-surgical treatment is available?

To summarise, how should patients with upper GI haemorrhage be managed?

Endoscopy and upper GI haemorrhage

It is generally accepted that endoscopy is a more accurate guide to the diagnosis of the site of bleeding following upper GI haemorrhage than are barium studies, particularly if it is performed within a few hours of haemorrhage (Thomas et al 1980, Forrest et al 1981). However, even this belief is not shared by all investigators (Dronfield et al 1977). After initial great enthusiasm for the use of urgent emergency endocopy, current practice suggests that this should be performed following a possible upper GI bleed in only those patients for whom emergency surgery or other procedures are indicated. These include patients with known liver disease (varices versus ulcer/erosions?), patients with evidence of continued severe bleeding on admission to hospital, or patients who bleed again after admission to hospital. In the majority of patients, endoscopy may be carried out at a convenient time within 24 hours of admission, but not necessarily as an urgent emergency procedure. There is controversy over the diagnostic value of endoscopy in relation to the time after bleeding: a bleeding site is identified in about 60–90% of patients if endoscopy is carried out within 12h of bleeding (thus, as an urgent emergency procedure), whereas the figures fall to 32–79% after 48h and lower still thereafter (Foster et al 1978). The main point is that urgent emergency endoscopy does not seem to improve prognosis or alter management significantly other than in those groups already mentioned. The identification of a visible vessel in relation to an ulcer, assumed to be the bleeding site, suggests that there is a high likelihood of rebleeding or continued haemorrhage (Griffiths et al 1979). Fresh bleeding from a lesion or an adherent clot in the base of an ulcer are also pointers towards this increased risk.

Treatment

Since most deaths occurring after upper GI haemorrhage are associated with surgery, the main management problem has always been to try to minimise the number of patients who receive emergency operations, while ensuring that those who do need operative intervention get it at an appropriate time and when they are in the best possible condition to undergo surgery. The identification of rebleed risk factors, such as a visible vessel or fresh clot in an ulcer, has helped to identify those patients in whom a high risk of rebleeding exists (Gilbert et al 1979). In a centre in which a more conservative attitude to surgery was adopted, so that the operation rate for bleeding peptic ulcers fell from 39% to 16.5% over 5 years, the mortality from both gastric and duodenal ulcer bleeding was halved. The operative mortality remained constant over the 5-year period at about 20% (Vellacott 1981).

Cimetidine

Because of its efficacy in the healing of duodenal ulcer and following the report of its beneficial effect in stopping bleeding from gastric erosions in patients with fulminant hepatic failure (MacDougall et al 1977), most patients with upper GI bleeding have, in recent years, received cimetidine virtually from the moment of entry into hospital. There is little evidence that this has any effect upon the likelihood of rebleeding or upon mortality. Hoare et al (1979) in a controlled trial showed that there was some reduction in rebleeding from gastric ulcer, but this has not been confirmed in other, larger, studies (LaBrooy et al 1979, Macklon et al 1979; Pickard et al 1979), or by clinical experience. Kayasseh and colleagues (1980) have suggested that somatostatin may control peptic ulcer bleeding more effectively than cimetidine. As somatostatin inhibits gastric acid and pepsin secretion and may reduce splanchnic blood flow (Keller et al 1978), this form of treatment certainly deserves further investigation.

Laser photocoagulation

There has recently been considerable interest in the use of endoscopic laser photocoagulation for the treatment of bleeding in peptic ulcer disease, particularly in the very patients most likely to require surgery — those with a protruding vessel or blood clot in relation to an ulcer seen at diagnostic endoscopy. The initial report of an uncontrolled study suggested that argon laser photocoagulation stopped active bleeding from 48/60 peptic ulcers treated (Laurence et al 1980). Subsequently, one randomised controlled trial of photocoagulation in bleeding peptic ulcer did not show any statistically confirmed benefit (Vallon et al 1981). In a second study, Swain et al (1981) identified 52 patients out of 330 consecutively admitted with upper GI haemorrhage, in whom a visible vessel was seen in relation to an ulcer. Eight out of 24 patients treated with argon laser bled again, whereas 17 of 28 control patients had a further haemorrhage. More important, 7 of these 28 control patients died after an episode of rebleeding, whereas none of the treated patients died. This difference is significant.

As in studies of other methods of treatment for bleeding, numerous patients must be assessed in order to confirm that benefit is actually conferred, because mortality rates are already relatively low, apart from those in patients with liver disease or malignancy. Laser equipment is extremely expensive; it is, therefore, important that further clinical trials are carried out to confirm this possible benefit in selected patients before the equipment is purchased by every 'self-respecting' district general hospital.

Summary

In the light of the information which has been presented, the answers to the questions posed in the discussion on mortality from upper GI haemorrhage may be as follows: the place of endoscopy in the management of upper GI haemorrhage is to identify the site of bleeding in patients in whom active haemorrhage continues; to identify lesions in which rebleeding seems likely; and possibly to treat selected lesions, notably prominent vessels, particularly in elderly patients where surgical risk is high.

Surgery should still be carried out in the presence of continued and uncontrolled bleeding or after a rebleed from a lesion close to an endoscopically identified blood vessel, particularly if other treatment (argon laser, somatostatin) has failed. Probably in elderly patients in whom haemodynamic equilibrium has been re-established and who have needed prolonged transfusion, surgery should also be carried out if a definite bleeding point has been identified in relation to a peptic ulcer. Surgery should be carried out in those hospitals where laser photocoagulation is not under trial.

It seems that, while the value of neither argon laser treatment nor of intravenous somatostatin has yet been confirmed, either or both of these over the next few years may be shown to be effective, at least in selected patients.

GALLSTONES AND THEIR DISSOLUTION

Formation

Because over 80% of gallstones found in patients from Western Europe and the United States are predominantly composed of cholesterol, and because we understand the physiology of the formation of cholesterol gallstones much more clearly than the physiology of non-cholesterol stones, it is only the former which will be considered here.

Small (1980) summarised the stages in the formation of cholesterol gallstone disease as follows:

1. There is a genetic and metabolic stage at which the genetic propensity or metabolic abnormality that can lead to the production of supersaturated bile is present but not yet manifest
2. There is a chemical stage, during which gall bladder bile becomes supersaturated with cholesterol
3. Next is a physical stage during which the supersaturated bile is nucleated and growth of cholesterol monohydrate crystals is initiated
4. Microscopic crystals grow or agglomerate into macroscopic stones
5. Macroscopic stones cause symptoms by initiating cholecystitis or by blocking the cystic duct, common duct or both.

The natural history of gallstone disease is not clear. An intensive study of the Pima Indians (Sampliner et al 1970, Shaffer & Small 1976, Bennion et al 1979) has shown that, in this highly susceptible race, about 70% of the women ultimately develop gallstones and approximately half have symptoms from the stones within 20 years. In a series of 123 American (mainly white male) subjects initially found to have completely asymptomatic and previously unsuspected gallstones on routine pre-employment cholecystography, Gracie & Ransohoff (1981) found that only 16 developed symptoms of gallstones in a follow-up of 10–20 years; in only three of these did complications occur. In Sweden, Wenckert & Robertson (1966) followed up 781 patients found on oral cholecystography to have gallstones and who did not have a cholecystectomy within 1 year of the X-ray examination. Half of these patients had no symptoms or only mild symptoms in a follow-up over 1–11 years. One-third of patients had severe symptoms, most requiring cholecystectomy, and complications (obstructive jaundice, cholangitis) developed in 18% of patients.

In Britain, the prevalence of gallstones at necropsy in subjects under 60 years of age was about 10% in men and 15% in women. This rose to 17% and 25% respectively, after the age of 75 years (Barker et al 1979). The vast majority of these subjects were asymptomatic of gallstone disease. Other post-mortem studies in several European countries suggest that 25–55% of individuals will have had a cholecystectomy or be found to have gallstones at the time of necropsy. Thus, the proportion of individuals who will ultimately develop gallstones varies from country to country and race to race (variability of stage 1 in the genesis of cholesterol gallstone disease). The proportion of patients who will develop symptoms (arrival at stage 5 from stage 4), is also poorly documented.

Few would argue that patients with severe symptoms or complications from gallstones should have cholecystectomy (Editorial, Lancet 1980), despite the risk of death from cholecystectomy — about 0.4% in elective operations (McSherry & Glenn 1980) and the probably increased risk of carcinoma of the colon in subjects who have had a cholecystectomy (Linos et al 1981, Vernick & Kuller 1981).

It is in the management of patients with mild or very infrequent symptoms, or with asymptomatic stones found by chance, that controversy still exists. It is 10 years since Danzinger and colleagues (1972) first demonstrated the dissolution of cholesterol gallstones by chenodeoxycholic acid (CDCA). It should therefore be possible to suggest whether gallstone dissolution is likely to be of benefit for such patients.

Dissolution

Many studies have now shown that only radiolucent gallstones in a functioning gallbladder have any chance of dissolution with bile acid treatment — CDCA or ursodeoxycholic acid (UDCA) (James 1979). Furthermore, gallstones in obese subjects, and those stones over about 15 mm in diameter, are probably resistant to treatment (Maton et al 1980).

Despite claims that CDCA and UDCA may, in time, dissolve gallstones in over 50% of patients treated after the above criteria have been met (Dowling 1981, Salen et al 1981), a large and well-conducted controlled study of CDCA has reported that, in 916 patients with radiolucent stones in functioning gallbladders, only 13.5% of patients taking 750 mg CDCA for up to 2 years (always for at least one year) showed complete dissolution of stones. Perhaps this dose was too low; nevertheless, this is a disappointing result (Schoenfield et al 1981). Higher doses of CDCA lead to diarrhoea but there have been no serious irreversible side effects after treatment with either bile acid. However, in the American National Cooperative Gallstone Study 'significant' hepatotoxicity was reported in 3% of patients receiving 750 mg CDCA per day. Although UDCA treatment only very rarely causes diarrhoea, in about 10% of patients treated with this agent stones may calcify, thus rendering dissolution impossible (Bateson et al 1981). A further nail in the coffin of current oral bile acid treatment is that in the best-available follow-up study, gallstones recurred in 22/28 patients within 5 years of dissolution (Ruppin & Dowling 1981). This means either that maintenance treatment may be necessary or that there should be considerable alteration of the diet by increased intake of dietary fibre and restriction of cholesterol consumption (Pomare et al 1976, Maudgal et al 1978). At present therefore, despite the continued optimism of gallstone-dissolving enthusiasts, it would seem that the following strategem is most sensible in dealing with this disease:

1. Complications or severe symptoms — cholecystectomy
2. Mild symptoms. Consider bile acid treatment in thin patients with small radiolucent stones in a functioning gallbladder, particularly if (a) the patient is anxious to obtain treatment without operation; (b) there is some contraindication to surgery
3. Asymptomatic. Masterly inactivity; alternatively, bile acid treatment if the patient might be at extra risk from complications or surgery at a later date.

VIRAL HEPATITIS

In no other area of medicine has there been a greater explosion of knowledge than in the field of viral hepatitis. We are beginning to understand the contributions which the three or four principal viruses responsible for these infections make, not only to acute but to chronic liver disease, cirrhosis and primary liver cancer.

Hepatitis A (infectious hepatitis)

The virus

It was not until 1973 that the virus responsible for hepatitis A (HAV) was isolated in the stools of volunteer patients who developed acute hepatitis (Feinstone et al 1973). The identity of the virus was confirmed on several continents within 3 years. HAV is a small cubic particle of 27–30 nm; the nucleic acid is a linear single-stranded RNA. The weight of evidence favours the classification of HAV as a Picornavirus, probably of the enterovirus group (Maynard & Bradley 1980). Immunofluorescent studies have shown that the virus is detectable in the liver only during the acute clinical phase of an HAV infection. Most of the virus is excreted via the faeces before the activity of hepatic enzymes becomes increased (Murphy et al 1978). The diagnosis of an acute HAV infection may be made by the detection of specific HAV antibodies of the IgM class (IgM anti-HAV) which is invariably present during an acute attack. This IgM diminishes over succeeding weeks after the onset of the attack and IgG anti-HAV increases. We may thus conclude that (1) if IgM anti-HAV is present in the serum of a patient, this is evidence of a recent infection with HAV: (2) if IgM anti-HAV is absent from the serum of a patient with an acute attack of hepatitis, then the HAV is not the virus responsible (Frosner et al 1980).

The clinical illness

The clinical expression of an acute HAV episode is changing. It is no longer predominantly a disease of children, possibly because of improved sanitation, but is now commonly seen in adults (Frosner et al 1979). Whereas in Germany the disease is found very rarely in persons above the age of 40 years and a high percentage show immunity to the disease, a recent outbreak amongst mainly elderly and distinguished doctors in Britain in which acute HAV hepatitis developed in over 25%, suggests that a higher proportion of older individuals are achieving years of maturity before exposure to the virus, thus rendering them susceptible to an acute HAV attack at what has hitherto been thought of as an unlikely advanced age. A similar trend has been observed in Scandinavia and in the United States. No case of chronic liver disease attributable to HAV infection has been recorded, nor has a 'carrier state' of the virus been recognised.

Hepatitis B (serum hepatitis)

The virus

The hepatitis B virus (HBV) is a 42 nm sphere (the Dane particle); this has an outer coat, where the antigenic determinant HBsAg is expressed, and an inner 27 nm core. The core is released from the virion by treatment with detergents and is associated with a unique antigenic activity, HBcAg. Within the core there is a small circular double strand of DNA and an enzyme, DNA polymerase; a further antigen found in the serum of some patients with HBV infection is also found inside the virus core, this is the HBeAg. (see Fig. 10.1). In addition, the serum of patients infected with HBV contains small spherical particles, 22 nm in diameter, and long filamentous

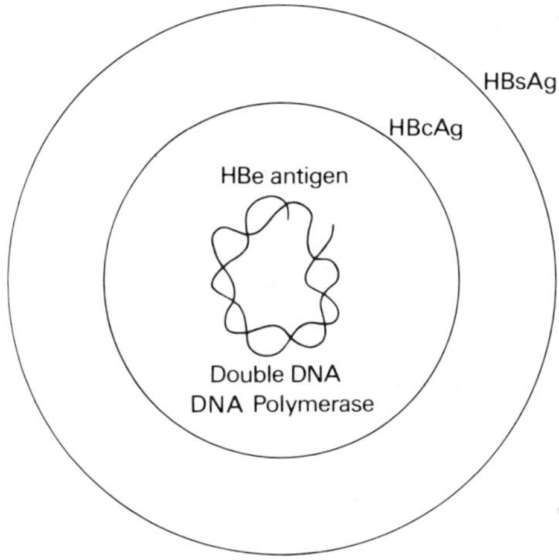

Fig. 10.1 The hepatitis B virus

structures. These carry HBsAg determinants on their surfaces but contain no nucleic acid. There are thus three antigenic components associated with the HBV, to each of which an antibody may be produced. I will deal with each antigen/antibody in turn and try to assess its significance.

HBsAg and anti-HBs. After an infection with the HBV, HBsAg appears in the blood within an incubation period of 6 months. This HBs antigenaemia usually precedes overt jaundice by about 1 week. In up to 10% of patients the HBsAg has already been cleared from the blood by the time that overt symptoms develop (Hoofnagle et al 1979); in a further 50% it has been cleared within 2 months. After 4 months the HBsAg has disappeared from the serum in almost all patients in whom an acute HBV attack has occurred without progression to chronic liver disease. Antibody to HBsAg (anti-HBs) appears only during convalescence, usually several weeks after the disappearance of HBsAg; rarely are HBsAg and anti-HBs detectable simultaneously. Anti-HBs is usually present in only low titre; indeed, in about 10% patients it never appears after an acute HBV infection. The antibody signifies immunity from the HBV and marks recovery from an HBV infection; it is not present in chronic HBV disease (Hoofnagle 1980). Persistence of HBsAg in the blood following an acute HBV infection indicates the likelihood of progression to chronic liver disease and the presence of a carrier state (Nielsen et al 1971).

HBeAg/anti HBe. HBeAg is found only during the period of HBs antigenaemia. It appears at about the time of onset of symptoms in patients with an acute HBV attack, and usually disappears after about 2 weeks. It is followed by an antibody, anti-HBe, which remains detectable in the serum for many months. If HBeAg is not replaced by anti-HBe during an acute attack of HBV infection but persists for more than 10 weeks in the serum, then progression to chronic liver disease is likely (Nielsen 1980). In a follow-up study of patients with HBsAg-positive chronic liver disease, Realdi et al (1980) showed that HBeAg was more likely to be associated with chronic active hepatitis without cirrhosis, whereas anti-HBe was found in patients with established cirrhosis: seroconversion from HBeAg to anti-HBe was found in 10 of 29 subjects and was associated with decrease in serum transaminase and progression to cirrhosis. The presence of HBeAg was thought to indicate active replication of whole HB viruses and thus to be a marker of infectivity. Patients who are HBsAg-positive with anti-HBe are thought to be producing only the HBsAg coat, not the whole Dane particle, and thus they are either non-infectious or have only very low infectivity. This may reflect incorporation of the HBV genome into the liver cell genome; thus the liver cell may produce the HBsAg independent of viral replication.

HBcAg/anti-HBc. The HBcAg is a unique antigenic determinant displayed on the core of the HBV. This core contains DNA polymerase. Thus the presence of HBcAg or this enzyme in the serum indicates that whole virus particles are present in the serum, and implies high infectivity (Robinson 1975). During acute HBV infection the antibody to HBcAg (anti-HBc) is detected at about the time of onset of the illness. The titre of this antibody, once elevated, may not fall for several years after an acute attack; it always remains elevated in patients who have persistent HBV infection. The level of specific anti-HBcIgM also rises at the outset of clinical infection. This disappears from the serum within a year after acute infection, but persists in chronic HBV disease. The detection of anti-HBc or anti-HBcIgM may be used to confirm recent HBV infection in the 'window' between the disappearance of HBsAg and the appearance of anti-HBs. Very occasionally, patients whose serum is negative for HBsAg but contains anti-HBc, or more specifically anti-HBcIgM, may be infectious.

The spectrum of clinical illness following HBV infection (Fig. 10.2)

The prevalence of HBsAg carriers in the apparently healthy population varies from 0.1% in the UK through about 5% in Greece to over 15% in Hong Kong and Singapore. Among chronic asymptomatic HBsAg carriers with normal liver function tests, about a quarter have changes of chronic persistent hepatitis; only 3 of 68 patients in a recent study by De Franchis et al (1980) had chronic active hepatitis on liver biopsy. During follow-up only one further patient developed abnormal liver function tests and progressed to chronic active hepatitis on biopsy; in this study the presence or absence of HBeAg or anti-HBe was of no prognostic value in follow-up. The histological abnormalities in the liver do not reflect serum biochemistry in asymptomatic carriers with abnormal LFTs but a considerable proportion have significant liver disease, even cirrhosis.

The clinical course of acute HBV viral hepatitis is familiar, the most important questions at the outset of an acute attack being (1) will this patient develop fulminant hepatic failure? and (2) will the patient develop chronic liver disease? Less than 5% of patients with acute type B hepatitis develop fulminant hepatic failure (FHF); in the majority of cases this is within a few days of the onset of symptoms. HB virus infection probably accounts for about 20% of patients in Britain with hepatic coma (Grade 4 or 5) from FHF. Survival, once unrousable (Grade 4) coma is reached, is about 10–20%. If serum albumin remains normal and thrombotest is over 25% of control then death from FHF is very unlikely indeed. Although support measures are vital, whatever the cause of FHF, there is no evidence from controlled trials that any treatment improves survival from FHF. This does not, and should not, stop the search continuing (Opolon et al 1978, Jenkins & Williams 1980).

The risk of developing chronic liver disease after acute HBV infection is closely, but not completely, related to the persistence of HBsAg in the serum. HBsAg persists

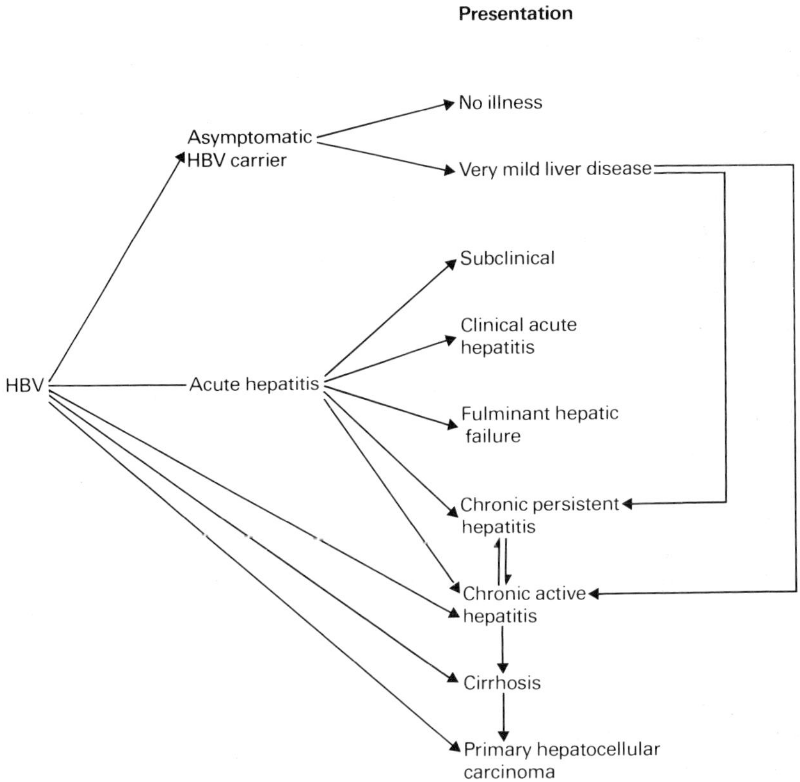

Fig. 10.2 Spectrum of clinical illness following infection with hepatitis B virus

in the serum for more than 4 months in 7–10% of patients and, of these, Norkrans et al (1976) showed that 86% developed chronic active hepatitis or chronic persistent hepatitis. In this study of 440 patients, only 18 (4%) who were only transiently HBsAg-positive, developed chronic liver disease. An identifiable acute attack does not seem important in the development of HBV-associated chronic liver disease. There are two histological precirrhotic forms: chronic persistent hepatitis (CPH) in which inflammation with plasma cells and lymphocytes is virtually confined to the portal tracts, and chronic active hepatitis (CAH) in which inflammation extends into the parenchyma of the liver with active destruction of liver cells and consequent fibrosis. The former rarely progresses to the latter and equally rarely does it apparently progress to cirrhosis, whereas HBsAg-associated chronic active hepatitis usually does progress to cirrhosis.

There is a striking geographical correlation between the frequency of primary hepatocellular carcinoma (PHC) and the prevalence of HBsAg carriers in the population. HBsAg carriers are rare in Britain and the USA, and PHC is also a fairly uncommon tumour: however, in South-East Asia, where over 10% of the population are HBsAg-positive, PHC is the second commonest malignant tumour. This has led to the hypothesis that infection with HBV is required for the development of most cases of PHC (Blumberg & London 1981). It is hypothesised that the genomes of the

HBV DNA become integrated into the host liver cells, ultimately producing malignant transformation of the cells. One other possible association between HBV infection and liver disease deserves mention. Mills et al (1981) have suggested that there is a relationship between serological evidence of previous HBV infection and alcoholic cirrhosis, particularly with portal hypertension. They suggest that previous HBV infection could be a risk factor in selecting those among a population of heavy drinkers who are particularly susceptible to alcohol-induced liver damage.

Treatment of chronic HBsAg-associated liver disease

Two main questions must be answered in discussion of treatment of HBsAg-associated chronic liver disease: (1) which patients should be treated? and (2) should treatment be aimed at the liver, the virus, or both?

If the main histological lesion is chronic persistent hepatitis (CPH), then the prognosis appears to be good without treatment, whether presentation is following acute HBV infection or because of chronic mild liver disease or following detection as an asymptomatic carrier. Few, if any, patients with this histological grade have developed serious symptoms or complications of liver disease after follow-up for as long as 19 years (Chadwick et al 1979). The treatment of HBsAg-positive chronic active hepatitis is an area of controversy. Treatment of 'lupoid' chronic active hepatitis (HBsAg-negative but with positive serum markers of autoimmunity) with corticosteroids has been shown to be very effective in improving survival and reducing complications of liver disease: as the histological appearance of the liver (liver cells and portal tracts being 'attacked' by lymphocytes and plasma cells) is so similar in HBsAg-positive and HBsAg-negative CAH, the temptation to use steroids to treat the former is clear. Although small uncontrolled studies have suggested benefit from such treatment, the recent control study of Lam et al (1981) suggested that treatment of HBsAg-positive CAH with prednisolone was disastrous. Prednisolone treatment led to increase in death rate, increase in complications and poorer liver function tests. It has been suggested that immunosuppressant treatment in HBV CAH causes increased viral replication, thus cancelling the beneficial effects which could otherwise ensue from damping-down inflammation. More hope for the future for the treatment of HBV liver disease in general, and of HBV CAH in particular, may be offered by the use of antiviral agents. Human leucocyte interferon has been shown to be of some benefit in large amounts (Greenberg et al 1976) but of no benefit in smaller quantities (Weimar et al 1980). Treatment with adenine arabinoside has been shown to reduce indices of viral replication and thus to reduce infectivity of some carriers (Bassendine et al 1981). It seems likely that antiviral therapy in future may not only reduce infectivity but may halt further liver injury.

Vaccination agains HBV infection

During 1980 and 1981 the results of a number of studies of vaccination using several different inactivated hepatitis B vaccines, particularly in high-risk groups of subjects, have been reported (Stevens et al 1980, Szmuness et al 1980, Crosnier et al 1981, Maupas et al 1981). It can be concluded, even at this early stage, that vaccination appears to be safe, even in young children and haemodialysis patients. After two booster doses, vaccination produced appreciable titres of anti-HBs in over 90% of patients tested in all studies so far, except in one French report of haemodialysis patients, only 60% of whom achieved satisfactory titres (Crosnier et al 1981). The evidence appears to be that, after 60 d following the first passive vaccination, fresh HBV infections are very rare indeed even in high-risk populations, although absolute immunity is not acquired. Vaccination appears to be least effective in male haemodialysis patients. Current HBV vaccines are expensive and before vaccination is considered on a wide scale in areas of the world of high endemicity, costs must fall very considerably. This advance does hold the hope of substantially reducing morbidity from chronic liver disease and even mortality from PHC in the future.

Non-A, non-B hepatitis

The emergence of viruses associated with clinical viral hepatitis resembles the British obsession with spies within its own Secret Service. With specific serological tests for HAV and HBV it has become clear that a further virus or viruses (non-A non-B) must be responsible for many cases of clinical hepatitis.

In the USA, non-A non-B hepatitis is said to be responsible for up to 89% of patients with post-transfusion hepatitis (Alter et al 1975), thus implying a parenteral means of transmission. Such non-A non-B hepatitis occurs in perhaps 10% of patients receiving blood transfusions in the USA (Aach et al 1981). In that country, non-A non-B hepatitis probably accounts for about 25% of hospital admissions for acute sporadic hepatitis (Dienstag et al 1977). In Britain the proportion is a little lower — perhaps about 16% (Bamber et al 1981). In Britain the importance of non-A non-B hepatitis following transfusion is unknown (Medical Research Council 1974) but is becoming recognised as a serious hazard in treatment of patients with factor VIII or factor IX concentrates which are prepared from large pools of donor plasma Editorial, Lancet 1981). In India however, where outbreaks of water-borne acute hepatitis are not uncommon, it appears that, contrary to previous belief, the virus responsible for a number of such outbreaks is not HAV but a non-A non-B organism (Wong et al 1980).

The incubation period of non-A non-B infection may be even less than 10 d (Kim et al 1980) although it is often 35–40 d; this adds weight to the belief that more than one virus is responsible. While non-A non-B hepatitis has been transmitted in chimpanzees and a candidate virus identified (Alter et al 1978), no virus irrefutably causing non-A non-B hepatitis has been identified in man. A number of immune reactions, notably the production of immune precipitin lines, have been described in the serum of patients with non-A non-B hepatitis: Suh et al (1981) have shown that such reactions may be due to the detection of immune complexes rather than of specific viral components. Serological tests for non-A non-B viruses will greatly assist our evaluation of the disease or diseases which they produce.

Non-A, non-B clinical course

Both sporadic and post-transfusion cases appear to have a similar spectrum. About half the patients who develop post-transfusion non-A, non-B hepatitis continue to have abnormal LFTs at least 1 year after the initial illness. Histological evidence of CPH, CAH and, more rarely, cirrhosis has been seen to develop. Cirrhosis may develop over several years and in a clinically inapparent fashion (Koretz et al 1980). On the other hand, recovery to normality may take over a year (Bamber et al 1981).

Evidence of a chronic non-A non-B carrier state in humans is scant up to now, although it is well documented in a few cases (Tabor et al 1980).

The 'silent' development of chronic liver disease after a clinically not very apparent post-transfusion infection of non-A, non-B hepatitis, and the possible frequency with which the disease occurs, suggest that here may be the clue to the major remaining cause of cryptogenic chronic liver disease — CAH or cirrhosis (Berman et al 1979).

CHRONIC ACTIVE HEPATITIS (CAH)

Definition

This condition has had many names: it was originally (and misleadingly) called lupoid hepatitis because of the occurrence of the LE cell phenomenon in some 15% of patients, notably younger women with an aggressive autoimmune form of illness. The 'disease' (CAH) is really a description of a histological appearance of the liver which has a wide variety of different causes. It may be defined as an inflammation of the liver, continuing for longer than 6 months, with histological features of (1) portal inflammation with lymphocytes and plasma cells, (2) aggressive formation of septa from portal tracts and (3) 'attack' upon liver cells with piecemeal necrosis and rosette formation (Anthony et al 1978, Editorial, British Medical Journal 1980). Redeker (1981) has pointed out that the distinction between CAH and chronic persistent hepatitis (CPH) is worth making because of the belief that chronic active hepatitis is a progressive disorder leading, in many instances, to the complications of liver cell failure or portal hypertension, whereas CPH is a non-progressive milder inflammatory lesion.

Diagnostic categories

The definition of the diagnostic sub-groups of CAH has become increasingly important as implications for treatment and prognosis clarify themselves. The diagnostic categories are shown in Figure 10.3.

Viral CAH

Most patients presenting with clinical CAH have been classified into one of two groups — HBsAg-positive CAH or HBsAg-negative, autoantibody-positive (autoimmune) CAH. A further group of patients comprises those who have clinical and biochemical features of CAH and have a compatible histological picture but who have no markers of past or present HBV infection or of autoimmunity. These may well turn out to be associated with persistent non-A non-B viral infection (Alter 1980). The management of these patients is at present ill-defined. Some suggestion exists from post-transfusion studies that the natural course of non-A non-B chronic liver disease is 'benign' in that, while some may progress to a relatively inactive cirrhosis, few patients develop progressive liver disease leading to liver cell failure in the manner of patients with autoimmune (lupoid) hepatitis (Berman et al 1979, Sampliner 1981).

I have already discussed the controversy over the use of steroids in the treatment of HBsAg-positive patients with CAH. This issue is further confused by the fact that

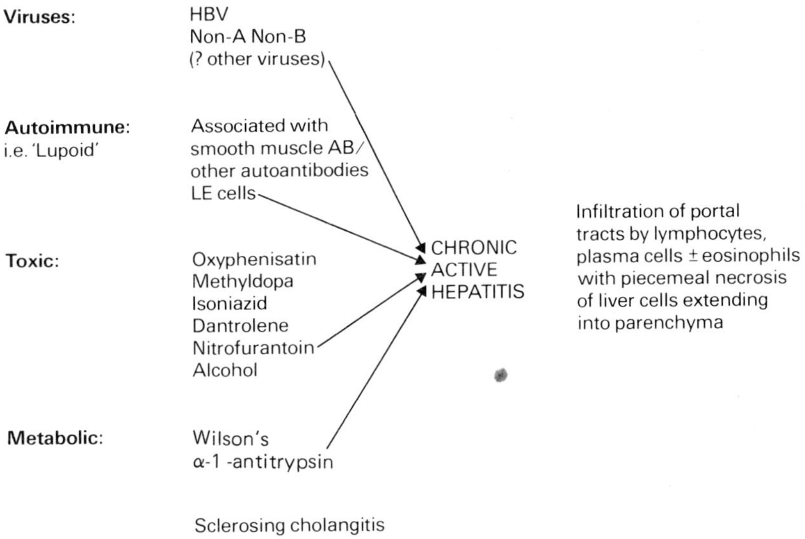

Fig. 10.3 Classification of the causes of chronic active hepatitis

HBsAg-positive CAH appears to be usually a fairly innocuous disease in Britain, whereas in the Far East, where it is much commoner, the clinical course is often more serious (Dudley et al 1972).

Autoimmune CAH

The mechanism by which autoimmune CAH arises is still poorly understood. The clinical correlation of CAH with thyroid disease, inflammatory bowel disease and sicca syndrome, the histological appearance of the liver with its lymphocytic infiltration, and the response to treatment with steroids with or without azathioprine, all lead to the belief that immunological factors must be important. It appears likely that an initial liver cell injury causes expression on the surface of the liver cell membrane of antigenic determinants which may cause a self-perpetuating cell-mediated immune reaction to occur. While such non-specific markers as smooth muscle or antimitochondrial antibodies (usually in low titre), and antinuclear antibodies, as well as the LE cell phenomenon, are found in the serum of patients with CAH, a more specific liver membrane protein or proteins have been described on the liver cell surface (Tage-Jensen et al 1977). At present it is difficult to distinguish cause from effect in immunological studies of CAH.

Effective treatment of CAH over a period of up to 5 years with prednisone or prednisolone with or without azathioprine in moderate doses has been demonstrated in three control trials during the early 1970s. Despite the fact that faults were subsequently found in these trials, their results have not been challenged (Wright et al 1977). From a recent long-term (10+ years) follow-up study of the original Royal Free Hospital controlled trial of prednisolone treatment, Kirk et al (1980) drew the following conclusions: 63% of prednisolone-treated patients were alive 10 or more years after diagnosis, compared with only 27% of the control group (two of whom had received prednisolone 5 or more years after the onset of symptoms). The beneficial effect of corticosteroids was most evident in the first 5 years from diagnosis; this was because untreated patients who survived for 6 years were all alive after 10 or more years. This finding supported the concept of the disease as being self-limiting, progressing to an inactive macronodular cirrhosis. Kirk et al (1980) finally suggested that the required duration of treatment is about 5 years.

Despite the thoroughness of the studies to which I have already referred, a number of questions still need consideration:

1. Which patients need treatment?
2. When should treatment be stopped and in whom?
3. How can relapse after cessation of treatment be predicted?

Wright et al (1977) have drawn attention to the diversity of criteria used before selecting patients for the trials of treatment. In an individual case it would seem sensible to start treatment (prednisolone about 20mg/day falling to about 10mg/day), plus azathioprine 75mg/day) on the basis of

1. liver histology showing CAH
2. one or more positive autoantibodies
3. serum transaminase elevated to twice normal or more and some elevation in gammaglobulin
4. HBsAg-negative
5. lack of presumptive evidence for an aetiology of CAH other than autoimmune.

In patients with clinically severe CAH who fail to respond to the doses of prednisolone and azathioprine mentioned, Schalm and colleagues (1976) found that the majority did respond to prednisolone 30mg and azathioprine 150mg daily.

The question of when to stop treatment is difficult. When liver function tests have returned to, or near, normal and the patient is clinically well, is this because of the effect of treatment? If so, on stopping the treatment the disease will flare again. Or has the disease burnt itself out, in which case the treatment is no longer needed? The best predictors of those patients still on treatment who will relapse if treatment is withdrawn, appear to be the level of serum bile acids (Korman et al 1974) and the persistence or disappearance of autoimmune markers in the serum (Dooley et al 1979). Liver biopsy is also important in the assessment of treatment and the likelihood of relapse. In general, if the liver biopsy has returned to normal or has progressed to an inactive cirrhosis, and LFTs have been normal for a year or more, then relapse is unlikely. If histology shows continuing CAH, then relapse after withdrawal of treatment is likely despite normal LFTs at the time of biopsy. The Mayo Clinic Group have shown that, if the biopsy appearance is that of chronic persistent hepatitis following treatment, then there is an even chance that the patient will relapse to more serious chronic active hepatitis within 2 years of stopping treatment (Czaja et al 1981). They suggest that the appearance of CPH seen after treatment of CAH with steroids is an unstable one — unlike CPH seen following HBV or non-A non-B infections.

Toxic CAH

It is of interest that a number of drugs together with alcohol may cause chronic liver disease in which the histological appearance of the liver is identical to that seen in lupoid hepatitis. Even serum markers of immune-mediated CAH may appear. The principal drugs implicated have been oxyphenisatin, methyldopa, isoniazid, dantrolene and nitrofurantoin (Maddrey & Boitnott 1977, Zimmerman & Ishak 1979, Sharp et al 1980); these are rare causes of CAH in Britain. Occasionally a patient with clinically 'cast iron' alcoholic liver disease turns out to have typical CAH on liver biopsy (Goldberg et al 1977). The reason is not clear but the emergence of cytotoxic lymphocytes sensitised towards alcoholic hyalin may be important in the progression of alcoholic liver disease in some patients (Kakumu & Leevy 1977). It may be appropriate to mention in this section that, in a recent study by Chapman et al (1980), the hepatic histology of two-thirds of 29 patients in whom a diagnosis of primary sclerosing cholangitis had been made, showed piecemeal necrosis suggesting a possible diagnosis of CAH. Seventy-two per cent of these patients also had ulcerative proctocolitis, although the connection between the conditions is not clear. It appears that this is yet another stimulus to which the hepatic response is that of a histological picture of CAH. Corticosteroid treatment was not effective in this series.

Metabolic CAH

Until recently it was thought that α-1-antitrypsin deficiency was an extremely rare cause of liver disease in adults, although it was an important cause of neonatal hepatitis (Fisher et al 1976, Triger et al 1976), but Hodges and colleagues (1980) have now suggested that as many as 20% of adults with non-HBV CAH may be heterozygous MZ α-1-antitrypsin patients. These subjects are older (mean age about 60 years) and meticulous examination of liver biopsies reveals PAS-positive diastase-resistant inclusions characteristic of α-1-antitrypsin within the liver. The importance of this finding remains to be assessed.

While at present there is no therapeutic implication to the detection of mild α-1-antitrypsin deficiency as a cause of liver disease, this is certainly not the case with Wilson's disease. One estimate was that up to 6% of patients presenting with CAH have Wilson's disease, but this is probably a gross exaggeration (Sternlieb & Scheinberg 1972). Nevertheless, in patients under 30 years of age presenting with CAH and with negative serum autoantibodies and markers of HBV infection, Wilson's disease must be excluded because early treatment gives a good prognosis for survival, whereas once features of portal hypertension or liver cell failure have developed, rapid demise is almost inevitable despite treatment with D-penicillamine. Prednisolone is of no benefit (Scott et al 1978). Kayser–Fleischer rings are usually present but may be absent in young patients in whom the disease has presented in acute form. In these patients, high urinary copper excretion and low serum ceruloplasmin levels should be looked for. Although liver copper estimation is useful (it is almost always over 250 μg per gram dry liver weight) it is not practical to wait for this result, which often takes months to be returned.

PRIMARY BILIARY CIRRHOSIS

Occurrence

Primary biliary cirrhosis (PBC) was once thought to be a rare disease of middle-aged women presenting with cholestatic jaundice, pruritus or complications of portal hypertension. Several studies have suggested, in Britain at least, that the disease is far from rare, point prevalence being about 50 per million (Hislop 1980, Triger 1980, James et al 1981); nevertheless, Saunders et al (1981) maintain that it *is* still very rare.

Aetiology

As with so many diseases of the gastrointestinal tract and its appendages, theories of the aetiology of PBC abound. These may be drawn into three strands: (1) immunological, (2) relation to other diseases and (3) infective/environmental.

The immunological aspects of PBC have been the subject of much speculation. The following appear to be relatively undisputed facts. The early histological lesion in PBC shows a monocytic inflammation with prominent accumulation of lymphocytes and granulomata in relation to portal tracts (Scheuer 1973). There is increased catabolism of complement (Jones et al 1979) and there are circulating complement-fixing immune complexes in the serum (Thomas et al 1978, Wands et al 1978) at several stages of the disease. Sandilands et al (1980) have also demonstrated IgG non-complement-fixing immune complexes which probably bind to the lymphocyte Fc receptors, thus in some way controlling the activity of these lymphocytes in the disease. Whether these and other immunological phenomena are a cause or an effect of the disease is far from clear. The mystery of the presence in virtually all patients with PBC of antibodies to the inner surface of mitochondrial membranes of several tissues (AMA) in several species is also not clear (Munoz et al 1981). Berg and colleagues (1980) have characterised the PBC-specific AMA as a trypsin-sensitive ATPase-associated antigen of the inner mitochondrial membrane, but the relationship of this antibody to the aetiology of PBC has not been elucidated.

The relationship between PBC and a number of other possibly immunologically mediated diseases — thyroid disease and sicca syndrome (Crowe et al 1980a), rheumatoid arthritis and connective tissue disorders (Schaffner 1979) — further strengthens the belief that PBC has some 'autoimmune' pathogenesis. Epstein et al (1980) drew the parallel between the 'dry gland' manifestations of PBC together with some of its hepatic histological features and the chronic graft-versus-host disease following bone-marrow transplantion.

While there is no direct evidence to support an infective cause for PBC, the finding of significant clustering in relation to water supply (Triger 1980) in one area and the occurrence of PBC in a mother, daughter and close friend (Douglas & Finlayson 1979) suggest that some environmental factor could be important, possibly in a person with increased susceptibility to the disease.

Finally, there is an accumulation of copper in PBC. By analogy with Wilson's disease it has been suggested that the copper may play a part in the pathogenesis, or at least in the continuing liver damage, of PBC (Fleming et al 1974). Certainly, copper is present in the liver at an early precirrhotic stage of the disease, although it is not localised within lysosomes. As the disease progresses, hepatic copper content increases and this does localise to lysosomes in a similar pattern to that seen in Wilson's disease; nevertheless, this accumulation probably still merely reflects impaired biliary excretion rather than a prime event in the pathogenesis of the condition (Weisner et al 1979, James et al 1981).

Clinical course

With the advent of widespread autoantibody screening for patients with possible autoimmune diseases, and with biochemical profiles including LFTs, it has become clear that patients with PBC may be asymptomatic for many years (Long et al 1977, Roll et al 1980). Indeed, a number of patients with diagnostic hepatic histology and positive AMA but with no symptoms of liver disease and normal LFTs have now been described. Some patients may, therefore, never develop a clinical illness associated with liver disease, but those who do, usually present with non-specific symptoms or pruritus rather than with jaundice (Christensen et al 1980). About 10% present for the first time with symptoms of portal hypertension (Sherlock & Scheuer 1973). In the later stages of the illness, serum bilirubin gives the best indication of prognosis. Shapiro et al (1979) showed that, when two serum bilirubin levels 6 months apart exceeded 34 μmol/l, the patient had entered a late phase of the disease with a mean survival of about 4 years. Presymptomatic patients have a life expectancy similar to that of the general population.

Signs of piecemeal necrosis and aggressive fibrosis are hepatic histological features suggesting a poor prognosis (Roll et al 1980). Epstein and colleagues (1981a) have found that the presence of granulomas in the biopsy is a very good prognostic sign, whatever the stage of the disease.

Treatment

By analogy with CAH and in view of the marked evidence of immunological disturbance in this disease, immunosuppressant treatment would seem logical. Because patients with advanced disease have osteomalacia associated with chronic cholestasis, corticosteroids are said to be contraindicated (Sherlock 1981), but no satisfactory control study has been carried out using prednisolone in the treatment of PBC. In two well-conducted controlled trials azathioprine has been shown to have no beneficial effect on liver function tests, hepatic histology or mortality (Heathcote et al 1976, Crowe et al 1980b). The potent immunosuppresant cyclosporin A has been shown to improve liver function tests markedly over a short period of treatment, but nephrotoxicity of this drug precludes long-term use (Routhier et al 1980).

Because of its ability to reduce hepatic copper concentration and perhaps because of its immunological and antifibrotic actions, D-pencillamine has also been used in the treatment of PBC. The full results of only one trial extending over 6 years are available (Epstein et al 1981b) and these are supported by some suggestions from other studies still in progress (Fleming et al 1978), although one trial was abandoned because of lack of response (Matloff et al 1979). It appears that D-penicillamine in a dose of about 600 mg daily significantly prolongs survival of patients with PBC, but this improvement in survival becomes apparent only after 18 months' treatment. Thus, patients dying before this time probably had liver disease too advanced to be influenced by treatment; treatment does not appear to prevent the changes in liver structure which lead to cirrhosis. About one-third of patients with PBC treated with D-penicillamine develop serious side effects, notably thrombocytopoenia, proteinuria and an SLE-like syndrome (Macklon et al 1982) so that treatment should not be undertaken lightly. At present it would appear reasonable to reserve D-penicillamine treatment for symptomatic patients with a later histological liver lesion since early asymptomatic patients have such an excellent prognosis.

In addition to definitive treatment, support measures with cholestyramine or possibly sun-ray lamp treatment for pruritus and fat-soluble vitamins plus calcium should be given. A few patients develop marked steatorrhea with weight loss for reasons which are not clear — such patients should receive a low-fat diet with added medium-chain triglyceride oil (Beckett et al 1980).

ALCOHOLIC LIVER DISEASE (Table 10.1)

More white males in the United States under 50 years of age die of alcoholic liver disease than from any other cause. The death rate from cirrhosis is closely related to the per capita consumption of alcohol among different European countries. In Britain the annual incidence of alcoholic cirrhosis in one city increased four-fold between 1959 and 1974 (Saunders et al 1981). Alcoholic cirrhosis now accounts for over 50% of patients with cirrhosis in Britain (Hamlyn & James 1978); deaths from cirrhosis rose by over 50% and per capita alcohol consumption doubled in the 20 years up to 1978 in Britain (Office of Population Censuses and Surveys 1979). Alcoholic liver disease may therefore now be regarded as epidemic in Britain although the number of deaths is probably grossly underestimated as all must be reported to H.M. Coroner and an inquest with its attendant publicity is then almost invariably carried out.

Table 10.1 Alcohol-induced liver damage (adapted from Occasional Survey, Lancet 1981)

Stage	Reversibility	Features
Fatty liver	Reversible	Clinical complications may include cholestatic episodes, acute liver failure, Zieve's syndrome
Alcoholic hepatitis	Transitional; without cirrhosis probably reversible	Essential lesion is liver cell necrosis with related polymorphonuclear-leucocyte infiltrate; may also show chronic active hepatitis-like picture; may be focal, diffuse, or massive; may cause acute liver failure and portal hypertension without cirrhosis
Cirrhosis	Irreversible	Nearly always micronodular in early stages; complications of liver failure or portal hypertension often develop
Hepatocellular carcinoma	Very occasionally resectable, almost always in cirrhotic liver	May present with deterioration in a previously stable cirrhotic

Susceptibility

The questions of individual susceptibility to liver damage by alcohol remain mostly unanswered. Women appear to be more susceptible than men (Pecquignot & Tuyns 1975). There may be a genetic susceptibility to alcoholic liver damage, at least in women, since there is an association between the HLA blood group HLA B8 and women with alcoholic liver disease (Bailey et al 1976). There may be a connection between infection with HBV and susceptibility to alcoholic liver disease, which I have already mentioned, for Mills et al (1981) found that among 250 patients with alcoholic liver disease, 47% of those with portal hypertension had HBsAb versus 5% control subjects, although none were HBsAg-positive.

It is generally accepted that men may drink up to 80 g ethanol per day (equivalent to ¼ bottle spirits or almost a 700 ml bottle of wine) without greatly increasing their risk of developing liver disease; women may drink perhaps half that amount. Pequignot suggests pessimistically that these figures should be reduced to 40–60 g per day for men and 20 g per day for women. Consumption of an increased quantity of alcohol is associated with a log linear increase in the likelihood of developing cirrhosis, but consumption of 1 bottle whisky (240 g alcohol)/day for 20 years leads to only a 50% chance of cirrhosis (Lelbach 1975). The proportion of women with alcoholic liver disease has increased to a quarter of all patients (Morgan & Sherlock 1977), and possibly as many as one-third of patients currently attending our alcoholic liver disease clinic are women.

Mechanism of alcoholic liver damage

Although the mechanisms by which ethanol causes liver damage are still poorly understood, a number of factors are emerging as being of importance. These may be rather arbitrarily divided into acute metabolic effects on the liver cell and slower effects upon the whole liver (Table 10.2). Ethanol is oxidised in the liver to acetaldehyde, which itself causes damage to liver cell membranes and mitochondrial damage. This conversion of ethanol to acetaldehyde is via two pathways: (1) the normal pathway, using the enzyme alcohol dehydrogenase and causing increased production of NADH from NAD, thus altering the redox state of the liver and (2) the inducible pathway, using the microsomal ethanol-oxidising system (MEOS). The increased quantities of NADH 'donate' hydrogen ion which decreases the activity of the citric acid cycle; pyruvate is converted to lactate rather than glucose; this may lead to metabolic acidosis and hypoglycaemia following an alcohol binge; lipoprotein synthesis is also increased and fatty acid oxidation is diminished (Lieber 1978).

Over a longer time-scale, alcohol appears to stimulate fibrogenesis within the liver with increased collagen formation (Rojkind & Dunn 1979). This fibrosis is initially pericellular producing a 'chicken wire' appearance; later, fibrosis around hepatic

Table 10.2 Mechanisms in the production of alcoholic liver damage

Acute metabolic effects	Slower effects
Accumulation of acetaldehyde	Increased fibrogenesis (↑ new collagen formation)
Increased synthesis of fatty acids	Inhibition of liver cell regeneration (↓ protein synthesis)
Decreased degradation of fatty acids	Perivenular fibrosis
	Increased oxygen consumption → centrizonal liver cell necrosis
	Stimulation of autoimmune liver damage (production of anti-LSP in some patients)
	Possible decreased intake and malabsorption of nutrients

venules may indicate the likelihood of progression to cirrhosis (Van Waes & Lieber 1977).

The demonstration of impaired hepatic regeneration in experimental animals after toxic liver injury, the in vitro inhibition of liver-cell protein synthesis by ethanol, and the appearance of the cytoplasm in some liver cells showing ballooning degeneration thought to result from impaired protein secretion (Occasional Survey, Lancet 1981) together with the beneficial effects claimed for infusions of insulin and glucagon (thought to stimulate hepatic regeneration in alcoholic hepatitis (Baker et al, 1981)) all suggest that liver protein synthesis and cellular regeneration are impaired following damage to the liver by ethanol.

Increased oxygen consumption, leading to hypoxia particularly around centrizonal terminal hepatic venules, may lead to centrizonal liver cell necrosis (Israel et al 1979).

Although immunological mechanisms may not be important in every patient who develops alcoholic liver disease, Perperas et al (1981) have shown a close association between the presence of antibodies to liver membrane lipoprotein (LSP) in serum and infiltration of portal tracts by lymphocytes, with other histological features suggesting an autoimmune disorder. This occurred in about a quarter of the patients they investigated. It is postulated that in some patients with active alcoholic liver damage there is loss of immune tolerance with production of antibodies to LSP, causing continuing liver damage.

A final factor of possible importance in the progress of alcoholic liver disease is that of malnutrition, which is common in alcoholics. Certainly, malnutrition leads to impaired immunity (O'Keefe et al 1980), but no firm evidence exists as to the contribution of deficiency of specific dietary components to the progress of alcoholic liver disease (Mezey 1980).

Treatment of alcoholic liver disease

Abstinence

The first and most important treatment for patient with alcoholic liver disease must be to get them to stop drinking, at least for several months. Borowsky et al (1981) have shown that, of 54 male alcoholic cirrhotic patients who were discharged from hospital after initial admission with ascites, 15 continued to drink heavily; 12 of these 15 had died after a mean of 7 months. Of 23 patients who remained abstinent for at least 1 year, only one patient had died after a mean follow-up of almost 3 years. Interestingly, survival amongst the 16 moderate or binge drinkers was not different from that in the abstainers (13/16). Other studies in patients with severe alcoholic liver disease (hepatitis or cirrhosis) have confirmed these results, if less dramatically. Brunt et al (1974) showed that the chance of survival for 5 years after diagnosis of alcoholic liver disease doubled in abstainers compared with continuing drinkers (64% versus 34%). Powell & Klatskin (1968) also reported improved survival following abstinence.

Conventional treatment

Whatever additional therapy is considered, the conventional treatment of patients with severe acute alcoholic liver disease should be followed. Intravenous vitamins, particularly vitamin B complex and folic acid, should be given. Blood glucose should be carefully monitored and kept above about 6 mmol/l by intravenous infusion if necessary. A high-protein diet should be given to patients who do not have encephalopathy and treatment for portosystemic encephalopathy is administered if necessary. If acute alcohol withdrawal causes restlessness, then chlordiazepoxide, usually 60 mg/d for several days, may be necessary. If restlessness is not rapidly controlled, intravenous chlormethiazole must be given to prevent the onset of delirium tremens.

Additional treatment

Maddrey (1981) has observed that 'the search continues for a therapy or therapies to improve survival and decrease the rate of progression to cirrhosis in patients with severe alcoholic liver disease'. This search has produced two recent studies of acute alcoholic hepatitis which both claim very promising results. Nasrullah & Galambos (1980) performed a controlled trial of intravenous amino-acid treatment in acute alcoholic hepatitis; they used a conventional, (not branched chain-enriched) solution of amino-acids giving 70–85 g amino acid daily. Mortality was reduced in the treatment group and serum bilirubin and albumin levels were improved. It is possible that the group of patients studied were not as severely ill at the outset of treatment as those in some other studies, for only four out of 18 patients in the control group died — a low mortality figure for severe alcoholic hepatitis. In a controlled study of the effect of intravenous insulin and glucagon on alcoholic hepatitis (Baker et al 1981) among 24 severely ill patients (with bilirubin levels greater than 6 mg/dl and a prolonged prothrombin time of over 3 s) one out of nine treated patients died versus five out of 12 control patients who received conventional treatment. The rationale of this latter treatment was to promote hepatic regeneration. Although there is still only limited evidence that factors in the portal blood, probably from the pancreas, do improve hepatic regeneration, several studies of this role of insulin and glucagon in experimental animals are convincing (Maddrey 1981).

Studies of the use of steroids in acute alcoholic liver disease are conflicting, but in severely ill patients 40 mg prednisolone/day for 4 weeks was shown by Maddrey et al (1978) to improve the likelihood of survival, possibly by decreasing the inflammatory component of the injury. Longer-term treatment with steroids increased mortality.

In summary, the management of serious alcoholic liver disease rests upon two pillars: (1) get patients over the acute illness, possibly with the addition of insulin and glucagon or steroids to conventional treatment for a short period and (2) stop or substantially reduce alcohol consumption for at least 6 months after discharge from hospital. The patient will need a great deal of support during this latter phase of treatment.

TREATMENT OF PORTAL HYPERTENSION

The two end-results of chronic liver disease are liver cell failure and portal hypertension. Despite the increasing number of patients with bleeding from oesophageal varices, there are still no clear-cut courses of action which have been proved to be of benefit to patients either at the stage of acute bleeding or in prevention of further bleeding. Graham & Smith (1981) have graphically shown that comparison of different modes of treatment for bleeding varices must be made from the same moment of entry into a study. A 1-year survival rate of 34% for all medically treated patients could be raised to 52% by eliminating from consideration all who failed to survive the first 2 weeks. In this study of American patients, the vast majority of whom had alcoholic cirrhosis, the survival of patients who lived for 2 weeks after a variceal haemorrhage was not different from that according to published data on unselected cirrhotics without bleeding. Thus, the area in which there is substantial room for improvement in survival is the early period after a bleed. There was no difference in overall survival of 85 patients with endoscopically confirmed variceal haemorrhage treated in an excellent American centre in the period 1975–1980, compared with a similar group of patients treated in the years up to 1955 (Nachlas et al 1955). As Graham and Smith aptly remark, 'It is apparent that ... in spite of 40 years of improved understanding of the pathophysiology involved and advances in therapy we have learned much and accomplished little'.

A further difficulty in assessment of methods of treatment for portal hypertension is in the patient groups selected. Johnston & Rodgers (1973) reported mortality after admission of only 18% using rigid oesophagoscopic sclerotherapy for the treatment of acute variceal haemorrhage in 117 patients; the majority of these patients had good hepatic function, many having non-cirrhotic portal hypertension due to portal vein block. In contrast, the mortality after admission for patients in Britain with poor liver function, usually with alcoholic liver disease, following a bleed from oesophageal varices is over 50% (Sherlock 1981). Thus, trials of treatment must take into account the clinical state of patients at presentation. The grading of Child & Turcott (1964), based on the presence or absence of ascites and encephalopathy together with serum bilirubin and albumin levels, is still widely used, A being the best and C the worst prognostic group.

Recommended management

With great diffidence, which the above remarks show is very appropriate, I would suggest that the management pathway outlined in Figure 10.4 is now appropriate, at least in Britain, unless a control trial of other management is being carried out.

Endoscopy

The proportion of patients bleeding from varices among all upper gastrointestinal haemorrhage patients admitted to hospital in Britain is rising, from the very low 2–3% seen perhaps 30 years ago (Jones et al 1968) towards the 16% now seen in the USA. Up to one-third of the episodes of upper gastrointestinal bleeding in patients with alcoholic cirrhosis with confirmed oesophageal varices are not attributable to bleeding from the varices but to mucosal tear, gastritis or peptic ulcer (Novis et al 1976, Terblanche et al 1979). Thus, endoscopic verification that an episode of bleeding is from varices is vital as treatment of bleeding duodenal ulcer with a Sengstaken tube is, of course, quite inappropriate. If bleeding has stopped but it appears very probable that the source was from varices (no other obvious lesion seen, clot on a varix), the patient should be anaesthetised, an endotracheal tube inserted and the varices injected with sclerosant (ethanolamine oleate) via a fibreoptic oblique-viewing endoscope. The injection sclerotherapy is repeated every 3–4 weeks until the varices have been obliterated or are too small to inject (Clark et al 1980).

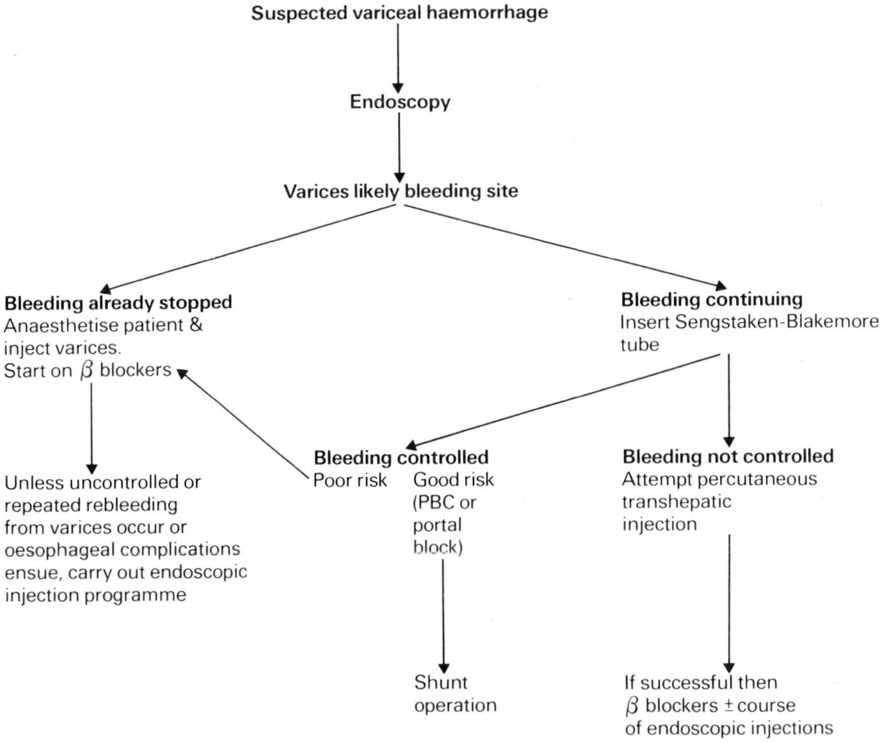

Fig. 10.4 Management of suspected haemorrhage from oesophageal varices

If bleeding is seen to be continuing at endoscopy, then after pitressin has been administered a four-lumen Sengstaken-Blakemore tube is passed and inflated to control haemorrhage. Once bleeding has been controlled and the clinical picture is stabilised, a more definitive treatment must be carried out because over 60% of patients admitted with bleeding oesophageal varices rebleed on the same admission and 90% do so within a year. The choice of treatment at present appears to be almost arbitrary since it is a truism that patients with good liver function (Child's grade A) do well and patients with poor liver function (Child's B and C) do poorly, whichever treatment is adopted. The good results from two centres using injection sclerotherapy (Terblanche et al 1979, Clark et al 1980) suggest that this may be the treatment of choice in patients with poor liver function or patients with alcoholic liver disease.

Shunt operations

Reynolds et al (1981) have compared the results obtained in a randomised trial of portacaval shunt versus medical management in 89 patients with alcoholic liver disease and severe upper gastrointestinal haemorrhage, with three other controlled trials of portacaval shunt also in rather poor-risk alcoholic patients. Although faults can be found in all four studies, the conclusions seem to be that portacaval shunt provided good protection from further gastrointestinal bleeding. Unfortunately, whereas non-surgically treated patients (who received no injection of varices) die of bleeding and its complications, surgically treated patients die of liver failure. Reynolds and colleagues confirm that they would no longer advise portacaval shunt in a patient with alcoholic liver disease after a single episode of gastrointestinal bleeding. They could not identify patients likely to do well or badly after surgery rather than medical treatment — presumably because the vast majority of patients continued to drink alcohol. A shunt operation, which virtually guarantees that there will be no recurrence of bleeding, is perhaps preferable in good-risk subjects. The results of portal decompression surgery seem to be particularly good in patients with primary biliary cirrhosis. Spinsi et al (1981) found that not one of 20 patients surviving the postoperative period following shunt surgery developed portal-systemic encephalopathy. All 15 patients in Child's grade A or B at the time of operation were alive 5 years later, with no rebleeding or encephalopathy. Although initially enthusiastic claims were made that the selective distal spleno-renal shunt resulted in less long-term encephalopathy than conventional portacaval shunt (Rikkers et al 1978), this view is now open to doubt.

Transhepatic venography

Although the scheme which I have outlined seems, to me at least, reasonable there are patients who have severe bleeding from varices in whom endoscopic injection or even placement of the Sengstaken tube proves to be impossible. After pitressin has been administered, Smith-Laing et al (1981) have used percutaneous transhepatic venography to demonstrate the vessels contributing to the oesophago-gastric varices and then to obliterate them using an injection of gelatin foam. This method, reserved for desperately ill patients, may stop bleeding temporarily and allow more definitive treatment, although rebleeding within a few months almost always occurs if no further treatment is offered.

β-blockers

Since prevention is better than cure, the observation of Lebrec et al (1980, 1981) that propranolol not only reduced portal pressure in cirrhotic patients but, in a control study, dramatically reduced the incidence of recurrence of upper gastrointestinal bleeds, is of considerable interest. They reported a one-year control study of propranolol versus placebo in preventing recurrence of bleeding from oesophageal varices. Eighteen of 36 patients who received placebo had bled again within periods up to 1 year after an initial bleeding episode had been controlled. Only one of 38 patients who received oral propranolol in doses that reduced the heart rate by 25% had bled again within the same period. These observations, if confirmed and extended over a longer follow-up period, will be of very great importance.

REFERENCES

Duodenal ulcer

Blackett R L, Johnston D 1981 Cimetidine and duodenal ulcer: can surgery cure the failures? Gut 22: A434

Burland W L, Hawkins B W, Beresford J 1980 Cimetidine treatment for the prevention of recurrence of duodenal ulcer; an international collaborative study. Postgraduate Medical Journal 56: 173–176

Centre for Ulcer Research and Education 1980 Is duodenal ulcer recurrence more common after cimetidine treatment? Gastroenterology 78: 1152
Editorial 1981 Cimetidine now. Lancet 1: 875–877
Editorial 1981a Does cimetidine cause gastric cancer? British Medical Journal 1: 1178–1179
Editorial 1981b Antacids for duodenal ulcer. British Medical Journal 1: 1495–1496
Elder J B, Ganguli P C, Gillespie I E 1979 Cimetidine and gastric cancer. Lancet 1: 1005–1006
Henry D A, Macdonald I A, Kitchingman G, Bell G D, Langman M J S 1980 Cimetidine and ranitidine: comparison of effects on drug metabolism. British Medical Journal 2: 775–777
Korman M G, Shaw D G, Hansky J, Schmidt G T, Stern A I 1981 Influence of smoking on healing rate of duodenal ulcer in response to cimetidine and high-dose antacid. Gastroenterology 80: 1451–1453
Lam S K, Lam K C, Lai C L, Yeung C K, Yam L Y C, Wong W S 1979 Treatment of duodenal ulcer with antacid and sulpiride. Gastroenterology 76: 315–322
Martin D 1981 Author's reply to 'prevention of duodenal ulcer recurrences'. Gastroenterology 81: 188
Martin D F, May S J, Tweedle D E F, Hollanders D, Ravenscroft M M, Miller J P 1981 Difference in relapse rates of duodenal ulcer after healing with cimetidine or tripotassium dicitrato bismuthate. Lancet 1: 7–10
Moshal M G, Gregory M A, Pillay C, Spilaela D J M 1979 Does the duodenal cell ever return to normal? A comparison between treatment with cimetidine and DeNol. Scandinavian Journal of Gastroenterology 14 (supplement 54): 48–51
Muscroft T J, Burdon D W, Youngs D J, Keighley M R B 1981 Cimetidine is unlikely to increase formation of intragastric N-nitroso-compounds in patients taking a normal diet. Lancet 1: 408–410
Peterson W L, Sturdevant R A L, Frankl H D, Richardson C T, Isenberg J I, Elashoff J D et al 1977 Healing of duodenal ulcer with an antacid regime. New England Journal of Medicine 297: 341–345
Pounder R E 1981 Model of medical treatment for duodenal ulcer. Lancet 1: 29–30
Roberts R K, Grice J, Wood L, Petroff V, McGuffie C 1981 Cimetidine impairs elimination of theophylline and antipyrine. Gastroenterology 81: 19–21
Robson R H, Heading R C 1978 Obsolete but dangerous antacid preparations. Postgraduate Medical Journal 54: 36–37
Serfontein W J, Meckel R 1979 Bismuth toxicity in man. Research Communications. Chemistry Pathology and Pharmacology 26: 391–411
Spencer H, Lender M 1979 Adverse effects of aluminium-containing antacids on mineral metabolism. Gastroenterology 76: 603–606
Thompson M R 1981 Effect of cimetidine on the surgical management of peptic ulcer disease. Gut 22: A433
Vantrappen G, Rutgeerts P, Broeckaert L, Janssens J 1980 Randomised open controlled trial of colloidal bismuth subcitrate tablets and cimetidine in the treatment of duodenal ulcer. Gut 21: 329–333
Walt R P, Trotman I F, Frost R, Golding P L, Shepherd T H, Rawlings J et al 1981 Comparison of twice daily ranitidine with standard cimeditine treatment of duodenal ulcer. Gut 22: 319–322

Upper GI haemorrhage

Allen R, Dykes P 1976 A study of the factors influencing mortality from gastrointestinal haemorrhage. Quarterly Journal of Medicine 1: 533–550
Birnie G G, Kennedy F, Mackay C, Watkinson G 1981 Experience of an upper gastrointestinal bleeding team. Gut 22: A416
Bulmer E 1927 The mortality from haematemesis. Lancet 2: 168–171
Conybeare J J 1934 Discussion on the prognosis of peptic ulcers. Proceedings of the Royal Society of Medicine 228–233
Dronfield M W, McIllmurray M B, Ferguson R, Atkinson M, Langman M J S 1977 A prospective randomised study of endoscopy and radiology in acute upper gastrointestinal tract bleeding. Lancet 1: 1167–1169
Forrest J A H, Zambartas C, Cregeen R J, Finlayson N D C 1981 Accuracy of urgent endoscopy in acute upper gastrointestinal bleeding. Gut 22: A416
Foster D N, Miloszewski K J A, Losowsky M S 1978 Stigmata of recent haemorrhage in diagnosis and prognosis of upper gastrointestinal bleeding. British Medical Journal 1: 1173–1177
Gilbert D A, Silverstein F E, Tedesco F J, Buengo N K et al 1979 Prognosis of upper gastrointestinal bleeding. Gastroenterology 76: 1138
Griffiths W J, Neumann D A, Welsh J D 1979 The visible vessel as an indicator of uncontrolled or recurrent gastrointestinal haemorrhage. New England Journal of Medicine 300: 1411–1413

Hoare A M, Bradby G V H, Hawkins C F, Kang J Y, Dykes P W 1979 Cimetidine in bleeding peptic ulcer. Lancet 2: 671–673
Jones F A 1947 Haematemesis and melaena. British Medical Journal 2: 441–446
Kayasseh L, Gyr K, Keller U, Stalder G A, Wall M 1980 Somatostatin and cimetidine in peptic ulcer haemorrhage; a randomised controlled trial. Lancet 1: 844–846
Keller U, Sonnenberg G E, Kayasseh L 1978 Effect of therapeutic doses of somatostatin on splanchnic blood flow in man. European Journal of Clinical Investigation 8: 335
LaBrooy S J, Misiewicz J J, Edwards J, Smith P M, Haggie S J, Libman L et al 1979 Controlled trial of cimetidine in upper gastrointestinal haemorrhage. Gut 20: 892–895
Laurence B H, Vallon A G, Cotton P B, Miro J R A, Oses J C S, Le Bodic L et al 1980 Endoscopic laser photocoagulation for bleeding peptic ulcers. Lancet 1: 124–125
MacDougall B R D, Bailey R J, Williams R 1977 H_2-receptor antagonists and antacids in the prevention of acute gastrointestinal haemorrhage in fulminant hepatic failure. Lancet 1: 617–619
Macklon A F, Roberts S H, James O F W 1979 Cimetidine in bleeding peptic ulcer. Lancet 2: 1135–1136
Pickard R G, Sanderson I, South M, Kirkham J S, Northfield T C 1979 Controlled trial of cimetidine in acute upper gastrointestinal bleeding. British Medical Journal 1: 661–662
Swain C P, Bown S G, Storey D W, Kirkham J S, Northfield T C, Salmon P R 1981 Controlled trial of argon laser photocoagulation in bleeding peptic ulcers. Lancet 2: 1313–1316
Thomas G E, Cotton P B, Clark C G, Boulos P B 1980 Survey of management of acute upper gastrointestinal haemorrhage. Journal of the Royal Society of Medicine 73: 90–95
Vallon A G, Cotton P B, Laurence B H, Miro J R A, Oses J C S 1981 Randomised trial of endoscopic argon laser photocoagulation in bleeding peptic ulcers. Gut 22: 228–233
Vellacott K D, Dronfield M W, Atkinson M, Langman M J S 1981 Comparison of surgical and medical management of bleeding peptic ulcers. Gut 22: A415–416

Gallstones

Barker D J P, Gardner M J, Power C, Hutt M S R 1979 Prevalence of gall-stones at necropsy in nine British towns. British Medical Journal 2: 1389–1392
Bateson M C, Maudgal D P, Trash D B, Northfield T C, Bouchier I A D 1981 Gallstone calcification caused by ursodeoxycholic acid. Gut 22: A432
Bennion L J, Knowler W C, Mott D M, Spagnola A M, Bennett P H 1979 Development of lithogenic bile during puberty in Pima Indians. New England Journal of Medicine 300: 873–876
Danzinger R G, Hofmann A F, Schoenfield L J, Thistle J L 1972 Dissolution of cholesterol gallstones by chenodeoxycholic acid. New England Journal of Medicine 286: 1–8
Dowling R H 1981 Medical treatment of gallstones with chenodeoxycholic acid and ursodeoxycholic acid. In: Paumgartner G, Stiehl A, Gerok W (eds) Bile acids and lipids. MTP Press, Lancaster, p 329–339
Editorial 1980 Stones without fire. Lancet 1: 403–404
Gracie W A, Ransohoff D F 1981 The natural history of silent gallstones: the innocent gallstone is not a myth. Gastroenterology 80: 1161
James O F W 1979 Bile acids and the dissolution of gallstones. In: Davies D M, Rawlins M D (eds) Topics in therapeutics 5. Pitman Medical, London, p 79–90
Linos D A, Beard C M, O'Fallon W M, Dockerty M B, Beart R W, Kurland L T 1981 Cholecystectomy and carcinoma of the colon. Lancet 2: 379–381
McSherry C K, Glenn F 1980 The incidence and causes of death following surgery for non-malignant biliary tract disease. Annals of Surgery 191: 271–275
Maton P N, Murphy G M, Dowling R H 1980 Lack of response to chenodeoxycholic acid in obese and non-obese patients. Gut 21: 1082–1086
Maudgal D P, Bird R, Blackwood W S, Northfield T C 1978 Low-cholesterol diet: enhancement of effect of CDCA in patients with gallstones. British Medical Journal 2: 851–853
Pomare E W, Heaton K W, Low-Beer T S, Espiner H J 1976 The effect of wheat bran upon bile salt metabolism and upon the lipid composition of bile in gallstone patients. American Journal of Digestive Diseases 21: 521–526
Ruppin D C, Dowling R H 1981 Is recurrence inevitable on withdrawing treatment after complete gallstone dissolution with chenodeoxycholic and ursodeoxycholic acids? Gut 22: A432–433
Salen G, Colalillo A, Verga D, Bagan E, Tint G S, Shefer S 1981 Effect of high and low doses of ursodeoxycholic acid on gallstone dissolution in humans. Gastroenterology 78: 1412–1418
Sampliner R E, Bennett P H, Comess L J, Rose F A, Burch T A 1970 Gallbladder disease in Pima Indians. New England Journal of Medicine 283: 1358–1364
Schoenfield L J, Lachin J M and the Steering Committee, The National Cooperative Gallstone Study Group 1981 Chenodiol (chenodeoxycholic acid) for dissolution of gallstones: the National

Cooperative Gallstone Study. A controlled trial of efficacy and safety. Annals of Internal Medicine 95: 257–282
Small D M 1980 Cholesterol nucleation and growth in gallstone formation. New England Journal of Medicine 302: 1305–1307
Shaffer E A, Small D M 1976 Gallstone disease: pathogenesis and management. Current Problems in Surgery 13(7): 1–72
Vernick L J, Kuller L H 1981 Cholecystectomy and right-sided colon cancer: an epidemiological study. Lancet 2: 381–383
Wenckert A, Robertson B 1966 The natural course of gallstone disease. Gastroenterology 50: 376–381

HAV and HBV hepatitis

Bassendine M F, Chadwick R G, Salmeron J, Shipton U, Thomas H C, Sherlock S 1981 Adenine arabinoside therapy in HBsAg-positive chronic liver disease. A controlled study. Gastroenterology 80: 1016–1022
Berman M, Alter H J, Ishak K G, Purcell R H, Jones E A 1979 The chronic sequelae of non-A, non-B hepatitis. Annals of Internal Medicine 91: 1–6
Blumberg B S, London W T 1981 Hepatitis B virus and the prevention of primary hepatocellular carcinoma. New England Journal of Medicine 304: 782–784
Chadwick R G, Galizzi J Jr, Heathcote J, Lyssiotis T, Cohen B J, Scheuer P J et al 1979 Chronic persistent hepatitis: hepatitis B virus markers and histological follow-up. Gut 20: 372–377
Crosnier J, Jungers P, Courouce A M, Laplanche A, Benhamou E, Degos F et al 1981 Randomised placebo-controlled trial of hepatitis B surface antigen vaccine in French haemodialysis units. II. Haemodialysis patients. Lancet 1: 797–800
De Franchis R, D'Arminio A, Vecchi M, Rouchi G, Del Ninno E, Parravicini A et al 1980 Chronic asymptomatic HBsAg carriers: histological abnormalities and diagnostic and prognostic value of serological markers of the HBV. Gastroenterology 79: 521–527
Feinstone S M, Kapikian A Z, Purcell R H 1973 Hepatitis A: detection by immune electron microscopy of a virus-like antigen associated with acute illness. Science 182: 1026–1028
Frosner G G, Deinhardt F, Roggendorf M, Scheid R, Bayerl B, Zachoval R 1980 Laboratory diagnosis of hepatitis A infection. In: Bianchi L, Gerok W, Sickinger K, Stalder G A (eds) Virus and the liver. MTP Press, Lancaster, p 17–26
Frosner G G, Papaevangelon G, Butler R, Iwarson S, Lindholm A, Courouce-Pauty A et al 1979 Antibody against hepatitis A in seven European countries. American Journal of Epidemiology 110: 63–69
Greenberg H B, Pollard R B, Lutwick L I, Gregory P B, Robinson W S, Merigan T C 1976 Effect of human leucocyte interferon on hepatitis B virus infection in patients with chronic active hepatitis. New England Journal of Medicine 295: 517–523
Hoofnagle J H 1980 Hepatitis B surface antigen (HBsAg) and antibody (anti-HBs). In: Bianchi L, Gerok W, Sickinger K, Stalder G A (eds) Virus and the liver. MTP Press, Lancaster, p 27–37
Hoofnagle J H, Seef L B, Bales Z B, Geretz R J, Tabor E 1979 Serological responses in HB. In: Vyas G N, Cohen S N, Schmid R (eds) Viral hepatitis. Franklin Institute Press, Philadelphia, p 219–242
Jenkins P J, Williams R 1980 Fulminant viral hepatitis. Clinical Gastroenterology 9: 171–189
Kim H C, Saidi P, Ackley A M, Bringelsen K A, Gocke D J 1980 Prevalence of type B and non-A non-B hepatitis in hemophilia: relationship to chronic liver disease. Gastroenterology 79: 1159–1164
Koretz R L, Stone O, Gitnick G L 1980 The long-term course of non-A, non-B post-transfusion hepatitis. Gastroenterology 79: 893–898
Lam K C, Lai C L, Ng R P, Trep C, Wu P C 1981 Deleterious effect of prednisolone in HBsAg-positive chronic active hepatitis. New England Journal of Medicine 304: 380–386
Maupas P, Chiron J P, Bann F, Coursaget P, Goudeau A, Perrin J et al 1981 Efficacy of hepatitis B vaccine in prevention of early HBsAg carrier state in children. Lancet 1: 289–292
Maynard J, Bradley D 1980 The hepatitis A virus. In: Bianchi L, Gerok W, Sickinger K, Stalder G A (eds) Virus and the liver. MTP Press, Lancaster, p 9–15.
Mills P R, Follett E A C, Urquhart G E D, Clements G, Watkinson G, MacSween R N M 1981 Evidence for previous hepatitis B virus infection in alcoholic cirrhosis. British Medical Journal 1: 437–438
Murphy B L, Maynard J E, Bradley D W, Ebert J W, Mathiesen L R, Purcell R H 1978 Immunofluorescence of hepatitis A virus antigen in chimpanzees. Infection and Immunity 21: 663–665

Nielsen J O 1980 Prognostic markers in acute hepatitis. In: Bianchi L, Gerok W, Sickinger K, Stalder G A (eds) Virus and the liver. MTP Press, Lancaster, p 241–246

Nielsen J O, Dietrichson O, Elling P, Christoffersen P 1971 Incidence and meaning of persistence of Australia antigen in patients with acute viral hepatitis: development of chronic hepatitis. New England Journal of Medicine 285: 1157–1160

Norkrans G, Hermodsson S, Lundin P, Iwason S 1976 The long-term outcome of hepatitis B. Infection 4: 70–72

Opolon P, Denis P, Damis F 1978 Assistance extra-corporelle par hemofiltration continue au cours des hepatites graves. Nouvelle Presse Medecine 7: 2473

Perillo R P, Gelb L, Campbell C 1979 Hepatitis BHe antigen, DNA polymerase activity and infection of household contacts with hepatitis B virus. Gastroenterology 76: 1319–1325

Realdi G, Alberti A, Rugge M, Bortolotti F, Rigoli A M, Tremolada F 1980 Seroconversion from hepatitis Be antigen to anti-HBe in chronic hepatitis B virus infection. Gastroenterology 79: 195–199

Reincke V, Dybkjaer E, Poulsen H, Banke O, Lylloff K, Nordenfelt D L 1972 A study of Australian-antigen-positive blood donors and their recipients with special reference to liver histology. New England Journal of Medicine 286: 867–870

Robinson W S 1975 DNA and DNA polymerase in the case of the Dane particle of hepatitis B. American Journal of Medical Science 270: 151–159

Sherlock S 1981 Virus hepatitis. In: Diseases of the liver and biliary system. Blackwell, Oxford, p 254.

Skelly J, Howard C R, Zuckerman A J 1979 Analysis of hepatitis B surface antigen components solubilised with Triton X-100. Journal of General Virology 44: 679–689

Stevens C E, Szmuness W, Goodman A I, Weseley S A, Fotino M 1980 Hepatitis B vaccine: immune responses in haemodialysis patients. Lancet 2: 1211–1213

Szmuness W, Stevens C E, Harley E J, Zang E A, Oleszko W R, William D C et al 1980 Hepatitis B vaccine. New England Journal of Medicine 303: 833–841

Weimar W, Ten Kate F J P, Masurel N, Heijtink R A, Schalm S W, Schellekens H et al 1980. Double-blind study of leucocyte interferon administration in chronic HBsAg-positive hepatitis. Lancet 1: 336–338

Non-A, non-B hepatitis

Aach R D, Szmuness W, Mosley J W, Hollinger F B, Kahn R A, Stevens C E et al 1981 Serum alanine aminotransferase of donors in relation to the risk of non-A, non-B hepatitis in recipients. New England Journal of Medicine 304: 989–994

Alter H J, Purcell R H, Holland P V, Popper H 1978 Transmissable agent in non-A, non-B hepatitis. Lancet 1: 459–463

Alter H J, Purcell R H, Holland P V, Feinstone S M, Morrow A G, Moritsugu Y 1975 Clinical and serological analysis of transfusion-associated hepatitis. Lancet 2: 838–841

Bamber M, Murray A, Bannister B, Thomas H C, Sherlock S 1981 Prospective study of acute non-A, non-B hepatitis in a London population. Gut 22: A427

Dienstag J L, Alaama A, Mosley J W, Redeker A G, Purcell R H 1977 Etiology of sporadic hepatitis B surface antigen-negative hepatitis. Annals of Internal Medicine 87: 1–6

Editorial 1981 Screening of blood donors for non-A, non-B hepatitis. Lancet 2: 73

Kim H C, Saidi P, Ackley A M, Bringelsen K A, Gocke D J 1980 Prevalence of type B and non-A, non-B hepatitis in hemophilia: relationship to chronic liver disease. Gastroenterology 79: 1159–1164

Medical Research Council Working Party on post-transfusion hepatitis. 1974. Post-transfusion hepatitis in a London hospital: results of a two-year prospective study. Journal of Hygiene 73: 173–188

Suh D J, White Y, Eddleston A L W F, Amini S, Tsiquaye K, Zuckerman A J et al 1981 Specificity of an immunoprecipitin test for non-A, non-B hepatitis. Lancet 1: 178–180

Tabor E, Seeff L B, Gerety R J 1980 Chronic non-A, non-B hepatitis carrier state. New England Journal of Medicine 303: 140–143

Wong D C, Purcell R H, Sreenivasan M A, Prasad S R, Pavri K M 1980 Epidemic and endemic hepatitis in India. Evidence for a non-A non-B hepatitis virus aetiology. Lancet 2: 876–878

Chronic active hepatitis

Alter H J 1980 The dominant role of non-A non-B with pathogenesis of post-transfusion hepatitis: a clinical assessment. Clinical Gastroenterology 9: 155–170

Anthony P P, Ishak K G, Nayak N C, Poulsen H E, Scheuer P J, Sobin L H 1978 The morphology of cirrhosis: recommendations on definition, nomenclature and classification by a working group sponsored by the WHO. Journal of Clinical Pathology 31: 395–414

Berman M, Alter H J, Ishak K G, Purcell R H, Jones E A 1979 The chronic sequelae of non-A non-B hepatitis. Annals of Internal Medicine 91: 1–6

Chapman R W G, Arborgh B A M, Rhodes J M, Summerfield J A, Dick R, Scheuer P J et al 1980 Primary sclerosing cholangitis: a review of its clinical features, cholangiography, and hepatic histology. Gut 21: 870–877

Czaja A J, Ludwig J, Baggenstoss A H, Wolf A 1981 Corticosteroid treated chronic active hepatitis in remission: uncertain prognosis of chronic persistent hepatitis. New England Journal of Medicine 304: 5–9

Dooley J S, Kirk A P, Thomas H C, Sherlock S 1979 Prediction of relapse following withdrawal of treatment in hepatitis B surface antigen negative chronic active liver disease. Gut 20: A954

Dudley F J, Scheuer P J, Sherlock S 1972 Natural history of hepatitis-associated antigen positive chronic liver disease. Lancet 2: 1388–1393

Editorial 1980 Chronic active hepatitis. British Medical Journal 2: 258–259

Fisher R C, Taylor L, Sherlock S 1976 α-1-antitrypsin deficiency in liver disease: the extent of the problem. Gastroenterology 71: 646–651

Goldberg S J, Mendenhall C L, Connell A M, Chedid A 1977 'Nonalcoholic' chronic hepatitis in the alcoholic. Gastroenterology 72: 598–604

Hodges J R, Milward-Sadler G H, Wright R 1980 Heterozygous MZ alpha-l-antitrypsin (AAT) deficiency, an important subgroup of cryptogenic cirrhosis and chronic active hepatitis (CAH) in adults. Gut 21: A901

Kakumu S, Leevy C M 1977 Lymphocyte cytotoxicity in alcoholic hepatitis. Gastroenterology 72: 594–597

Kirk A P, Jain S, Pocock S, Thomas H C, Sherlock S 1980 Late results of the Royal Free Hospital prospective controlled trial of prednisolone therapy in hepatitis B surface antigen negative chronic active hepatitis. Gut 21: 78–83

Korman M G, Hofmann A F, Summerskill W H J 1974 Assessment of activity in chronic active liver disease, serum bile acids compared with conventional tests and histology. New England Journal of Medicine 290: 1399–1402

Maddrey W C, Boitnott J K 1977 Drug-induced chronic liver disease. Gastroenterology 72: 1348–1353

Redeker A G 1981 Editorial. Treatment of chronic active hepatitis. New England Journal of Medicine 304: 420–421

Sampliner R E 1981 Editorial. Chronic non-A, non-B liver disease. Archives of Internal Medicine 141: 1581

Scott J, Gollan J L, Samourian S, Sherlock S 1978 Wilson's disease, presenting as chronic active hepatitis. Gastroenterology 74: 645–651

Schalm S W, Ammon H V, Summerskill W H J 1976 Failure of customary treatment in chronic active liver disease: causes and management. Annals of Clinical Research 8: 221–227

Sharp J R, Ishak K G, Zimmerman H J 1980 Chronic active hepatitis and severe hepatic necrosis associated with nitrofurantoin. Annals of Internal Medicine 92: 14–19

Sternlieb I, Scheinberg I H 1972 Chronic hepatitis as a first manifestation of Wilson's disease. Annals of Internal Medicine 76: 59–64

Tage-Jensen U, Amold W, Dietrichson O, Hardt F, Hopf U, Meyer Zum Buschenfelde K H et al 1977 Liver-cell-membrane autoantibody specific for inflammatory liver diseases. British Medical Journal 1: 206–208

Triger D R, Milward-Sadler G H, Czaykowski A A, Trowell J, Wright R 1976 Alpha-l-antitrypsin deficiency and liver disease in adults. Quarterly Journal of Medicine 45: 351–372

Wright E C, Seeff L B, Berk P D, Jones E A, Plotz P H 1977 Treatment of chronic active hepatitis: an analysis of three controlled trials. Gastroenterology 73: 1422–1430

Zimmerman H J, Ishak K G 1979 Hepatic injury due to drugs and toxins. In: MacSween R N, Anthony P P, Scheuer P J (eds) Pathology of the liver. Churchill Livingstone, Edinburgh, p 335–386

Primary biliary cirrhosis

Beckett G J, Dewhurst N, Finlayson N D C, Percy-Robb I W 1980 Weight loss in primary biliary cirrhosis. Gut 21: 734–737

Berg P A, Wiedmann K H, Sayers T, Kloppel G, Lindner H 1980 Serological classification of chronic cholestatic liver disease by the use of two different types of antimitochondrial antibodies. Lancet 2: 1329–1332

Christensen E, Crowe J, Doniach D, Popper H, Ranek L, Rodes et al 1980 Clinical pattern and course of disease in primary biliary cirrhosis based on an analysis of 236 patients. Gastroenterology 78: 236–246

Crowe J P, Christensen E, Butler J, Wheeler P, Doniach D, Kennan J et al 1980 Primary biliary cirrhosis: the prevalence of hypothyroidism and its relation to thyroid antibodies and sicca syndrome. Gastroenterology 78: 1437–1441

Crowe J, Christensen E, Smith M, Cochrane M, Ranek L, Watkinson G et al 1980 Azathioprine in primary biliary cirrhosis. A preliminary report of an international trial. Gastroenterology 78: 1005–1010

Douglas J G, Finlayson N D C 1979 Are increased individual susceptibility and environmental factors both necessary for the development of primary biliary cirrhosis? British Medical Journal 2: 419–420

Epstein O, Thomas H C, Sherlock S 1980 Primary biliary cirrhosis is a 'dry gland' syndrome with features of chronic graft versus host (GVH) disease. Lancet 1: 1166–1168

Epstein O, Lee R G, Jauregi H O, Sherlock S, Scheuer P J 1981a Granulomas in primary biliary cirrhosis a prognostic feature. Gut 22: A419

Epstein O, Lee R G, Boss A M, Jain S, Cook D G, Scheuer P J et al 1981b D-penicillamine treatment improves survival in primary biliary cirrhosis. Lancet 1: 1275–1277

Fleming C R, Ludwig J, Dickson E R 1978 Asymptomatic primary biliary cirrhosis. Presentation, histology and results with D-penicillamine. Mayo Clinic Proceedings 53: 587–593

Fleming C R, Dickson E R, Baggenstoss A H, McCall J T 1974 Copper and primary biliary cirrhosis. Gastroenterology 67: 1182–1187

Heathcote E J, Ross A, Sherlock S 1976 A prospective controlled trial of azathioprine in primary biliary cirrhosis. Gastroenterology 70: 656–660

Hislop W S 1980 Primary biliary cirrhosis: an epidemiological study. British Medical Journal 2: 1069–1070

James O F W, Macklon A F, Watson A J 1981 Primary biliary cirrhosis — a revised clinical spectrum. Lancet 1: 1278–1281

Jones E A, Frank M M, Jaffe C J, Vierling J M 1979 Primary biliary cirrhosis and the complement system. Annals of Internal Medicine 90: 72–84

Long R G, Scheuer P J, Sherlock S 1977 Presentation and course of asymptomatic primary biliary cirrhosis. Gastroenterology 72: 1204–1207

Macklon A F, Bassendine M, James O F W 1982 Incidence and severity of side effects of D-penicillamine treatment for primary biliary cirrhosis. Hepatology 2: (in press)

Matloff D, Resnick R, Alpet E, Kaplan M 1979 D-penicillamine does not alter the course of primary biliary cirrhosis. Gastroenterology 77: A26

Munoz L E, Thomas H C, Scheuer P J, Doniach D, Sherlock S 1981 Is mitochondrial antibody diagnostic of primary biliary cirrhosis? Gut 22: 136–140

Roll J, Boyer J, Klatskin G 1980 Long-term survival of asymptomatic and symptomatic patients with primary biliary cirrhosis. Gastroenterology 79: A1050

Routhier G, Janossy G, Epstein O, Thomas H C, Sherlock S, Kung P C et al 1980 Effects of cyclosporin A on suppressor as inducer T lymphocytes in primary biliary cirrhosis. Lancet 2: 1223–1226

Sandilands G P, Galbraith I, Reid F M, Mills P R, MacSween R N M 1980 Immune-complex inhibition of lymphocyte Fc-receptors in primary biliary cirrhosis. Lancet 2: 9–13

Saunders J B, Walters J R F, Davies P, Paton A 1981 A 20-year prospective study of cirrhosis. British Medical Journal 1: 263–266

Schaffner F 1979 Primary biliary cirrhosis as a collagen disease. Postgraduate Medical Journal 65: 97–102

Scheuer P J 1973 Primary biliary cirrhosis. In: Scheuer P J (ed) Liver biopsy interpretation. Ballière Tindall, London, p 33–39

Shapiro J M, Smith H, Schaffner F 1979 Serum bilirubin a prognostic factor in primary biliary cirrhosis. Gut 20: 137–146

Sherlock S 1981 Primary biliary cirrhosis. In: Sherlock S (ed) Diseases of the liver and biliary system. Blackwell Scientific Publications, Oxford, p 227–239

Sherlock S, Scheuer P J 1973 The presentation and diagnosis of 100 patients with primary biliary cirrhosis. New England Journal of Medicine 289: 674–678

Thomas H C, De Villiers D, Potter B, Hodgson H, Jain S, Jewell D P et al 1978 Immune complexes in acute and chronic liver disease. Clinical and Experimental Immunology 31: 150–157

Triger D R 1980 Primary biliary cirrhosis: an epidemiological study. British Medical Journal 2: 772–775

Wands J R, Dienstag J L, Bhan A K, Feller E R, Isselbacher K J 1978 Circulating immune complexes and complement activation in primary biliary cirrhosis. New England Journal of Medicine 298: 233–237

Weisner R H, Barham S S, Dickson E R 1979 hepatic copper elevation, subcellular distribution and progression of primary biliary cirrhosis. Gastroenterology 78: 1326

Alcoholic liver disease

Bailey R J, Krasner N, Eddleston A L W F, Williams R, Tee D E H, Doniach D et al 1976 Histocompatibility antigens, autoantibodies and immunoglobulins in alcoholic liver disease. British Medical Journal 2: 727–729
Baker A L, Jaspan J B, Haines N W, Hatfield G E, Krager P S, Schneider J F 1981 A randomized clinical trial of insulin and glucagon infusion for treatment of alcoholic hepatitis. Gastroenterology 80: 1410–1414
Borowsky S A, Strome S, Lott E 1981 Continued heavy drinking and survival in alcoholic cirrhotics. Gastroenterology 80: 1405–1409
Brunt P W, Kew M C, Scheuer P J, Sherlock S 1974 Studies in alcoholic liver disease in Britain. Gut 15: 52–58
Hamlyn A N, James O 1978 Can we believe the figures? Deaths from cirrhosis and hospital prevalence. Gut 18: A968
Israel Y, Videla L, Bernstein J 1979 Liver hypermetabolic state after chronic ethanol consumption: hormonal interrelationships and pathogenic implications. Federation Proceedings 34: 2052–2059
Lelbach W K 1975 Cirrhosis in the alcoholic and its relation to the volume of alcohol albuse. Annals of the New York Academy of Sciences 252: 85–105
Lieber C S 1978 Pathogenesis and early diagnosis of alcoholic liver injury. New England Journal of Medicine 298: 888–893
Maddrey W C 1981 Insulin and glucagon therapy for alcoholic hepatitis. Gastroenterology 80: 1596–1598
Maddrey W C, Boitnott J K, Bedine M S, Weber F L, Mezey E, White R I 1978 Corticosteroid therapy of alcoholic hepatitis. Gastroenterology 75: 193–199
Mezey E 1980 Alcoholic liver disease: roles of alcohol and malnutrition. American Journal of Clinical Nutrition 33: 2709–2718
Mills P R, Follet E A C, Urquhart G E D, Clements G, Watkinson G, MacSween R N M 1981 Evidence for previous hepatitis B virus infection in alcoholic cirrhosis. British Medical Journal 1: 437–438
Morgan M Y, Sherlock S 1977 Sex-related differences among 100 patients with alcoholic liver disease. British Medical Journal 1: 939–941
Nasrullah S M, Galambos J T 1980 Amino acid therapy of alcoholic hepatitis. Lancet 2: 1276–1277
Occasional Survey 1981 Alcoholic liver disease: morphological manifestations. Lancet 1: 707–711
Office of Population Censuses and Surveys 1979 Mortality statistics. Review of the Registrar General on deaths in England and Wales 1974 et seq. HMSO, London
O'Keefe S J, Carraher T E, El-Zayadi A R, Davis M, Williams R 1980 Malnutrition and immunocompetence in patients with liver disease. Lancet 2: 615–617
Pecquignot G, Tuyns A 1975 Rations d'alcool declarées et risques pathologiques. In: Symposium Franco-Britannique sur l'alcoolisme. INSERM, Paris, p 117–128
Perperas A, Tsantoulas D, Portmann B, Eddlestone A L W F, Williams R 1981 Autoimmunity to a liver membrane lipoprotein and liver damage in alcoholic liver disease. Gut 22: 149–152
Powell W J, Klatskin G 1968 Duration of survival in patients with Laennec's cirrhosis. American Journal of Medicine 44: 406–420
Rojkind M, Dunn M A 1979 Hepatic fibrosis. Gastroenterology 76: 849–863
Saunders J B, Walters J R F, Davies P, Paton A 1981 A 20-year prospective study of cirrhosis. British Medical Journal 1: 263–266
Van Waes L, Lieber C S 1977 Early perivenular sclerosis in alcoholic fatty liver: an index of progressive liver injury. Gastroenterology 73: 646–650

Variceal haemorrhage

Child C G III, Turcott J G 1964 Surgery and portal hypertension. In: Major problems in clinical surgery: the liver and portal hypertension. W B Saunders, Philadelphia, vol 1, p 1–85
Clark A W, Macdougall B R D, Westaby D, Mitchell K J, Silk D B A, Strunin L et al 1980 Prospective controlled trial of injection sclerotherapy in patients with cirrhosis and recent variceal haemorrhage. Lancet 2: 552–554
Graham D Y, Smith J L 1981 The course of patients after variceal haemorrhage. Gastroenterology 80: 800–809
Johnston G W, Rodgers H W 1973 A review of 15 years' experience in the use of sclerotherapy in the control of acute haemorrhage from oesophageal varices. British Journal of Surgery 60: 797–800

Jones F A, Gummer J W P, Lennard-Jones J E 1968 Gastrointestinal haemorrhage. In: Clinical gastroenterology. Blackwell, Oxford, p 348
Lebrec D, Nouel O, Corbic M, Benhamou J P 1980 Propranolol — a medical treatment for portal hypertension? Lancet 1: 180–182
Lebrec D, Poynard T, Hillon P, Benhamou J P 1981 Propranolol for prevention of recurrent gastrointestinal bleeding in cirrhotic patients. New England Journal of Medicine 305: 1371–1374
Nachlas M M, O'Neil J E, Campbell A J A 1955 The life history of patients with cirrhosis of the liver and bleeding oesophageal varices. Annals of Surgery 141: 10–23
Novis B H, Duys P, Barbezat G O, Clain J, Bank S, Terblanche J 1976 Fibreoptic endoscopy and the use of the Sengstaken tube in acute gastrointestinal haemorrhage in patients with portal hypertension and varices. Gut 17: 258–263
Reynolds T B, Donovan A J, Mikkelsen W P, Redeker A G, Turrill F L, Weiner J M 1981 Results of a 12-year randomised trial of portacaval shunt in patients with alcoholic liver disease and bleeding varices. Gastroenterology 80: 1005–1011
Rikkers L F, Rudman D, Galambos J T, Fulenwider T, Millikan W J, Kutner M et al 1978 A randomized controlled trial of the distal splenorenal shunt. Annals of Surgery 188: 271–282
Sherlock S 1981 The portal venous system and portal hypertension. In: Sherlock S (ed) Diseases of the liver and biliary system. Blackwell, Oxford, p 135–176
Smith-Laing G, Scott J, Long R G, Duk R, Sherlock S 1981 Role of percutaneous transhepatic obliteration of varices in the management of haemorrhage from gastroesophageal varices. Gastroenterology 80: 1031–1036
Spinsi R, Smith-Laing G, Epstein O, Sherlock S 1981 Results of portal decompression in patients with primary biliary cirrhosis. Gut 22: 345–349
Terblanche J, Northover J M A, Bomman P, Kahn D, Barbezat G O, Sellars S L et al 1979 A prospective evaluation of injection sclerotherapy in the treatment of acute bleeding from oesophageal varices. Surgery 85: 239–245

11

Connective tissue diseases

M. J. Walport and G. R. V. Hughes

INTRODUCTION

There are major degrees of overlap, both clinical and pathological, between the connective tissue diseases. They are linked by a thread of immunological abnormalities of cellular and humoral responses. The enormous amount of scientific interest devoted to them has given an insight into the mechanisms of ordered and disordered immune responsiveness and regulation. The groups of diseases to be considered are Sjögren's syndrome, systemic lupus erythematosus, polymyositis, scleroderma, systemic vasculitis and relapsing polychondritis.

SJÖGREN'S SYNDROME

Introduction

Sjögren's syndrome (SS) occupies a central position among the connective tissue diseases. As originally defined, it represents the triad of keratoconjunctivitis sicca, xerostomia and a connective tissue disease. Recently, it has been recognised that primary Sjögren's syndrome may exist in the absence of another connective tissue disorder.

Pathology

Lymphocytic and plasma-cell infiltration of exocrine glands, particularly salivary and lacrimal glands, is the pathological hallmark of Sjögren's syndrome.

Immunology

Immunogenetic studies have shown that Sjögren's syndrome occurs in conjunction with two genetic backgrounds associated with a differing profile of autoantibodies. Up to 75% of patients with SS have histocompatibility antigen DR3, and in 55% B8 is also present (Chused et al 1977). These antigens are associated with primary SS, and with SS in association with SLE. Precipitating antinuclear and anticytoplasmic antibodies found with this background of SS are SS-A and SS-B (identical to Ro and La, discussed below) (Alspaugh et al 1976). In contrast, of the 20% of patients with rheumatoid arthritis who have SS, the histocompatibility antigen DR4 is found in 64% (Moutsopoulos et al 1979). A precipitating antibody SS-C (renamed RAP — rheumatoid arthritis precipitin) occurs in these patients (Alspaugh et al 1976), and this reacts with rheumatoid arthritis nuclear antigen (RANA) (Alspaugh et al 1978).

The lymphocytic infiltrates of salivary glands contain both B and T cells (Talal et al 1974). B-cell hyperactivity is manifested by polyclonal hypergammaglobulinaemia seen in most patients with SS. Hyperviscosity may result from macroglobulinaemia or rheumatoid factor complexes. Elkon and colleagues (1981) have demonstrated secretion of IgA rheumatoid factor within salivary lymphocytic infiltrates and shown IgA in circulating immune complexes. Cryoglobulinaemia may occur, with occasional vasculitis and glomerulonephritis.

Of a series of 136 patients with SS followed at the National Institute of Health for an average of 8 years, 23 developed lymphoproliferative disorders (Kassan et al 1978). A fall in previously increased gammaglobulin levels, lymphadenopathy and splenomegaly, should raise suspicion that lymphoma is developing.

Clinical features

Most symptoms relate to dryness of the mucosal surfaces of the eye, mouth and vagina. Grittiness of the eyes with recurrent conjunctivitis is the commonest complaint of patients with keratoconjunctivitis sicca. Slit-lamp examination with Rose Bengal staining may reveal punctate keratitis and keratitis filamentosa. Xerostomia is manifested by difficulty in eating dry foods, and the time taken to eat a dry biscuit is a useful index of disease severity. Many patients drink excessive fluids and may present with polyuria associated with low serum and urinary osmolalities. Dental caries is a common problem, requiring meticulous dental hygiene. Salivary gland swelling with sialectasis occurs commonly and may be associated with infection or calculus. Pancreatic exocrine involvement probably occurs more frequently than has been documented.

Pulmonary involvement includes interstitial lymphocytic infiltration, small-airways obstruction from lymphocytic accumulations (Newball & Brahim 1977), and recurrent chest infections, possibly associated with dryness of the airways (bronchitis sicca). Renal abnormalities are seen in up to 25% of patients with SS (Whaley et al 1972). Renal tubular acidosis is the most common problem, but other tubular defects include diabetes insipidus, amino-aciduria and phosphaturia. Glomerulonephritis is rare and should suggest the additional diagnosis of SLE.

Peripheral neuropathy and, more unusually, cranial nerve palsies, are signs of SS involving the nervous system. The aetiology of these complications is believed to be vasculitic. Organ-specific antibodies are fairly commonly found. Graves' disease, primary biliary cirrhosis, myasthenia gravis and pernicious anaemia have all been associated with SS. Drug allergy, as with SLE, is common in SS and Bloch et al (1965) found that 71 of 83 patients with SS treated with gold salts developed an allergic skin rash.

Diagnosis

Diagnosis can be difficult, as most tests in SS have low sensitivity (high incidence of false-negative results). Keratoconjunctivitis should be identified by Schirmer's test and slit-lamp examination. Xerostomia can be very difficult to document. Salivary scintigraphy using $^{99}Tc^{m}$ pertechnetate has been claimed to be a sensitive test of salivary function (Cummings et al 1971), but is expensive and time-consuming. Lip gland biopsy is probably the most useful investigation, providing a minor salivary gland for histological assessment of the degree of lymphocytic infiltration (Chisholm & Mason 1968). False-negative results can occur with this test.

Treatment

Symptomatic relief provides the mainstay of treatment. Ocular dryness responds to methylcellulose eye drops, with prompt treatment of bacterial infections. Xerostomia may be helped by sialogogues such as unsweetened lemon juice, and by liberal fluid intake.

Systemic steroids or cytotoxic agents are very rarely indicated and only for patients with severe symptomatic involvement or major pulmonary or renal disease.

SYSTEMIC LUPUS ERYTHEMATOSUS

The spectrum of autoantibodies (Table 11.1) in systemic lupus erythematosus (SLE) is the subject of much current interest (Reichlin 1981). The most commonly identified antibodies to double-stranded and single-stranded DNA (ds and ss DNA) are widely believed to have a major pathological role when complexed with antigen. Both DNA and anti-DNA (aDNA) antibodies have been demonstrated in glomeruli of SLE patients with nephritis (Koffler et al 1973). Work by Izui et al (1977) showed that denatured DNA has an affinity for glomerular basement membrane, suggesting that in situ complex formation may be important. Miniter et al (1979) have suggested that the ability of aDNA antibodies to fix complement is correlated with the presence of nephritis. Studies from our own laboratory (Gharavi et al 1981) have failed to confirm this.

Antibodies to nuclear ribonucleoprotein (nRNP) in high titre are strongly associated with Raynaud's phenomenon. Sharp et al (1972) noted that patients possessing such antibodies to nRNP shared a number of additional clinical features (good prognosis, low incidence of cerebral and renal disease) and suggested that they be classified as having a distinct disease — mixed connective tissue disease.

Table 11.1 Principal antinuclear and anticytoplasmic antibodies

Antigen	Comment
dsDNA	Highly specific for SLE
ssDNA	Found in many connective tissue diseases
RNP	High titre in MCTD, low titre in SLE, dermatomyositis
Sm	Acidic nuclear glycoprotein, 30% of SLE patients
SS-A (Ro)	Cytoplasmic glycoprotein. ANA-negative SLE, Sjögren's syndrome
SS-B (La) (Ha)	Cytoplasmic and nuclear RNA protein, SLE, Sjögren's syndrome
Histone	Basic nuclear proteins, drug-induced SLE
RANA	Nuclear antigen related to E-B virus transformation of cell lines, rheumatoid arthritis
Scl-1 and centromere	Scleroderma
PM-1 and Jo-1	Polymyositis

Review of Sharp's original series of 25 patients (Nimelstein et al 1980) suggested that many subsequently evolved features characteristic of another connective tissue disease — usually scleroderma. On the basis of these data, combined with reports of both renal and cerebral disease in patients with MCTD, doubt has been expressed about whether MCTD is a genuine entity. Nevertheless, antibody to nRNP remains a striking marker of Raynaud's phenomenon and in a 7-year follow-up of 300 patients with MCTD, only 7% have died (Sharp & Anderson 1980).

The antibodies Ro and La are found with a lupus subset which may be ANA-negative, has an 80% incidence of rheumatoid factor, and is commonly associated with severe photosensitivity dermatitis (Bell & Maddison 1980). These two antibodies (immunologically identical to SS-A and SS-B) are also associated with Sjögren's syndrome. The association of Sm with neuropsychiatric disease (Winfield et al 1978) has not yet been confirmed. Antibody to the nuclear acidic protein, MA, is claimed to be a marker for severe SLE (Winn et al 1979).

The observation of Alarcon-Segovia et al (1978), that antibody to nRNP may penetrate living mononuclear cells by their surface Fc receptors and react with their nuclear RNP, is intriguing but unconfirmed.

Molecular biologists are taking advantage of these naturally occurring reagents. Lerner et al (1980) have shown that a RNP antibodies recognise small nuclear RNA species which may serve as recognition units for RNA splicing. The protein component of the RNA antigen may be splicing enzymes.

Lafer et al (1981) have exploited the hybridoma technique to examine the antigenic specificity of murine aDNA antibodies. One of the monoclonal aDNA antibodies formed by this technique showed marked cross-reactivity with cardiolipin, and acted as a lupus anticoagulant. DNA backbone contains a regular array of carbon atoms equally spaced with phosphodiester-linked phosphate groups. A similar group occurs in cardiolipin, and probably in a phospholipid involved in the activation of the intrinsic coagulation pathway. It seems probable that the hybridoma antibody cross-reacts with these apparently diverse substrates by virtue of specificity for a common phosphodiester-bond grouping.

The mechanisms underlying the origin of these autoantibodies are the subject of an enormous research effort. New Zealand Black (NZB) and New Zealand Black/White F_1 (NZB/W) mice are the prototypic animal models for SLE, and have now been joined by the MRL/1 and BXSB strains (Murphy & Roths 1979). A colony of Beagle dogs also develops a disease strikingly similar to human SLE (Lewis et al 1973).

From the immunological standpoint, virtually the only common feature of these animal models is early B-cell hyperactivity. In the apparent absence of previous stimulation, these cells produce spontaneous polyclonal antibodies to a variety of

Table 11.2 Proposed immunoregulatory abnormalities in murine SLE (Theofilopoulos & Dixon 1981)

Primary genetic B-cell malfunction
Acquired B-cell malfunction
Endogenous or exogenous polyclonal B-cell activators
Lack of negative influence by suppressor T cells
Enhanced positive influence by helper T cells
Defects in regulatory function of T-cell subjects (eg. Ly 123^+)
Lack of acceptor sites for suppressor messages on B cells

antigens including haptens and autoantigens, with resulting hypergammaglobulinaemia. A large number of possible immunoregulatory malfunctions have been proposed to explain this excessive B-cell activity (Table 11.2).

From careful immunological and genetic analysis of these mice, a number of points have emerged:

1. Murine SLE probably has a number of different aetiologies with common final manifestations.

2. In the NZB/W strain many genes independently control different facets of disease, demonstrated by segregation studies.

3. Genetic studies have dissociated the coexistence of retrovirus and autoimmune markers (Datta & Schwarz 1976). Group 70 retroviral envelope antigens have been found in a number of apparently normal strains of mice. The pronounced antibody response to these antigens in NZB/W mice is probably a reflection of polyclonal B cell activation.

4. A number of accelerating factors can modify the time of onset and severity of disease in mice. These include:

a. Viral factors: neonatal LCM virus infection accelerates the onset of disease in NZB/W mice.

b. Hormonal factors: male NZB/W mice are relatively resistant to the onset of lupus, which can be accelerated by castration. Equally, administration of androgen to female NZB/W mice ameliorates disease (Roubinian et al 1977).

c. Y chromosome: in BXSB mice the presence of the Y chromosome hastens the onset of disease from 15 months to 6 months (Murphy & Roths 1979).

Human SLE is equally complex and probably also has a number of differing aetiologies. Risk factors include being female, possessing the histocompatibility antigens DR2 and DR3, and having a family member with SLE. Evidence in favour of a viral aetiology includes the finding of a high incidence of lymphocytotoxins in household contacts of patients with SLE (DeHoratius & Messner 1975). Two families have been described in whom not only several family members but also the family dog had SLE (Beaucher et al 1977).

Hydralazine-induced lupus illustrates well that independent risk factors can summate to produce disease. In a study by Batchelor et al (1980), these risk factors were: female sex, HLA DR4, genetically slow acetylation of hydralazine and a daily intake of 200 mg of hydralazine. When all these factors were present in this study, all patients had hydralazine-induced lupus.

Immunodeficiency of individual complement components and of IgA has been described in association with SLE-like disease. This may relate to another immunological facet of SLE — the abnormal handling of immune complexes. Macrophages bear receptors for the Fc portion of immunoglobulins and for C3b. These seem to be important for the clearance of circulating soluble immune complexes (Arend & Mannik 1971).

Using IgG-coated erythrocytes as a model for clearance of Fc-coated particles, Frank et al (1979) showed that this clearance was impaired in patients with active SLE. The significance of this observation remains to be clarified.

Clinical

SLE is not an uncommon disease. Among a population of 121 444 in San Francisco, Fessel (1974) found a prevalence of 1 in 2000. In women aged 15–64 years the prevalence was 1 in 700, and rose to 1 in 245 among Negro women.

With the advent of more specific serological tests, many milder cases of SLE are now being recognised. Five-year survival in most series now exceeds 95% (Grigor et al 1978).

Skin

It is a fallacy that butterfly facial rash occurs in every patient with SLE, and that all patients should avoid direct exposure to the sun. The presence of precipitating antibodies to Ro and La may predict a small group likely to suffer from photosensitivity (Bell & Maddison 1980), but most affected patients discover this through bitter experience.

Alopecia can be an extremely useful clinical guide to disease activity and occurs in up to 65% of patients (Grigor et al 1978).

Musculoskeletal

Tendonitis is a common feature of SLE, affecting particularly finger flexors. This may result in tendon shortening with resulting characteristic hand deformity (Bywaters 1975). Deforming arthritis is exceptional, and the presence of erosions suggests rheumatoid arthritis.

Aseptic necrosis of the hip (Zizic et al 1980) is a potential major problem, usually ultimately requiring hip replacement. Aseptic necrosis in SLE is unfortunately more likely to be caused by steroid therapy than by the disease itself.

Lungs

Pulmonary involvement may occur in 80% of patients, although it is usually mild (Gibson et al 1977). The most common abnormality is a minor reduction in lung volume associated with reduced carbon monoxide diffusing capacity. Gas transfer is usually normal when corrected for lung volume. Occasionally severe loss of lung volume occurs ('shrinking lungs'), and measurements have demonstrated impairment of diaphragmatic function (Gibson et al 1977). Significant interstitial fibrosis is rare in SLE.

Pulmonary emboli, usually associated with signs of deep venous thrombosis, may occur in up to 10% of patients (Gladman & Urowitz 1980).

Pleural involvement, with symptomatic pleurisy and occasional effusion, affects about 50% of patients. After an attack of pleurisy some patients notice recurrent poorly localised pain around the costal margins, and this pain may persist for years (Gibson et al 1977).

Cardiovascular system

An increasing problem is coronary artery disease and myocardial infarction. This is more likely to be secondary to long-term corticosteroid therapy, associated with raised levels of triglycerides and with hypertension, than to SLE itself (Urowitz et al 1976). Pericarditis is common, often associated with pleurisy.

Kidneys

Investigation and management of lupus nephritis remains a controversial problem. The improvement in survival of patients with lupus nephritis over the past 20 years is attributable less to a reduction in those dying of uraemia, than to a lower incidence of death from sepsis occurring at high dose levels of prednisolone (Baldwin et al 1977, Cameron et al 1979).

Of 71 patients reviewed by Cameron et al (1979), the 5-year survival was 75% and was independent of the initial histological pattern of nephritis. Treatment was graded according to the severity of the histological picture. Those with minimal change, mesangial and minor focal glomerulonephritis were given steroids alone. In the presence of membranous or diffuse proliferative changes or a falling glomerular filtration rate, a combination of a corticosteroid and an immunosuppressive agent, usually azathioprine, was administered. It is in the latter group that the improvement in survival has been most striking, and is almost certainly due to the steroid-sparing effect of azathioprine. Nevertheless, Decker et al (1979) at the National Institutes of Health have *not* found that the addition of oral azathioprine and cyclophosphamide reduces the incidence of infection, arrests the progress of renal disease, or reduces the mortality rate. The reason for this difference is not obvious.

Nervous system

Central nervous system (CNS) lupus is manifest in up to two-thirds of patients with SLE (Estes & Christian 1971). This is a major cause of morbidity, although more conservative steroid therapy has made it a declining cause of mortality. It poses major problems of diagnosis and treatment.

Minor psychiatric abnormalities and migrainous headaches are the commonest signs of CNS involvement. Florid and focal neuropsychiatric abnormalities are more easily diagnosed.

The pathology of the CNS disease varies from extensive small-vessel involvement with microinfarcts, resembling the changes of thrombotic thrombocytopenic purpura, to a transverse myelitis with demyelination resulting in paraparesis.

The choroid plexus resembles the glomerular basement membrane and is a site of deposition of immune complexes (Atkins et al 1972). The presence of lymphocytotoxic antibodies cross-reacting with neuronal tissues has been found to correlate with CNS involvement (Bluestein & Zvaifler 1976). Abnormal metabolic brain scans have been reported in patients with cerebral lupus (Pinching et al 1978).

Most authors favour conservative management of CNS lupus with appropriate symptomatic treatment of psychiatric manifestations. In the absence of controlled trials, it is difficult to withhold high-dose corticosteroids and immunosuppressive agents from patients with severe disease manifest by convulsions, focal neurological signs, and retinal vasculitis.

Reticuloendothelial system and blood

Abnormalities of the reticuloendothelial system are very common in SLE (Table 11.3). Thrombocytopenia and haemolytic anaemia may present years before other features of SLE develop. Alger et al (1977) have suggested that haematological disease is associated with a more benign subset of lupus.

Table 11.3 Abnormalities of the reticuloendothelial system

	Patients affected (%)
Normochromic, normocytic anaemia	75
Positive direct Coomb's test	25
Haemolysis	15
Leucopenia (WBC $< 4.5 \times 10^9$/l (especially lymphocytopenia)	65
Thrombocytopenia (platelets $< 100 \times 10^9$/l	20
Lymphocytotoxins	75
Circulating anticoagulant	10

Pregnancy

It is not true that SLE is a contraindication to pregnancy. There is a high incidence of spontaneous abortion, in which context it is interesting to note the cross-reactivity of some lymphocytotoxic antibodies with placental trophoblast (Bresnihan et al 1977). The only major contraindications to pregnancy in this context are significant renal or cardiac disease.

Infection

In a computer-assisted survey of factors predisposing to infection in SLE (Ginzler et al 1978), the major factor was corticosteroid dosage. Prednisolone in doses above 40 mg per day was associated with an extremely high rate of infection. Other risk factors for infection were azathioprine-induced neutropenia, and renal failure. However, flares of disease activity and low C3 estimations did not correlate with a significantly increased risk of infection.

Laboratory investigations

Diagnostic tests

The value of a laboratory investigation in diagnosis depends on its specificity (100% minus the percentage of false-positive results) and sensitivity (100% minus the percentage of false-negative results). Tests for SLE are tabulated in terms of these two characteristics (Table 11.4).

LE cells. These represent mononuclear cells containing phagocytosed pyknotic nuclei. Their specificity is limited by their common occurrence in association with discoid lupus, chronic active hepatitis and, occasionally, with rheumatoid arthritis and Sjögren's syndrome.

Antinuclear antibodies (ANA). ANA are demonstrated by indirect immunofluorescence, usually using rat liver or kidney as substrate. Analysis of the pattern of nuclear staining has now largely been superseded by more precise identification of antibodies by precipitation with partly defined nuclear antigens. The ANA found in

Table 11.4 Tests for SLE in terms of specificity and sensitivity

	LE cells	ANA in high titre	Lupus band	DNA binding	*Crithidia*
Specificity	Moderate	Low	High	High	High
Sensitivity	High	High	Moderate	High	Moderate

association with rheumatoid arthritis, Sjögren's syndrome, scleroderma and mixed connective tissue disease are usually speckled and have been partly resolved by precipitation analysis (Table 11.1). In contrast, the pattern of ANA in SLE is usually homogeneous.

Lupus band test. Examination of skin by direct immunofluorescence may demonstrate immunoglobulins and complement components deposited at the dermoepidermal junction (positive lupus band test). If light-exposed skin without lesions is examined, a positive lupus band test has high specificity. Early claims, that the class of immunoglobulin deposited in the skin might reflect the class of aDNA antibody and the risk of development of lupus nephritis, have not been confirmed.

Antibodies to double-stranded DNA. These antibodies have a remarkable specificity for SLE and form the cornerstone of serological diagnosis of SLE. They are usually detected by a modifed Farr assay in which aDNA antibodies complexed to native double-stranded DNA are precipitated by ammonium sulphate (DNA-binding assay). Levels of aDNA antibody broadly correlate with disease activity. However, the recognition that high DNA-binding values do not necessarily indicate serious disease has led to a more conservative approach to the treatment of clinically well patients with serological abnormalitics alone (Hughes 1979).

Crithidia luciliae. This flagellate protozoan has a kinetoplast containing almost pure dsDNA. Utilizing indirect immunofluorescence, this is a quick and highly specific way to demonstrate aDNA antibodies. As this test detects high-titre antibody levels only, its sensitivity is limited.

Other investigations

Complement levels. Low levels of C3, C4 and CH50, together with increased levels of DNA-binding and circulating immune complexes, are evidence of active disease. A rapid fall in C3 levels, although not a specific indication for more active therapy, should act as a warning to watch the patient very carefully.

Immune complexes. Over 40 methods of measuring immune complexes are described (reviewed by Zubler & Lambert 1978). During active disease most patients with SLE can be shown to have circulating immune complexes by several of these assays. Identification of the composition of these complexes may provide valuable information about the pathogenesis of SLE. The measurement of immune complexes has not yet found a place in the clinical management of patients with SLE (Inman et al 1980).

C-reactive protein (CRP). CRP is an acute-phase reactant providing a useful marker of inflammation in many diseases. Patients with SLE have a striking inability to mount a CRP response, and frequently have barely detectable levels of CRP in the presence of a very high ESR. In SLE patients with infection the CRP may become raised, which can be a useful pointer in patients with pyrexia of unknown origin (Honig et al 1977, Becker et al 1980).

Treatment

Two major factors in the improved survival of patients with SLE are the identification of milder cases of disease and a more conservative approach to treatment (Cameron et al 1979, Hughes 1979).

In a recent survey, the mean daily prednisolone dosage was 7.5 mg daily over 1433 patient-months (Grigor et al 1978). Most authors agree that immunosuppressive agents such as azathioprine have a major place as steroid-sparing agents in severe systemic illness, and where vital organs are threatened, although there are few data from controlled studies to support their use.

Non-steroidal anti-inflammatory drugs have a useful place in the management of mild disease. Aspirin in full doses often causes hepatotoxicity and is best avoided (Seaman & Plotz 1976, Travers & Hughes 1978).

Antimalarial agents have again become fashionable in small doses which minimise the risks of retinal toxicity (reviewed by Dubois 1978). They are particularly useful for the control of cutaneous symptoms.

Plasma exchange seems to have a limited but useful role in patients with severe disease associated with high levels of circulating immune complexes, until disease activity can be controlled with corticosteroids and immunosuppressive agents (Verrier-Jones et al 1979).

Methylprednisolone administered slowly as bolus injections of 1 g is another therapy for severe exacerbations of SLE (Cathcart et al 1976) currently being evaluated in controlled trials.

POLYMYOSITIS AND DERMATOMYOSITIS

Introduction

Bohan & Peter (1975) classified polymositis and dermatomyositis into five subgroups (Table 11.5). Bohan et al (1977) analysed 153 patients and suggested a series of diagnostic criteria (Table 11.6). By classifying patients strictly according to these criteria it has been possible to dispel some of the myths about these diseases, especially their relationship to malignancy.

Table 11.5 Diagnostic criteria for polymyositis and dermatomyositis

1. Symmetrical proximal muscle weakness with or without dysphagia and respiratory muscle weakness
2. Elevation of serum enzyme activity: CPK, aldolase, transaminases, lactate dehydrogenase
3. Electromyographic triad of (a) fibrillation potentials, (b) polyphasic action potentials, (c) pseudomyotonic discharges
4. Muscle biopsy abnormalities of degeneration, regeneration, necrosis, phagocytosis and an interstitial inflammatory infiltrate
5. Typical skin rash of dermatomyositis

Malignancy and myositis

In Bohan's series, only 9% of patients had associated malignancy, usually carcinoma of the breast or stomach. The mean age of presentation of this group of patients was 62, compared with 47 for patients with idiopathic polymyositis or dermatomyositis.

Table 11.6 Classification of polymyositis and dermatomyositis

I	Primary idiopathic polymyositis
II	Primary idiopathic dermatomyositis
III	Dermatomyositis (or polymyositis) associated with neoplasia
IV	Childhood dermatomyositis (or polymyositis) associated with vasculitis
V	Polymyositis (or dermatomyositis) associated with collagen-vascular disease

Pathogenesis

There is increasing evidence for the importance of cell-mediated autoallergy in the pathology of this group of diseases. Lymphocytes from patients have been shown to adhere to monolayer muscle cultures and to cause their disruption (Currie et al 1971). This observation has formed the basis of a specific test for lymphocyte myotoxicity. The release of tritiated carnitine located in myotubes is measured following incubation of the patient's lymphocytes with a monolayer muscle culture. This myotoxicity appears to correlate with disease activity (Cambridge & Stern 1981).

Viruses have been implicated by a number of workers. Electron microscopy has shown the presence of inclusion bodies in muscle fibres. Increased Coxsackie B virus neutralisation titres have been noted in some patients. A Coxsackie A and an influenza A virus have been isolated from muscle specimens.

Drug-induced myositis is rare and is best described as a complication of penicillamine therapy (Lane & Mastaglia 1978).

Clinical features

Although proximal muscle weakness is the central feature of this group of diseases, in 30% of Bohan's series muscle strength was normal at the time of presentation.

The major adverse prognostic feature in polymyositis is pulmonary involvement, which may take two forms. Respiratory muscle weakness, often associated with dysphagia, may result in ventilatory failure or aspiration pneumonia. Fibrosing alveolitis has very occasionally been described in association with polymyositis and dermatomyositis (Schwarz et al 1976).

Cardiac involvement occurs in up to 20% of patients with polymyositis (Group I) and includes dysrhythmias and congestive cardiomyopathy.

In pure polymyositis and dermatomyositis (Groups I and II), arthralgia and myalgia occur in 25% of patients and Raynaud's phenomenon in 12% (Bohan et al 1977).

If possible, muscle weakness should be documented objectively by strain gauge myometry (Edwards & Hyde 1977). Pulmonary function should be followed sequentially. Levels of several muscle enzymes should be measured, and these may be useful in following the course of the disease. In up to 30% of patients, creatine phosphokinase (CPK) may be normal (Vignos & Goldwyn 1972). Electromyography (EMG) may be useful in establishing the diagnosis and in distinguishing steroid myopathy. There is no evidence that EMG abnormalities correlate with disease activity.

Sequential needle biopsy, which is superseding open biopsy, can be very helpful in following the progress of polymositis, and is a procedure with little morbidity

(Schwarz et al 1980). Ideally, interpretation of biopsy specimens requires special histochemical staining.

The clinical use of the lymphocyte myotoxicity test is currently undergoing evaluation in our laboratories. Other indices of muscle breakdown include urinary 3-methylhistidine excretion (Elia et al 1981), creatine excretion (Askari et al 1976) and serum myoglobin measurement (Kagen 1971).

Treatment

Most would agree with the impression of Medsger et al (1971) that prednisolone improves survival during the acute phase of polymyositis, but may operate adversely later in the disease if high-dose therapy is maintained for too long. The most important indicator of response is improvement in muscle strength, best documented by strain gauge myometry and by improvement in pulmonary function. Improvement in levels of muscle enzymes may be helpful but should be interpreted with great caution. In a recent study (Bunch et al 1980) 10 out of 16 patients had evidence of active myositis on biopsy 3 months after the start of therapy, although CPK levels had fallen into the normal range.

Steroid myopathy should always be considered in any patient who apparently relapses whilst taking steroids. In this situation, needle muscle biopsy is probably the most helpful investigation. Pronounced atrophy of type 2 muscle fibres in the absence of marked inflammation suggests this diagnosis.

A few patients seem to be resistant to steroid therapy and may benefit from an additional immunosuppressive agent. Bohan et al (1977) suggested that a lack of response to prednisone 40 mg daily for 4 months should be defined as steroid resistance, although many would add immunosuppressive agents at a far earlier stage.

Again, there is a disappointing lack of data from controlled studies. Indeed, the only controlled prospective randomised double-blind trial of any immunosuppressive agent in polymyositis (Bunch et al 1980) failed to show any benefit from the addition of azathioprine to steroids in the initial management of polymyositis. Open follow-up of these patients for 3 years has, however, revealed that the group taking azathioprine and steroids developed less functional disability and required smaller doses of prednisone (Bunch 1981).

Nevertheless, there are many reports of benefit of such immunosuppressive agents as methotrexate, cyclophosphamide, azathioprine, and chlorambucil given to steroid-resistant patients, in uncontrolled trials. Many consider that methotrexate is the agent of choice. Metzger et al (1974) reported improvement in 17 of 22 corticosteroid-resistant patients treated with an average of 42 mg of methotrexate i.v. weekly. They were able to reduce prednisone dosage in these patients from 47 mg daily to 12 mg daily. A recent case report has described how total body irradiation apparently produced remission in a case of severe polymyositis refractory to conventional therapy (Engel et al 1981).

Prognosis

In a series of 124 patients described by Medsger et al (1971), the 2-year mortality was 28% and at 7 years was 47%. In subsequent series the mortality has been much lower — 14% out of 153 patients reported by Bohan et al (1977). Contrary to initial reports, childhood dermatomyositis has a relatively good prognosis.

SCLERODERMA

Introduction

Scleroderma (progressive systemic sclerosis — PSS) is a disease characterised by thickening and fibrosis of skin, by abnormalities of small blood vessels, and by varying degrees of fibrosis of muscles, joints and viscera.

Similar cutaneous changes may be found in a variety of conditions (Table 11.7) which may be confused with scleroderma; some of these are discussed below.

Table 11.7 Classification of scleroderma (adapted from Rodnan 1981)

1.	Scleroderma a. with diffuse visceral involvement b. CREST syndrome c. in overlap with other connective tissue disease
2.	Localised scleroderma (no visceral involvement) a. morphoea — plaque-like, guttate, generalised b. linear scleroderma c. scleroderma 'en coup de sabre' with or without facial hemiatrophy
3.	Chemical-induced scleroderma-like conditions a. vinyl chloride disease b. pentazocine-induced fibrosis c. bleomycin-induced fibrosis
4.	Eosinophilic fasciitis
5.	Diseases with skin changes mimicking scleroderma a. scleroedema b. carcinoid syndrome c. phenylketonuria d. amyloid e. porphyria cutanea tarda

Pathology

Research into the pathogenesis of this obscure group of conditions is following three main avenues — studies of fibrosis, abnormalities of vasculature, and altered immunological mechanisms. There is ample evidence that the skin thickening in scleroderma is related to increased synthesis of collagen (Rodnan et al 1979). Herbert et al (1974) found an increase in the proportion of reducible aldimine-bond cross-links between tropocollagen molecules. These bonds are normally stabilised to a non-reducible form in mature collagen, and the presence of aldimine bonds is evidence of the presence of newly synthesised collagen.

In vitro studies (LeRoy 1974) have shown increased synthesis of collagen by fibroblasts. There is an unconfirmed report of reduced skin collagenase activity in scleroderma (Brady 1975).

Vascular abnormalities are mainly confined to small blood vessels. Histological studies of vessels show proliferation and thickening of the intima, little change in the media and fibrosis of the adventitia.

Maricq & LeRoy (1979), using wide-field microscopy, have emphasised abnormalities of the pattern of small vessels in the skin. They noted enlarged and distorted capillary loops occurring in clusters along the nailfolds and on other parts of the skin of the fingers. On cooling, standstill of capillary blood flow was a uniform feature in subjects with scleroderma (Maricq et al 1976).

It has been suggested that the primary lesion in scleroderma is vascular; however, most of the vascular lesions described in scleroderma may be found in patients with Raynaud's disease alone, in whom sclerosis does not follow the ischaemia induced by digital vasospasm.

Using conventional sections of rat liver and kidney as substrates for indirect immunofluorescence, the incidence of positive antinuclear antibodies (ANA) in scleroderma has been found to be around 50%. Tan and colleagues (1980), using a human epithelial cell line (HEp-2) in which the cells are rapidly dividing, demonstrated ANA in 96% of patients with scleroderma. Two antibodies seemed to have very high specificity for scleroderma. A precipitin against a saline extract of thymic nuclei (Scl-70) was found in 18% of scleroderma patients. An anticentromere antibody, identified by indirect immunofluorescence, seemed to be a selective marker for CREST syndrome (see below).

Accumulations of lymphocytes are often found in the dermis of patients with scleroderma. It is interesting to speculate that these secrete lymphokines which stimulate fibroblast division and secretion of collagen. A scleroderma-like condition may occur in human graft-versus-host disease following bone marrow transplantation (Lawley et al 1977).

Clinical

Raynaud's phenomenon

Raynaud's phenomenon occurs in more than 95% of patients with scleroderma. Indeed, the late onset of Raynaud's phenomenon suggests the possible development of either scleroderma or mixed connective tissue disease.

Cold-induced vasospasm can occur in organs other than the fingers. Pulmonary vasoconstriction with pulmonary hypertension in response to cold has been reported by Naslund et al (1981). Using xenon-133 washout curves, Cannon et al (1974) showed a reduction of renal cortical blood flow during cold-induced digital Raynaud's phenomenon.

Skin

Cutaneous involvement usually evolves through three phases. Initial oedema is followed by induration with a taut, shiny appearance and, finally, atrophic changes. Telangiectases may be widespread, although they rarely cause significant blood loss. Both increased skin pigmentation and vitiligo commonly occur, as does alopecia. Calcification of the skin and subcutaneous tissues is usually restricted to the finger tips, but may involve the extensor surface of the forearms, olecranon bursae, and prepatellar area.

Muscle and joints

A mild myositis, with slight proximal weakness and minor abnormalities on electromyography is common in scleroderma. Histological examination of muscle reveals predominantly interstitial changes with increased deposition of collagen and fat. Myofibrillar changes, if present, are degenerative in nature. Very occasionally a florid myositis with severe weakness develops, and biopsy of muscle at this stage reveals inflammatory changes with infiltrates of lymphocytes.

Polyarthritis may occur early in the course of the disease, mainly involving small joints. Later, limitation of joint movement secondary to periarticular fibrosis may become a major problem.

Gastrointestinal involvement

Oesophageal involvement occurs in up to 80% of patients with scleroderma, although it may be asymptomatic. Symptoms of heartburn and dysphagia for solid foods predominate. A hiatus hernia, and occasionally an oesophageal stricture, may develop.

A barium oesophagram is the simplest aid to diagnosis. Cineradiography reveals diminished peristalsis of the lower oesophagus, which may be confirmed by manometry. A combination of diminished distal oesophageal peristalsis and reduced oesophageal sphincter pressure was found in 73% of patients with scleroderma and was highly specific (Turner et al 1973).

The aetiology of these oesophageal abnormalities is not clear. Oesophageal histology may be normal, or may reveal muscular atrophy with collagen deposition. The mechanism may be primarily neurogenic, and it is interesting in this context that there is a close correlation between the presence of Raynaud's phenomenon and oesophageal disease, suggesting a possible common neurogenic mechanism (Stevens et al 1964).

Management of oesophageal symptoms should include raising the head of the patient's bed, antacids as required, and multiple small meals. Ramirez-Mata et al (1977) have shown that metoclopramide may improve lower oesophageal function. Cimetidine may be very helpful in the management of acid reflux with oesophagitis.

Small-bowel involvement is less common, but can prove very difficult to manage. Troublesome symptoms include abdominal distension, pain, nausea and vomiting. Pseudo-obstruction sometimes results from atonic dilatation of segments of small bowel. Radiological changes of duodenal dilatation with flocculation of barium are characteristic. Very occasionally pneumatosis cystoides intestinalis may develop (Meihoff et al 1968).

Malabsorption can occur because of bowel sclerosis, lymphatic obstruction, ischaemia secondary to vascular disease, or bacterial overgrowth. The latter is most amenable to treatment and, if possible, should be confirmed by culture of a jejeunal aspirate. It may respond well to broad-spectrum antibiotics. Pseudo-obstruction should be managed conservatively, and only very rarely is surgical intervention indicated.

Large-bowel involvement may result in bloating, with either constipation or diarrhoea. The radiological appearance of wide-mouthed colonic diverticula is almost pathognomonic of scleroderma. A high-roughage diet may prove helpful.

Lungs

Dyspnoea on exertion is reported to occur in 20–50% of patients with scleroderma. The pathological basis of this seems to be a combination of interstitial fibrosis and vascular changes, including characteristic intimal hypertrophy of small vessels.

Clinical examination may reveal bilateral basal fine inspiratory crackles. Clubbing is surprisingly uncommon and the explanation for this is not clear.

Radiological changes are initially beneficial but, later in the course of pulmonary disease, chest X-ray usually shows increased interstitial markings. A honeycomb pattern may develop occasionally, with underlying cystic changes in the lungs. Pulmonary function tests show that there is an equal incidence of restrictive and obstructive disease patterns in patients with scleroderma. Small-airways obstruction in largely asymptomatic patients was demonstrated in 19 out of 45 patients studied by Guttadauria et al (1977). Impairment of diffusing capacity for carbon monoxide is usually found in patients with a restrictive pattern of pulmonary function.

The possibility of pulmonary hypertension should be considered in patients who are disproportionately breathless for the apparent degree of pulmonary function.

The possibility of pulmonary hypertension should be considered in patients who are disproportionately breathless for the apparent degree of pulmonary parenchymatous involvement. Up to 50% of patients with scleroderma may have increased pulmonary artery pressures (Sackner et al 1964) which does not necessarily correlate with the presence of parenchymatous disease. Alveolar-cell carcinoma occurring in areas of pulmonary fibrosis, often detected only at necropsy, seems to occur more frequently in patients with scleroderma (Richards & Milne 1958).

Heart

Myocardial involvement occurs in up to 50% of patients with scleroderma (Bulkley et al 1976). Congestive cardiac failure results from myocardial fibrosis and necrosis unrelated to coronary artery disease. Dysrhythmias may follow either fibrosis of conducting tissue or injury to working myocardium. Pericardial involvement is very common, and may occasionally be associated with large effusions.

Kidneys

Renal and cardiac involvement in scleroderma are indicators of a poor prognosis. About 50% of patients develop renal involvement, of which the cardinal signs are proteinuria, hypertension and impaired creatinine clearance. The dramatic onset of malignant hypertension associated with rapid renal failure and microangiopathic haemolytic anaemia is a common mode of presentation of renal failure.

The characteristic pathological lesion is intimal proliferation and thickening in small cortical interlobular arteries (Cannon et al 1974). Fibrinoid necrosis of small arteries follows the development of malignant hypertension. Hypertension appears to be mediated by renin (Cannon et al 1974) and may respond dramatically to bilateral nephrectomy or to the angiotensin-converting enzyme antagonist captopril (Lopez-Ovejero et al 1979).

Aggressive therapy of hypertension is essential for the successful management of scleroderma kidney. If this fails, bilateral nephrectomy followed by haemodialysis or transplantation may usefully prolong survival (Richardson 1973).

Management

There is no specific therapy for scleroderma but, fortunately, rapidly progressive disease is fairly uncommon.

The effects of Raynaud's phenomenon can be minimised by living in as warm an environment as possible. Tobacco smoking should be discouraged, as it may aggravate vasoconstriction. Many vasodilator and α-blocking drugs have been recommended, including guanethidine and phenoxybenzamine, with no clear results.

Surgical sympathectomy has largely been abandoned as ineffective. Claims for plasmapheresis therapy for Raynaud's phenomenon have been made (Talpos et al 1978), but this has not been evaluated in a controlled manner.

Physiotherapy, including active range-of-motion exercises, wax baths and rest splints, is an important part of management, but unfortunately seldom succeeds in preventing contractures. Non-steroidal anti-inflammatory drugs may markedly help musculoskeletal symptoms. True inflammatory myositis usually responds to corticosteroids and cytotoxic agents. D-pencillamine, if given during the active phase of disease, may slow the progression of cutaneous and possibly of pulmonary disease (reviewed by Nassonova & Ivanova 1979).

There are no controlled trials of corticosteroids in scleroderma, and in most patients they are not indicated. Occasionally, where early inflammatory features predominate, and in inflammatory myositis, corticosteroids may prove helpful.

Alarcon-Segovia et al (1979) studied the effects of colchicine in the management of scleroderma. Colchicine, by disrupting microtubules, blocks collagen extrusion from fibroblasts. It also enhances collagenase activity through an unknown mechanism. Cutaneous improvement was the most significant effect of treatment, although in some patients improvement was noted in dysphagia and Raynaud's phenomenon (Alarcon-Segovia et al 1979). However, some of the other studies, including one double-blind study (Steigerwald & Lynch 1977), have not confirmed these results.

Plastic surgery to calcified plaques has proved useful. Unfortunately, surgery to improve contractures has not been as satisfactory.

Prognosis

Bennett et al (1971) reviewed the prognosis of 67 scleroderma patients seen at Hammersmith Hospital. Adverse prognostic features included age, extensive cutaneous sclerodermatous involvement, and major visceral involvement. Five-year survival was 73%.

'CREST' syndrome

This benign subset of scleroderma is manifest by calcinosis, Raynaud's phenomenon, oesophagitis ('esophagitis'), sclerodactyly and telangiectasia. It affects around 15% of cases of scleroderma and is marked by the presence of antibodies to centromere (Tan et al 1980). The progression is slow and benign (Medsger et al 1971), although complications such as late development of pulmonary fibrosis, pulmonary hypertension, and occasionally, biliary cirrhosis, may be fatal (Reynolds et al 1971).

Vinyl chloride disease

Acro-osteolysis, with Raynaud's phenomenon, oesophageal abnormalities and pulmonary fibrosis, has been described in workmen who clean reactor vessels containing vinyl chloride (Dodson et al 1971).

Eosinophilic fasciitis

This uncommon condition is characterised by symmetrical inflammatory swelling and induration of the arms and legs, usually sparing the hands and feet. It often starts following a bout of heavy exercise. There is absence of Raynaud's phenomenon and visceral involvement. Blood eosinophilia, increased erythrocyte sedimentation rate and hypergammaglobulinaemia are found. Diagnosis is by deep fascial biopsy which shows an inflammatory infiltrate of lymphocytes, plasma cells and eosinophils. It is important to identify this condition as it is responsive to corticosteroids. The condition has been reviewed by Moore & Zuckner (1980).

VASCULITIS

Introduction

The understanding of vasculitis is obscured by the large number of non-overlapping classification systems in widespread use. A classification based solely on histological appearances, or on immunological abnormalities, has little apparent relationship to the clinical spectrum of disease. A useful classification of vasculitis depends on the assembly of many different features relating both clinical and pathological aspects.

Immunopathology

Most vasculitides are assumed to be mediated through immunopathogenetic mechanisms. The final common pathway of damage is inflammation of blood vessels mediated by immune complexes and sensitised lymphocytes (Gell and Coombs Type III and Type IV reactions).

The complexity of the potential immunological response to a single agent is illustrated by nine distinct syndromes that may be induced by the drug penicillamine (Table 11.9).

Histopathologists recognise the results of Type III immunological reactions as a leucocytoclastic vasculitis in which the remnants of degranulated polymorpho-

Table 11.8 Major systemic vasculitic syndromes

Syndrome	Vessel involvement	Histology	Treatment
Polyarteritis nodosa	Small and medium muscular arteries	Leucocytoclastic necrotising	Steroid-responsive may require cytotoxics
Churg–Strauss	Medium and small arteries	Eosinophilic, granulomatous, necrotising	Steroid-responsive may require cytotoxics
Wegener's granulomatosis	Small vessels	Necrotising, granulomatous	Steroids and cyclophosphamide
Hypersensitivity angiitis	Small vessels	Leucocytoclastic, necrotising	Self-limited, may require steroids
Lymphomatoid granulomatosis	Small and medium vessels	Angiodestructive infiltration by polymorphic lymphocytic and lymphocytoid cells	Steroids and cytotoxics
Temporal arteritis	Medium and large vessels	Panarteritis with giant-cell formation	Very steroid-responsive

nuclear leucocytes surround necrotic blood vessels. Lymphocytic infiltration and granuloma formation are evidence of Type IV reaction. These two histological pictures frequently coexist. Immunofluorescent techniques may reveal the presence of immunoglobulins, complement components and fibrin.

Many factors potentially influence the site of deposition of immune complexes. The size of immune complexes seems to be important. Small complexes may deeply penetrate the walls of large vessels and result in fibrinoid necrosis of the arterial elastic lamina. Changes in vascular permeability induced by amines from platelets and mast cells may have a major role. Depletion of circulating platelets, or the co-administration of histamine and 5-hydroxytryptamine antagonists, can prevent immune complex vasculitis in rabbits (Kniker & Cochrane 1968).

Aetiology

A large number of possible aetiological agents of vasculitis have been described. Where the disease appears to be mediated by immune complexes, identification of participating antigens may give a clue to the aetiology.

Hepatitis B antigenaemia in association with polyarteritis nodosa was first described by Gocke et al (1970). Estimates of this association vary from 6% (Sack et al 1975) to 41% in a series from New York (Christian & Sergent 1976). Hepatitis B antigen has also been found in the mixed cryoglobulins derived from the serum of patients with small-vessel 'hypersensitivity' vasculitis (Levo et al 1977).

Necrotising vasculitis commonly complicates subacute bacterial endocarditis. Other septic vasculitic illnesses are associated with chronic meningococcal, gonococcal and pseudomonal septicaemias and infected atrioventricular shunts.

Drugs implicated in causing vasculitis include hydralazine, thiazides, sulphonamides and penicillins. Polyarteritis nodosa has been described in abusers of amphetamines (Citron et al 1970), although some of these patients probably carried hepatitis B antigen.

Circulating immune complexes are found in most connective tissue diseases. Only occasionally has the antigen in these complexes been identified, but such antigens include immunoglobulins themselves in rheumatoid factors, and single- and double-stranded DNA in SLE. A wide spectrum of vasculitic syndromes occur in patients with primary connective tissue disease.

Malignancy may be complicated by vasculitis. Presumably tumour antigens are involved in the immune complexes circulating in patients with breast and visceral carcinomata. The mechanism is less apparent in tumours of the reticuloendothelial

Table 11.9 Penicillamine-induced diseases mediated by mechanisms which are assumed to be immunological

Nephritis
Vasculitis
SLE
Dermatomyositis
Pemphigus
Myasthenia
Goodpasture's syndrome
Morbilliform drug eruption
Lichen planus

system such as Hodgkin's disease, multiple myeloma and hairy cell leukaemia (Elkon et al 1980).

From the clinical standpoint it is important to recognise the high degree of overlap that may exist between the 'classic' vasculitis syndromes. It is helpful to think of systemic vasculitides in terms of size of vessels involved, target organ involvement, histological appearance, underlying immunological abnormalities and associated connective tissue disease. Within this framework certain vasculitic syndromes have distinctive patterns and, more important, distinctive responses to therapy (Table 11.8).

Clinical features

Vasculitic disease can masquerade as a wide variety of medical conditions. Almost any skin rash may be the sign of underlying vasculitis. Equally, fulminant vasculitis may occur in the total absence of cutaneous manifestations. Any organ system may be involved. In the context of a multisystem disease, useful pointers to an underlying vasculitis include a history of upper respiratory tract disease, otitis or conjunctivitis. Arthralgia and myalgia are frequent symptoms.

Asthma, haemoptysis, or pulmonary infiltrates are common signs of pulmonary involvement. Myocardial infarction or cardiac failure may follow coronary artery vasculitis. Mononeuritis multiplex is a very useful sign of nervous involvement. Small patches of anaesthesia should be carefully delineated as these may be the only sign of mononeuritis.

Abdominal emergencies are occasionally the presentation of a necrotising vasculitis and may follow perforation of a viscus, haemorrhage, or pancreatitis.

Polyarteritis nodosa (PAN)

Polyarteritis nodosa is a necrotising vasculitis involving predominantly small and medium-sized muscular arteries. Target organs include kidneys, liver, abdominal viscera, nervous system, skin, joints and coronary arteries. Severe hypertension is common and polyarteritis may cause malignant hypertension. Calf muscle pain is a characteristic feature of PAN occurring in 50% of our patients (Travers et al 1979). Cutaneous involvement is relatively uncommon, but includes livedo reticularis and subcutaneous nodules, from which the disease derives its name.

The finding of multiple small aneurysms is almost pathognomonic of PAN. These usually occur at the branches of medium-sized arteries and are best demonstrated by hepatic, renal and mesenteric angiography (Bron et al 1965). In 17 patients studied at Hammersmith, 60% had aneurysms (Travers et al 1979).

Investigation of a patient with PAN may prove surprisingly negative. There is usually neutrophilia, sometimes reaching 30–40 $\times$ 10^9/l. Autoantibodies and circulating immune complexes are usually not detected. Visceral angiography should be performed and, in the absence of aneurysms, biopsy of liver and kidney may be helpful if there is biochemical evidence of their involvement. Blind muscle biopsy has been demoted to the status of a second-line investigation since the more widespread use of angiography. Nerve conduction studies may confirm mononeuritis multiplex, and sural nerve biopsy may show vasculitis of the vasa nervorum.

Treatment of PAN, Churg–Strauss vasculitis and Wegener's granulomatosis follows the same general principles and is discussed below.

Adverse prognostic features of PAN include persistent tachycardia, renal involvement and severe hypertension. It seems that patients who survive the initial months of PAN have a good long-term prognosis and the disease may be self-limiting. Neuropathy and hypertension may persist long after active disease has died down; these symptoms probably reflect the presence of irreversible damage.

Churg–Strauss vasculitis

The very rare syndrome of allergic granulomatosis, described by Churg and Strauss, is closely related to polyarteritis nodosa. It affects medium and small vessels; histological examination demonstrates the presence of eosinophilic infiltrates and granulomata. The peripheral blood usually shows a marked eosinophilia.

Pulmonary involvement, with asthma and radiological evidence of pulmonary infiltrates, is a major feature of the disease. Cardiac involvement is common, as is neuropathy. In a series from the Mayo Clinic (Chumbley et al 1977) adverse prognostic features included a short antecedent history of asthma, and severe cardiac involvement.

There is a wide range of overlap between Churg–Strauss syndrome and polyarteritis nodosa, and they represent two extremes of a spectrum of disease.

Wegener's granulomatosis

Wegener's granulomatosis is a necrotising granulomatous vasculitis that affects predominantly small vessels of the upper and lower respiratory tract, and the kidney. Rhinitis and sinusitis, progressing to extensive destruction of the cartilage and soft tissues of the nose and palate, are the clinical hallmarks of Wegener's granulomatosis. Orbital involvement may result in unilateral proptosis. Serous otitis media may follow granulomatosis of the auditory tract. Pulmonary involvement is commonly associated with the presence of parenchymal nodules seen on chest X-ray. These may break down and cavitate. A necrotising glomerulonephritis occurs in 85% of patients with Wegener's granulomatosis and, in the past, has been responsible for the high mortality of this condition.

Investigations seldom reveal any salient abnormalities. As with other vasculitic syndromes, the ESR and C-reactive protein are greatly increased. There is normochromic anaemia, usually associated with marked neutrophilia and thrombocytosis. Biopsy of clinically involved nasal, pulmonary or renal tissue may reveal characteristic histological changes.

Treatment

If they are untreated, PAN, Churg–Strauss vasculitis and Wegener's granulomatosis pursue a malignant and rapidly fatal course. PAN has a 50% mortality rate in 6 months (Frohnert & Sheps 1967), and untreated Wegener's granulomatosis has an 80% mortality rate in one year (Walton 1958).

Corticosteroids have considerably improved the survival rate. Sack et al (1975) reported a 5-year survival in 57% of patients with PAN. The introduction of cytotoxic agents such as cyclophosphamide and azathioprine has resulted in further improvement in survival, particularly in patients with Wegener's granulomatosis. Leib et al (1979) found that the 5-year survival of patients with PAN improved from 53% to 80% with the addition of cytotoxic agents. Fauci et al (1978) have reported a remission rate of 90% among 47 patients with Wegener's granulomatosis treated with combination cyclophosphamide and corticosteroids.

Our own policy is as follows. Patients with life-threatening necrotising vasculitis are started immediately on prednisolone 60 mg per day and cyclophosphamide 2 mg/kg body weight per day. As soon as the disease is controlled, usually within 6–8 weeks, azathioprine is introduced at a dose level of 2.5 mg/kg and cyclophosphamide is stopped after an overlap period of 1 week. Subsequently, steroid therapy and azathioprine are slowly withdrawn with careful monitoring of clinical and laboratory evidence of disease activity. This management policy is less aggressive than that advocated by American authors (Fauci et al 1978, Fan et al 1980) who maintain cyclophosphamide treatment for 1 year, in cases of Wegener's granulomatosis.

Hypersensitivity vasculitis

Hypersensitivity vasculitis predominantly affects arterioles and venules; histologically, it is a leucocytoclastic vasculitis. The most commonly involved organ is the skin, with a rash varying from classic palpable purpura to ulcerative, and occasionally urticarial, lesions. The disease seems to represent the common response to a wide variety of stimuli and is found in association with a large number of underlying conditions (Table 11.10). Frequently it is a benign condition limited to the skin and requiring no treatment. A fulminant necrotising systemic vasculitis may occur which is poorly responsive to immunosuppressive therapy. It is this disease that is sometimes called 'microscopic polyarteritis nodosa'.

Management of this variable condition should be directed to assessing the extent and severity of organ involvement. The aggressiveness of the treatment should be guided by the aggression of the disease. Underlying conditions should be identified and, wherever possible, the stimulus to the vasculitis removed.

Table 11.10 Disease associations of hypersensitivity vasculitis

Cryoglobulinaemia
Henoch-Schonlein purpura
1° connective tissue disease
Carcinomata
Haematological malignancy
Drug reaction
Acute and chronic infection
Serum sickness
Chronic hepatitis
1° biliary cirrhosis
Ulcerative colitis

Lymphomatoid granulomatosis

Lymphomatoid granulomatosis is a rare vasculitis in which blood vessels are invaded and destroyed by a bizarre polymorphic infiltrate of lymphocytic and atypical lymphocytoid cells. Lung, skin, central nervous system and kidneys are commonly involved. Histologically, the appearances border on those of a lymphoproliferative disorder and lymphomas evolve in 13% of patients (Liebow et al 1972). This serious condition may respond to corticosteroids and cyclophosphamide if treated at an early stage.

Giant-cell arteritis and polymyalgia rheumatica

Two recent publications (Graham et al 1981, Jones & Hazleman 1981) have emphasised some of the problems in the management of these poorly understood syndromes.

The relationship between polymyalgia rheumatica (PMR) and giant-cell arteritis (GCA) remains controversial. Fauchald et al (1972) found positive temporal artery biopsies in 40% of patients with symptoms of polymyalgia alone. In a series of 85 patients at a polymyalgia rheumatica clinic, 42% developed clinical evidence of GCA with a mean time of onset 1 year after development of PMR. There were no features by which this group of patients could have been identified in advance. Of 90 patients presenting to ophthalmology and neurology departments with histological evidence of GCA, 33% had evidence of PMR (Graham et al 1981). The late presentation of PMR in patients with GCA seems to be uncommon, although it has been recorded.

PMR and GCA seem to represent a spectrum of disease with PMR at the benign end. In view of the significant risk of late progression of PMR to GCA, it is clear that patients require prolonged follow-up with clear warnings of the importance of early reporting of symptoms suggestive of GCA.

Diagnosis of polymyalgia and temporal arteritis

PMR can be very difficult to distinguish from early rheumatoid arthritis and, indeed, true synovitis may be a prominent feature. Major features of PMR include severe shoulder and pelvic girdle pain and early-morning stiffness. Muscle tenderness is not usually severe and EMG, muscle enzymes and muscle biopsy are all normal. Onset of illness is usually rapid. The ESR is greater than 30 mm in 1 hour in most cases, although it is notable that three out of 90 of Graham's patients with GCA had an ESR of less than 30 mm (Graham et al 1981) A rapid response to oral prednisolone usually confirms diagnostic suspicions. Other abnormal findings commonly include a normochromic normocytic anaemia and a raised hepatic alkaline phosphatase.

GCA may be asymptomatic and detected only by temporal artery biopsy. Symptomatic GCA is suggested by cranial artery or scalp tenderness, jaw tenderness or claudication, visual symptoms including diplopia, or more extensive signs of cerebrovascular insufficiency. Vascular involvement elsewhere is uncommon, but giant-cell aortitis is described.

Prognosis

Twenty-three per cent of patients in Jones & Hazleman's series with PMR went on later to develop potentially serious neurological or visual complications (Jones & Hazleman 1981); 10% developed permanent visual loss. In 50% of Graham's series, visual loss was the presenting symptom and seldom improved. Significantly, the two features associated with increased mortality were high-dose maintenance steroids and visual loss.

Management

All agree that immediate administration of corticosteroids in high dosage is the correct management of GCA, but there is some debate as to how long this should be maintained. In view of possible adverse effects, our policy is to reduce the dose over a period of 3 months to 10 mg of prednisolone daily and to continue to reduce it steadily thereafter, usually in 1 mg decrements with careful monitoring.

Patients with PMR usually respond to prednisolone 20 mg daily, but at the earliest sign of GCA this dose should be increased. There is, at present, no evidence that high-dose prednisolone treatment prevents the onset of GCA in PMR.

It is increasingly apparent that PMR and GCA are not benign illnesses. The physician is faced with the difficult task of balancing the danger of prednisolone therapy in old and vulnerable patients with the risks inherent in PMR and GCA.

Takayasu's arteritis

This uncommon large-vessel vasculitis predominantly affects young women, and occurs mainly in the Far East. The aortic arch and its branch vessels are the main sites of involvement although other large vessels, including pulmonary arteries, may be affected. From the clinical standpoint it is a disease with two phases. The first systemic phase, an acute illness with pyrexia, synovitis, polymyalgia rheumatica and sometimes erythema nodosum, is followed after an interval of weeks or months by symptoms of upper limb claudication, congestive cardiac failure, and cerebrovascular insufficiency. Characteristic clinical findings are absent pulses and proximal bruits. Diagnosis is confirmed by arch aortography.

Treatment is unsatisfactory, although there is some evidence that corticosteroids have improved the survival rate (Fraga et al 1972). As yet there are no reported trials of cytotoxic therapy.

Mucocutaneous lymph node syndrome (Kawasaki disease)

This disease of young children, assumed to be of infectious aetiology, has reached epidemic proportions in Japan since 1970, and over 650 cases have now been reported in the USA. It is an acute illness characterised by high spiking fever, rash, conjunctivitis, cervical lymphadenopathy and distinctive erythema of the oral cavity and palms, with desquamation of the fingertips. Laboratory findings include an initial anaemia, neutrophilia and thrombocytosis, associated with raised ESR, proteinuria, sterile pyuria and hepatic function abnormalities. The disease is usually self-limiting. However, a small proportion of patients die, usually suddenly from myocardial infarction during the convalescent phase of disease. At necropsy, coronary arteritis is a prominent feature. There is no specific treatment for this condition and it is not known how to identify those patients who are at risk from coronary arteritis.

Relapsing polychondritis

Up to 1976 only 159 cases of this rare and serious inflammatory condition of cartilagenous ground substance had been reported (reviewed by McAdam et al 1976). The aetiology is unknown, with both biochemical and immunological factors being implicated. Intravenous injection of papain protease into young rabbits results in collapse of their ears with diffuse depletion of cartilage matrix (McCluskey & Thomas 1958). Foidart and colleagues (1978) showed anti-cartilage antibodies with specificity for Type II collagen in five out of 15 patients with relapsing polychondritis (RP). The titres of these antibodies appeared to correlate with the activity of disease.

Clinical features include inflammation of the pinna of the ear, polyarthritis, nasal chondritis, ocular inflammation, respiratory tract chondritis and audiovestibular damage. Less commonly, involvement of the aortic media may result in aortic regurgitation and aneurysm formation. Very occasionally, vasculitis and glomerulonephritis complicate relapsing polychondritis. Corticosteroids may prove to be life-saving, with the addition of cytotoxic agents as necessary. Severe pulmonary and aortic involvement are the major adverse prognostic features.

REFERENCES

Sjögren's syndrome

Alspaugh M A, Talal N, Tan E M 1976 Differentiation and characterization of autoantibodies and their antigens in Sjögren's syndrome. Arthritis and Rheumatism 19: 216–222

Alspaugh M A, Jensen F C, Rabin H, Tan E M 1978 Lymphocytes transformed by Epstein-Barr virus. Journal of Experimental Medicine 147: 1018–1027

Bloch K J, Buchanan W W, Wohl M J, Bunim J J 1965 Sjögren's syndrome: a clinical, pathological and serological study of 62 cases. Medicine 44: 187–231

Chisholm D M, Mason D K 1968 Labial salivary gland biopsy in Sjögren's disease. Journal of Clinical Pathology 21: 656–660

Chused T M, Kassan S S, Opelz G, Moutsopoulos H M, Terasaki P I 1977 Sjögren's syndrome associated with HLA-Dw3. New England Journal of Medicine 296: 895–897

Cummings N A, Schall G L, Asofsky R, Anderson L G, Talal N 1971 Sjögren's syndrome – newer aspects of research, diagnosis and therapy (NIH conference). Annals of Internal Medicine 75: 937–950

Elkon K B, Caeiro F, Gharavi A E, Patel B, Ferjencik P P, Hughes G R V 1981 Radioimmunoassay profile of antiglobulins in connective tissue diseases: elevated levels of IgA antiglobulin in systemic sicca syndrome. Clinical and Experimental Immunology 46: 547–556

Kassan S S, Thomas T L, Moutsopoulos H M, Hoover R, Kimberly R P, Budman D R et al 1978 Increased risk of lymphoma in sicca syndrome. Annals of Internal Medicine 89: 888–892

Moutsopoulos H M, Mann D L, Johnson A H, Chused T M 1979 Genetic differences between primary and secondary sicca syndrome. New England Journal of Medicine 301: 761–763

Newball H H, Brahim S A 1977 Chronic obstructive airway disease in patients with Sjögren's syndrome. American Review of Respiratory Disease 115: 295–304

Talal N, Sylvester R A, Daniels T E, Greenspan J S, Williams R C Jr 1974 T and B lymphocytes in peripheral blood and tissue lesions in Sjögren's syndrome. Journal of Clinical Investigation 53: 180–189

Whaley K, Webb J, McAvoy B A, Hughes G R V, Lee P, MacSween R N M et al 1972 Sjögren's syndrome: clinical associations and immunological phenomena. Quarterly Journal of Medicine 42: 513–548

Systemic lupus erythematosus

Alarcon-Segovia D, Ruiz Arguelles A, Fishbein E 1978 Antibody to nuclear ribonucleoprotein penetrates live human mononuclear cells through Fc receptors. Nature 271: 67–69

Alger M, Alarcon-Segovia D, Rivero S J 1977 Hemolytic anaemia and thrombocytopenic purpura: two related subsets of systemic lupus erythematosus. Journal of Rheumatology 4: 351–357

Arend W P, Mannik M 1971 Studies of antigen—antibody complexes. II. Quantification of tissue uptake of soluble complexes in normal and complement-depleted rabbits. Journal of Immunology 107: 63–82

Atkins C J, Kondon J J Jr, Quismorio F P, Friou G J 1972 The choroid plexus in systemic lupus erythematosus. Annals of Internal Medicine 76: 65–72

Baldwin D S, Gluck M C, Lowenstein J, Gallo G R 1977 Lupus nephritis. American Journal of Medicine 62: 12–30

Batchelor J R, Welsh K I, Mansilla Tinoco R, Dollery C T, Hughes G R V, Bernstein R et al 1980 Hydralazine-induced systemic lupus erythematosus: influence of HLA-DR and sex on susceptibility. Lancet 1: 1107–1109

Beaucher W N, Garman R H, Condemi J J 1977 Familial lupus erythematosus: antibodies to DNA in household dogs. New England Journal of Medicine 296: 982–984

Becker G J, Waldburger M, Hughes G R V, Pepys M B 1980 Value of serum C-reactive protein measurement in the investigation of fever in systemic lupus erythematosus. Annals of the Rheumatic Diseases 39: 50–52

Bell D A, Maddison P J 1980 Serological subjects in systemic lupus erythematosus. Arthritis and Rheumatism 23: 1268–1273

Bluestein H G, Zvaifler N J 1976 Brain-reactive lymphocytotoxic antibodies in the serum of patients with systemic lupus erythematosus. Journal of Clinical Investigation 57: 509–516

Bresnihan B, Grigor R R, Oliver M, Hughes G R V, Lovins R E, Faulk W P 1977 Immunological mechanism for spontaneous abortion in systemic lupus erythematosus. Lancet 2: 1205–1207

Bywaters E G L 1975 Jaccoud's syndrome: a sequel to the joint involvement of systemic lupus erythematosus. Clinics in Rheumatic Diseases 1(1): 125–148

Cameron J S, Turner D R, Ogg C S, Williams D G, Lessof M H, Chantler C et al 1979 Systemic lupus with nephritis: a long-term study. Quarterly Journal of Medicine 48: 1–24

Cathcart E S, Idelson B A, Scheinberg M A, Couser W G 1976 Beneficial effects of methylprednisolone 'pulse' therapy in diffuse proliferative lupus nephritis. Lancet 1: 163–166

Datta S K, Schwartz R S 1976 Genetics of expression of xenotropic viruses and autoimmunity in NZB mice. Nature 263: 412–415

Decker J L, Steinberg A D, Reinertsen J L, Plotz P H, Balow J E, Klippel J H 1979 Systemic lupus erythematosus: evolving concepts (NIH conference). Annals of Internal Medicine 91: 587–604

De Horatius R J, Messner R P 1975 Lymphocytotoxic antibodies in family members of patients with systemic lupus erythematosus. Journal of Clinical Investigation 55: 1254–1258

Dubois E L 1978 Antimalarials in the management of discoid and systemic lupus erythematosus. Seminars in Arthritis and Rheumatism 8: 33–51

Estes D, Christian C L 1971 The natural history of systemic lupus erythematosus by prospective analysis. Medicine 50: 85–95

Fessel W J 1974 Systemic lupus erythematosus in the community. Archives of Internal Medicine 134: 1027–1035

Frank M M, Hamburger M I, Lawley T J, Kimberly R P, Plotz P H 1979 Defective reticuloendothelial system Fc-receptor function in systemic lupus erythematosus. New England Journal of Medicine 300: 518–523

Gharavi A E, Elkon K B, Schifferli J A, Hughes G R V 1981 Complement-fixing properties of antibodies to double-stranded DNA in systemic lupus erythematosus. Journal of Clinical and Laboratory Immunology 6: Pt 3: 251–255

Gibson G J, Edmonds J P, Hughes G R V 1977 Diaphragm function and lung involvement in systemic lupus erythematosus. American Journal of Medicine 63: 926–932

Ginzler E, Diamond H, Kaplan D, Weiner M, Schlesinger M, Seleznick M 1978 Computer analysis of factors influencing frequency of infection in systemic lupus erythematosus. Arthritis and Rheumatism 21: 37–44

Gladman D D, Urowitz M B 1980 Venous syndromes and pulmonary embolism in systemic lupus erythematosus. Annals of Rheumatic Diseases 39: 340–343

Grigor R, Edmonds J, Lewkonia R, Hughes G R V 1978 Systemic lupus erythematosus: a prospective analysis. Annals of Rheumatic Diseases 37: 121–128

Honig S, Gorevic P, Weissmann G 1977 C-reactive protein in systemic lupus erythematosus. Arthritis and Rheumatism 20: 1065–1070

Hughes G R V 1979 Systemic lupus erythematosus: treatment and prognosis. British Medical Journal 2: 1019–1022

Inman R D, Fong J K, Pussell B A, Ryan P J, Hughes G R V 1980 The Clq binding assay in systemic lupus erythmatosus: discordance with disease activity. Arthritis and Rheumatism 23: 1282–1286

Izui S, Lambert P H, Miescher P A 1977 In vitro demonstration of a particular affinity of glomerular basement membrane and collagen for DNA: a possible basis for a local formation of DNA/anti-DNA complexes in SLE. Journal of Experimental Medicine 144: 428–443

Koffler D, Agnello V, Kunkel H G 1973 Polynucleotide immune complexes in serum and glomeruli of patients with systemic lupus erythematosus. American Journal of Pathology 74: 109–124

Lafer E M, Rauch J, Andrzejewski C Jr, Mudd D, Furie B et al 1981 Polyspecific monoclonal lupus autoantibodies reactive with both polynucleotides and phospholipids. Journal of Experimental Medicine 153: 897–909

Lerner M R, Boyle J A, Mount S M, Wolin S L, Steitz J A 1980 Are snRNPs involved in splicing? Nature 283: 220–224

Lewis R M, André-Schwartz J, Harris G S, Hirsch M S, Black P H, Schwartz R S 1973 Canine systemic lupus erythematosus: transmission of serologic abnormalities by cell-free filtrates. Journal of Clinical Investigation 52: 1893–1907

Maddison P J, Provost T T, Reichlin M 1981 Serological findings in patients with 'ANA-negative' systemic lupuserythematosus. Medicine 60: 87–94

Miniter M F, Stollar B D, Agnello V 1979 Reassessment of the clinical significance of native DNA antibodies in systemis lupus erythematosus. Arthritis and Rheumatism 22: 959–968

Murphy E D, Roths J B 1979 Autoimmunity and lymphoproliferation: induction by mutant gene lpr, and acceleration by a male-associated factor in Strain BXSB mice. In: Rose N R, Bigazzi P E, Warner N (eds) Genetic control of autoimmune disease. Elsevier North Holland Inc. New York, p 207

Nimelstein S H, Brody S, McShane D, Holman H R 1980 Mixed connective tissue disease: a subsequent evaluation of the original 25 patients. Medicine 59: 239–248

Pinching A J, Travers R L, Hughes G R V, Jones T, Moss S 1978 Oxygen-15 brain scanning for detection of cerebral involvement in systemic lupus erythematosus. Lancet 1: 898–900

Reichlin M 1981 Current perspectives on serological reactions in SLE patients. Clinical and Experimental Immunology 44: 1–10

Roubinian J R, Papoian R, Talal N 1977 Androgenic hormones modulate autoantibody responses and improve survival in murine lupus. Journal of Clinical Investigation 59: 1066–1070

Seaman W E, Plotz P H 1976 Effect of aspirin on liver tests in patients with RA or SLE and in normal volunteers. Arthritis and Rheumatism 19: 155–160

Sharp G C, Anderson P C 1980 Current concepts in the classification of connective tissue diseases: overlap syndromes and mixed connective tissue disease. Journal of American Academy of Dermatology 2: 269–279

Sharp G C, Irvin W S, Tan E M, Gould R G, Holman H R 1972 Mixed connective tissue disease — an apparently distinct rheumatic disease syndrome associated with a specific antibody to an extractable nuclear antigen (ENA). American Journal of Medicine 52: 148–159

Theofilopiloulos A N, Dixon F J 1981 Etiopathogenesis of murine SLE. Immunological Reviews 55: 179–216

Travers R L, Hughes G R V 1978 Salicylate hepatotoxicity in SLE: a common occurrence? British Medical Journal 2: 1532–1533

Urowitz M B, Bookman A A M, Koehler B E, Gordon D A, Smythe H A, Ogryzlo M A 1976 The bimodal mortality pattern of systemic lupus erythematosus. American Journal of Medicine 60: 221–225

Verrier-Jones J, Cumming R H, Bacon P A, Evers J, Fraser I D, Bothamley J et al 1979 Evidence for a therapeutic effect of plasmapheresis in patients with systemic lupus erythematosus. Quarterly Journal of Medicine 48: 555–576

Winfield J B, Brunner C M, Koffler D 1978 Serological studies in patients with systemic lupus erythematosus and central nervous system dysfunction. Arthritis and Rheumatism 21: 289–294

Winn D M, Wolfe J F, Harmon D, Sharp G C 1979 Characterisation of a distinct nuclear acidic protein antigen (MA) and clinical findings in systemic lupus erythematosus patients with MA antibodies. Journal of Clinical Investigation 1979: 820–823

Zizic T M, Hungerford D S, Stevens M B 1980 Ischaemic bone necrosis in systemic lupus erythematosus. Medicine 59: 134–142

Zubler R H, Lambert P H 1978 Detection of immune complexes in human diseases. Progress in Allergy 24: 1–48

Polymyositis and dermatomyositis

Askari A, Vignos P J Jr, Mushowitz R W 1976 Steroid myopathy in connective tissue disease. American Journal of Medicine 61: 485–492

Bohan A, Peter J B 1975 Polymyositis and dermatomyositis. New England Journal of Medicine 292: 344–347, 403–407

Bohan A, Peter J B, Bowman R L, Pearson C M 1977 A computer-assisted analysis of 153 patients with polymyositis and dermatomyositis. Medicine 56: 255–286

Bunch T W 1981 Prednisone and azathioprine for polymyositis: long-term follow-up. Arthritis and Rheumatism 24: 45–48

Bunch T W, Worthington J W, Combs J J, Ilstrup D M, Engle A G 1980 Azathioprine with prednisone for polymyositis: a controlled, clinical trial. Annals of Internal Medicine 92: 365–369

Cambridge G, Stern C M M 1981 The uptake of tritium-labelled carnitine by monolayer cultures of human fetal muscle and its potential as a label in cytoxicity studies. Clinical and Experimental Immunology 43: 211–219

Currie S, Saunders M, Knowles M, Brown A E 1971 Immunological aspects of polymyositis: the in vitro activity of lymphocytes on incubation with muscle antigen and muscle cultures. Quarterly Journal of Medicine 40: 63–84

Edwards R H T, Hyde S A 1977) Methods of measuring muscle strength and fatigue. Physiotherapy 63: 51–55

Elia M, Carter A, Bacon S, Winearls C G, Smith R 1981 Clinical usefulness of urinary 3-methylhistidine excretion in indicating muscle protein breakdown. British Medical Journal 282: 351–354

Engel W K, Lichter A S, Galdi A P 1981 Polymyositis: remarkable response to total body irradiation. Lancet 2: 658

Kagen L J 1971 Myoglobinemia and myoglobinuria in patients with myositis. Arthritis and Rheumatism 14: 457–464

Lane R J M, Mastaglia F L 1978 Drug-induced myopathies in man. Lancet 2: 562–565

Medsger T A Jr, Robinson H, Masi A T 1971 Factors affecting survivorship in polymyositis. Arthritis and Rheumatism 14: 249–258

Metzger A L, Bohan A, Goldberg L S, Bluestone R, Pearson C M 1974 Polymyositis and dermatomyositis: combined methotrexate and corticosteroid therapy. Annals of Internal Medicine 81: 182–189

Schwarz H A, Slavin G, Ansell B M 1980 Histological and morphometric studies in polymyositis and dermatomyositis. Annals of the Rheumatic Diseases 39: 186

Schwartz M I, Matthay R A, Sahn S A, Stanford R E, Marmorstein B L, Scheinhorn D J 1976 Interstitial lung disease in polymyositis and dermatomyositis. Analysis of 6 cases and review of the literature. Medicine 55: 89–104

Vignos P J Jr, Goldwyn J 1972 Evaluation of laboratory tests in diagnosis and management of polymyositis. American Journal of the Medical Sciences 263: 291–308

Scleroderma

Alarcon-Segovia D, Ramos-Niembro F, Ibanez de Kasep G, Alcocer J, Perez Tamayo R 1979 Long-term evaluation of colchicine in the treatment of scleroderma. Journal of Rheumatology 6: 705–712

Bennett R M, Bluestone R H, Holt P J L, Bywaters E G L 1971 Survival in scleroderma. Annals of the Rheumatic Diseases 30: 581–588

Brady A H 1975 Collagenase in scleroderma. Journal of Clinical Investigation 56: 1175–1180

Bulkley B H, Ridolfi R L, Salyer W R, Hutchins G M 1976 Myocardial lesions of progressive systemic sclerosis. A cause of cardiac dysfunction. Circulation 53: 483–490

Cannon P J, Hassar M, Case D B, Casarella W J, Somners S C, LeRoy E C 1974 The relationship of hypertension and renal failure in scleroderma (progressive systemic sclerosis) to structural and functional abnormalities of the renal cortical circulation. Medicine 53: 1–46

Dodson V N, Dinman B D, Whitehouse W M, Nasr A N M, Magnuson H J 1971 Occupational acro-osteolysis. III. A clinical study. Archives of Environmental Health 22: 83–91

Guttadauria M, Ellman H, Emmanuel G, Kaplan D, Diamond H 1977 Pulmonary function in scleroderma. Arthritis and Rheumatism 20: 1071–1079

Herbert C M, Lindberg K A, Jayson M I V, Bailey A J 1974 Biosynthesis and maturation of skin collagen in scleroderma and effect of D-penicillamine. Lancet 1: 187–192

Lawley T J, Peck G L, Moutsopoulos H M, Gratwohl A A, Deisscrotin A B 1977 Scleroderma, Sjögren-like syndrome, and chronic graft-versus-host disease. Annals of Internal Medicine 87: 707–709

LeRoy E C 1974 Increased collagen synthesis by scleroderma skin fibroblasts in vitro. A possible defect in the regulation or activation of the scleroderma fibroblast. Journal of Clinical Investigation 54: 880–889

Lopez-Ovejero J A, Saal S D, D'Angelo W A, Cheigh J S, Stegel K H, Laragh J H 1979 Reversal of vascular and renal crisis of scleroderma by oral angiotensin-converting enzyme blockade. New England Journal of Medicine 300: 1417–1419

Maricq H R, LeRoy E C 1979 Progressive systemic sclerosis: disorders of the microcirculation. Clinics in Rheumatic Diseases 5(1): 81–101

Maricq H R, Downey J A, LeRoy E C 1976 Standstill of nailfold capillary blood flow during cooling in scleroderma and Raynaud's syndrome. Blood Vessels 13: 338–349

Medsger T A, Masi A T, Rodnan G P, Benedek T G, Robinson H 1971 Survival with systemic sclerosis (scleroderma). A life-table analysis of 309 patients. Annals of Internal Medicine 75: 369–376

Meihoff W E, Hirschfield J S, Kern F Jr 1968 Small intestinal scleroderma with malabsorption and pneumatosis cystoides intestinalis. Report of three cases. Journal of the American Medical Association 204: 854–858

Moore T L, Zuckner J 1980 Eosinophilic fasciitis. Seminars in Arthritis and Rheumatism 9: 228–235

Naslund M J, Pearson T A, Ritter J M 1981 A documented episode of pulmonary vasoconstriction in systemic sclerosis. Johns Hopkins Medical Journal 148: 78–80

Nassonova V A, Ivanova M M 1979 Progressive systemic sclerosis. Management: D-pencillamine. Clinics in Rheumatic Diseases 5(1): 277–288

Ramirez-Mata M, Ibanez G, Alarcon-Segovia D 1977 Stimulatory effect of metoclopramide on the esophagus and lower esophageal sphincter of patients with progressive systemic sclerosis. Arthritis and Rheumatism 20: 30–34

Reynolds T B, Denison E K, Frankl H D, Lieberman F L, Peters R L 1971 Primary biliary cirrhosis with scleroderma, Raynaud's phenomenon and telangiectasia. American Journal of Medicine 50: 302–312

Richards R L, Milne J A 1958 Cancer of the lung in progressive systemic sclerosis. Thorax 13: 238–245

Richardson J A 1973 Hemodialysis and kidney transplantation for renal failure from scleroderma. Arthritis and Rheumatism 16: 265–271

Rodnan G P 1981 When is scleroderma not scleroderma? The differential diagnosis of progressive systemic sclerosis. Bulletin on the Rheumatic Diseases 31: 7–10

Rodnan G P, Lipinski E, Luksick J 1979 Skin collagen content in progressive systemic sclerosis (scleroderma) and localized scleroderma. Arthritis and Rheumatism 22: 130–140

Sackner A M, Akgun N, Kimbel P, Lewis D H 1964 The pathophysiology of scleroderma involving the heart and respiratory system. Annals of Internal Medicine 60: 611–630

Steigerwald J C, Lynch D 1977 Colchicine therapy versus placebo. A double-blind study in progressive systemic sclerosis. In: Abstracts of the XIVth International Congress of Rheumatology, San Francisco, p 163

Stevens M B, Hookman P, Siegel C I, Esterly J R, Shulman L E, Hendrix T R 1964 Aperistalsis of the esophagus in patients with connective-tissue disorders and Raynaud's phenomenon. New England Journal of Medicine 270: 1218–1222

Talpos G, Horrocks M, White J M, Cotton L T 1978 Plasmapheresis in Raynaud's disease. Lancet 1: 416–417

Tan E M, Rodnan G P, Garcia I, Moroi Y, Fritzler M J, Peebles C 1980 Diversity of antinuclear antibodies in progressive systemic sclerosis: anti-cantromere antibody and its relationship to crest syndrome. Arthritis and Rheumatism 23: 617–625

Turner R, Lipschutz W, Miller W, Rittenberg G, Schumacher H R, Cohen S 1973 Esophageal dysfunction in collagen disease. American Journal of Medical Sciences 265: 191–199

Vasculitis and relapsing polychondritis

Bron K M, Strott C A, Shapiro A P 1965 The diagnostic value of angiographic observations in polyarteritis nodosa. Archives of Internal Medicine 116: 450–454

Christian C L, Sergent J S 1976 Vasculitis syndromes: clinical and experimental models. American Journal of Medicine 61: 385–392

Chumbley L C, Harrison E G Jr, DeRemee R A 1977 Allergic granulomatosis and angiitis (Churg-Strauss syndrome): report and analysis of 30 cases. Mayo Clinic Proceedings 52: 477–484

Citron B P, Halpern M, McCarron M, Lundberg G D, McCormick R, Pincus I J et al 1970 Necrotising angiitis associated with drug abuse. New England Journal of Medicine 283: 1003–1011

Elkon K B, Hughes G R V, Catovsky D, Clauvel J P, Dumont J, Seligman M et al 1980 Hairy-cell leukaemia with polyarteritis nodosa. Lancet 2: 280–282

Fan P T, Davis J A, Somer T, Kaplan L, Bluestone R 1980 A clinical approach to systemic vasculitis. Seminars in Arthritis and Rheumatism 9: 248–304

Fauchald P, Rygvold O, Øystese B 1972 Temporal arteritis and polymyalgia rheumatica: clinical and biopsy findings. Annals of Internal Medicine 77: 845–852

Fauci A S, Haynes B F, Katz P 1978 The spectrum of vasculitis: clinical, pathologic, immunologic and therapeutic considerations (NIH conference). Annals of Internal Medicine 89: 660–676

Foidart J-M, Abe S, Martin G R, Zizic T M, Barnett E V, Lawley T J et al 1978 Antibodies to type II collagen in relapsing polychrondritis. New England Journal of Medicine 299: 1203–1207

Fraga A, Mintz G, Valle L, Flores-Izquierdo G 1972 Takayasu's arteritis: frequency of systemic manifestations (study of 22 patients) and favourable response to maintenance steroid therapy with adrenocorticosteroids (12 patients). Arthritis and Rheumatism 15: 617–624

Frohnert P P, Sheps S G 1967 Long-term follow up study of periarteritis nodosa. American Journal of Medicine 43: 8–14

Gocke D J, Hsu K, Morgan C, Bombardieri S, Lockshin M, Christian C L 1970 Association between polyarteritis and Australia antigen. Lancet 2: 1149–1153

Graham E, Holland A, Avery A, Ross Russell R W 1981 Prognosis in giant-cell arteritis. British Medical Journal 282: 269–271

Jones J G, Hazleman B L 1981 Prognosis and management of polymyalgia rheumatica. Annals of the Rheumatic Diseases 40: 1–5

Kniker W T, Cochrane C G 1968 The localisation of circulating immune complexes in experimental serum sickness: the role of vasoactive amines and hydrodynamic forces. Journal of Experimental Medicine 127: 119–136

Levo Y, Gorevic P D, Kasab H J, Zucker-Franklin L D, Franklin E C 1977 Association between hepatitis B virus and essential mixed cryoglobulinemia. New England Journal of Medicine 296: 1501–1504

Lieb E S, Restivo C, Paulus H E 1979 Immunosuppressive and corticosteroid therapy of polyarteritis nodosa. American Journal of Medicine 67: 941–947

Liebow A A, Carrington C R B, Friedman P J 1972 Lymphomatoid granulomatosis. Human Pathology 3: 457–558

McAdam L P, O'Hanlan M, Bluestone R, Pearson C M 1976 Relapsing polychondritis: prospective study of 23 patients and a review of the literature. Medicine 55: 193–215

McCluskey R T, Thomas L 1958 The removal of cartilage matrix, in vivo, by papain. Journal of Experimental Medicine 108: 371–384

Sack M, Cassidy J T, Bole G G 1975 Prognostic factors in polyarteritis. Journal of Rheumatology 2: 411–420

Travers R L, Allison D J, Brettle R P, Hughes G R V 1979 Polyarteritis nodosa: a clinical and angiographic analysis of 17 cases. Seminars in Arthritis and Rheumatism 8: 184–199

Walton E W 1958 Giant cell granuloma of the respiratory tract (Wegener's granulomatosis). British Medical Journal 2: 265–270

12

Calcium and bone metabolism

B. E. C. Nordin and M. Peacock

This chapter describes recent advances in certain aspects of calcium metabolism and reviews progress in the understanding of metabolic bone and stone disease.

CALCIUM PHYSIOLOGY

Plasma calcium homeostasis

The concentration of calcium in plasma and extracellular fluid is a positive function of the rate of calcium flow through the plasma, a positive function of the rate of renal tubular reabsorption of calcium and a negative function of glomerular filtration rate (Nordin 1976a). In the normal state the calcium flow comprises *net* calcium absorption (i.e. the difference between dietary and faecal calcium) and *net* bone resorption (i.e. the difference between the rates of bone formation and resorption) (Fig. 12.1). In the fasting state, or where there is malabsorption of calcium, the calcium flow necessary to maintain the plasma calcium concentration within the normal range must be derived from the skeleton.

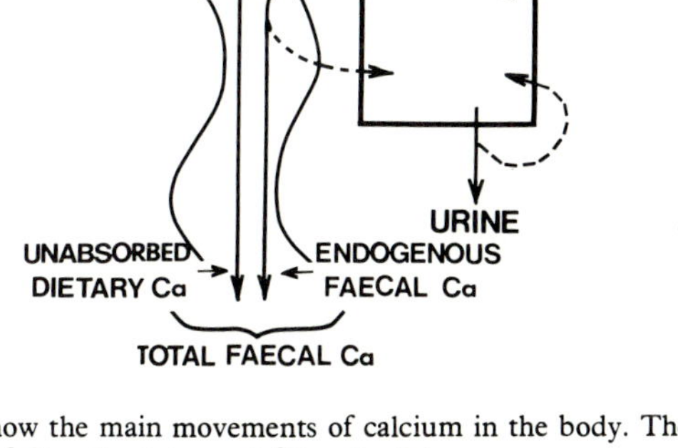

Fig. 12.1 Diagram to show the main movements of calcium in the body. The interrupted lines represent reabsorption of digestive juice and filtered calcium

The constancy of the plasma calcium concentration in normal subjects, despite wide variations in calcium intake and absorption, is largely accounted for by the negative feedback of the plasma (ionised) calcium concentration on the activation of the parathyroid hormone/vitamin D system (see below). This system responds by increasing calcium absorption from the gut and tubular reabsorption of calcium in the kidney and (if necessary) bone resorption when the plasma calcium falls, and decreasing these rates when it rises. Generally speaking, plasma calcium concentrations above or below the normal range results from disturbances in this parathyroid hormone/vitamin D system although there are other causes of hypocalcaemia and hypercalcaemia which will be discussed below.

Parathyroid hormone

Parathyroid hormone has been characterised in a variety of species. It is a polypeptide containing 84 amino acids with a molecular weight of about 9000. Measurement of this hormone in plasma depends upon radioimmunoassay, generally with antisera to bovine hormone, but for various reasons, including the circulation in plasma of parathyroid hormone fragments (particularly in renal failure), the assay is imprecise. Although it is useful in the diagnosis of hyperparathyroidism and the distinction of primary hyperparathyroidism from other forms of hypercalcaemia, it is generally not specific enough to measure variations in hormone concentration within or below the normal range. More precise and specific assays are under development (Manning et al 1980).

Parathyroid hormone acts to increase tubular reabsorption of calcium in the kidney and to increase bone resorption. Its apparent positive effect on calcium absorption is mediated through 1, 25-dihydroxycholecalciferol (1, 25 $(OH)_2D$), the synthesis of which in the kidney is stimulated by parathyroid hormone. The extent to which the actions of parathyroid hormone on bone resorption and on tubular reabsorption of calcium require the presence of vitamin D or its metabolites is uncertain.

Vitamin D

The vitamin D system can now be regarded as an endocrine system in the sense that the active metabolites are under feedback control and are secreted in parts of the body distinct from their target organs. 7-dehydrocholesterol is converted in the skin, under the influence of ultraviolet radiation, to vitamin D_3 which is converted in the liver to 25OHD which in turn is metabolised in the kidney to $1,25(OH)_2D$. Many other vitamin D metabolites have now been described but their physiological actions are uncertain. Considerable controversy surrounds the possible role of $24,25(OH)_2D$ in bone calcification (Malluche et al 1980).

As far as the principal vitamin D metabolites 25OHD and $1,25(OH)_2D$ are concerned, the latter is at least a thousand times as potent as the former in respect of its action on bone resorption (Peacock et al 1977) and calcium absorption (Parkes 1978) but because $1,25(OH)_2D$ circulates in the plasma in one thousandth of the concentration of 25OHD, it is possible that they are both contributing to the physiological actions of 'vitamin D' (Nordin et al 1979). Some uncertainty surrounds this concept, however, because it is not entirely clear what is the relationship between the free circulating concentrations of these two metabolites and the relative affinities of the cytosol carrier for them. What is reasonably well established is that the free 1,25$(OH)_2$D concentration is only about 1% of the total and the free 25OHD is only about 0.05% of the total, most of both being carried on the vitamin-D-binding protein (Bouillon & van Baelen 1979). However, whatever may be the situation in normal subjects, it is clear that both compounds can act independently on calcium absorption, for 25OHD therapy is effective in patients with renal failure (Rutherford et al 1975) and 1,25$(OH)_2$D therapy is effective in severe vitamin D deficiency (Peacock et al 1979a).

Calcitonin

Although no plasma calcium disturbance attributable to calcitonin excess or deficiency has yet been described in man, and the importance of calcitonin in adult humans therefore remains somewhat uncertain, sensitive assays have now been developed which permit the definition of a normal range. The hormone is a peptide comprising 32 amino acids with a molecular weight of about 3000. Its secretion is stimulated by an increase in plasma calcium concentration and by many other stimuli including alcohol and pentagastrin (Care & Bates 1972, Cohen et al 1973). The circulating concentration is higher in men than in women and is increased by oestrogen administration (Hillyard et al 1978). High calcitonin levels have been reported in pregnancy (Stevenson et al 1979) and in various types of malignancy (Coombs et al 1976), and calcitonin has been used in the treatment of various types of hypercalcaemia (Hosking 1980).

DIAGNOSTIC PROCEDURES

There have been a number of developments concerning diagnostic procedures in calcium disorders, which have been reviewed elsewhere (Nordin 1976b). They include the measurement of the *fasting* urine calcium/creatinine and hydroxyproline/creatinine ratios as indicators of bone resorption; the use of a single radioisotope of calcium to measure calcium absorption; the precise measurement of mean metacarpal cortical width to monitor sequential changes in cortical bone width; and the use of polyethylene glycol as a non-absorbable faecal marker for the determination of calcium balances on a daily basis. Other developments are the use of neutron-activation analysis to measure whole-body calcium (Nelp et al 1972), the increasing use of gamma-ray absorptiometry for the measurement of peripheral (Cameron & Sorenson 1963) and spinal (Lindquist et al 1979) bone density, and the introduction of computerised axial tomography for the same purpose (Exner et al 1979). In view of the importance of calcium absorption it is worth noting that this can be assessed quite easily by comparing the urinary calcium/creatinine ratio of a fasting patient with the 24-h ratio when the patient has a normal or high calcium intake, or by comparing the absolute 24-h calcium outputs on low and high calcium intakes. The difference between urinary calcium excretion in the fasting state or on a low calcium diet, and the excretion on a normal or high intake, is a measure of calcium absorptive status (Nordin 1976b).

CLINICAL DISORDERS

Osteoporosis

Definition and classification

It is generally agreed that the term 'osteoporosis' denotes a reduced quantity of bone associated with an increase in fracture risk. The steep rise in fracture rates with age, particularly in women, which accompanies the decline in bone mass in the population suggests that the mechanical safety margin in the skeleton is small and that the fracture risk rises as soon as relative bone mass falls below a certain 'fracture threshold' (Newton-John & Morgan 1968). Because there is uncertainty about the precise level of this 'fracture threshold', it has been suggested that it should be equated with the lower limit of bone mass in young normal adults; values below this 'young normal' range should be regarded as osteoporotic (Horsman et al 1981). Cortical and trabecular bone do not behave in precisely the same way and therefore osteoporosis must be qualified as being 'trabecular' or 'cortical', the reference bone being stated in any particular case and the reference standard derived from the 'young normal' range of the appropriate sex. The most widely used cortical reference bone is the second metacarpal of the right hand (Barnett & Nordin 1960) and the most popular measurement is the cortical area/total area ratio (CA/TA) (Garn 1970). The most usual trabecular reference bone is the iliac crest, the measurement being made on a biopsy sample; it remains to be seen whether non-invasive densitometry of the forearm or spine can be equally useful. Osteoporosis can be further subdivided into primary and secondary forms (according to whether a 'cause' can be identified or not) and into localised and generalised types.

If fractures in the elderly are in fact, attributable to the development of osteoporosis, the elderly subjects who suffer fractures would be expected to be osteoporotic. This is generally true in cases of vertebral and femoral-neck fractures but not always true in those of distal forearm fractures. Moreover, if the fracture risk is proportional to the severity of the osteoporosis, patients with fractures should be more osteoporotic than age-matched control patients. This is also true of vertebral and femoral-neck fracture patients, particularly if both cortical and trabecular bone values are taken into account. The best discriminant between crush fracture cases and age-matched controls is the iliac crest bone volume, and the best discriminant between femoral-neck fracture cases and age-matched controls is the Singh index (Singh et al 1970) but, with both fractures, discrimination is improved if a cortical measurement like the metacarpal CA/TA is also taken into account (Horsman et al 1981).

Pathogenesis

Primary osteoporosis. The onset of osteoporosis in women roughly coincides with the menopause: in men the loss of bone starts later and proceeds more slowly. The available data on pathogenetic mechanisms are derived mainly from observation of women.

The loss of bone which starts at the menopause in the female population must be caused by an increase in the rate of bone resorption, a reduction in the rate of bone formation, or a combination of the two. Histological evidence regarding which of these variables is disturbed is inconclusive, but there are probably more data in favour of accelerated bone resorption than of reduced bone formation (Fig. 12.2).

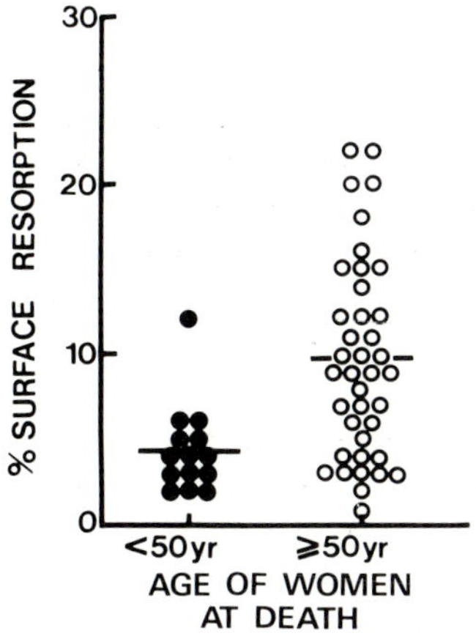

Fig. 12.2 Percentage of surface resorption in iliac crest samples obtained post mortem from women below and over the age of 50 years

This is compatible with the biochemical evidence, for the menopause is associated with a rise, not only in the fasting plasma and urine calcium and phosphate (which could be attributable to reduced bone formation or increased bone resorption), but also in plasma alkaline phosphatase and urinary hydroxyproline (Crilly et al 1980), which are impossible to reconcile with reduced bone formation. All these biochemical changes are reversible with oestrogen therapy (Fig. 12.3) which prevents

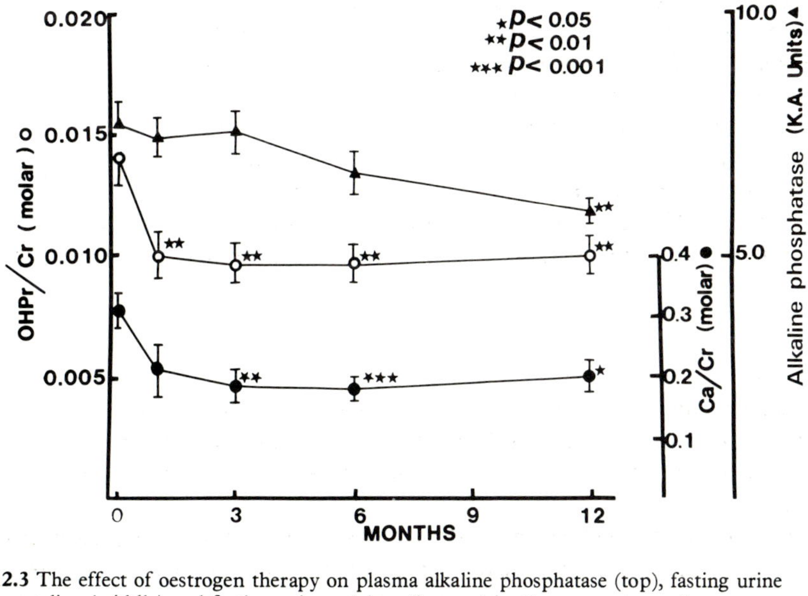

Fig. 12.3 The effect of oestrogen therapy on plasma alkaline phosphatase (top), fasting urine hydroxyproline (middle) and fasting urine calcium (bottom) in 61 postmenopausal women

postmenopausal bone loss (Lindsay et al 1980) (Fig. 12.4). These data are compatible with the concept that loss of bone after the menopause is due to increased sensitivity of the bone to bone-resorbing agents in the absence of oestrogen (Heaney 1965, Jasani et al 1965).

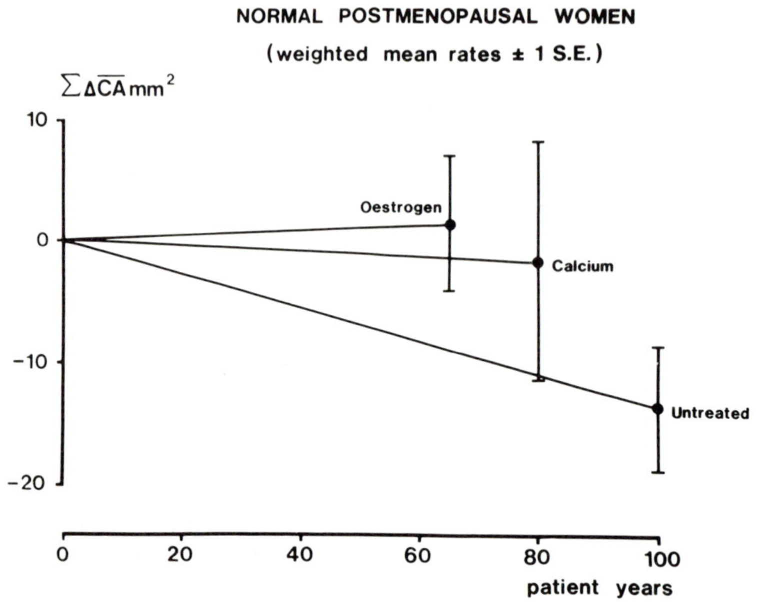

Fig. 12.4 The effect of oestrogen therapy and calcium supplements on mean metacarpal cortical area in postmenopausal women (30 subjects in each group) (mean values ± 1 S.E.)

Another way of looking at the effect of the menopause on calcium metabolism is to regard it as an increase in calcium requirement due to an increase in the obligatory urinary calcium (Nordin et al 1981a) and (possibly) a reduction in calcium absorption (Heaney et al 1977). This increased requirement can be met by giving calcium supplements, which also delay or prevent bone loss (Recker et al 1977, Horsman et al 1977) (Fig. 12.4). However, whereas oestrogens act by blocking the effect on bone of bone-resorbing agents such as parathyroid hormone and $1,25(OH)_2D$, calcium supplements probably act by suppressing the secretion of these agents. This may explain why withdrawal of oestrogens (which tend to stimulate the parathyroids) is followed by a relatively rapid loss of bone (Lindsay et al 1978) whereas withdrawal of calcium supplements (which tend to suppress the parathyroids) is not (Horsman et al 1979).

It has already been indicated that patients with fractures generally have a more severe bone deficiency than age-matched controls. Many of these actually suffer from accelerated osteoporosis, and some other factor in addition to the menopause must therefore be invoked to explain their bone status. In cases of crush fracture (trabecular osteoporosis) the main additional risk factor appears to be malabsorption of calcium – both in men and in women. Some workers have attributed this to a deficiency of $1,25(OH)_2D$ (Gallagher et al 1979) but others disagree (Nordin et al 1981a). In women with predominantly cortical osteoporosis, calcium absorption may be normal but plasma oestrogen levels are reduced (Nordin et al 1981b); however, no hormonal abnormality has been described in males. It is of interest, however, and may help to explain why men are less prone to osteoporosis than women, that plasma oestrogen levels are higher in men than in postmenopausal women (Nordin et al 1981b).

In cases of femoral-neck fracture, malabsorption of calcium is frequently present. In this population, however, it can be accounted for by vitamin D deficiency because these patients have significantly lower plasma 25OHD levels than controls (Baker et al 1979) and many of them also have osteomalacia (Aaron et al 1974). The cause of the vitamin D deficiency in these elderly patients is not dietary but is caused by inadequate exposure to sunlight. Most femoral-neck fractures occur in the home and affect a predominantly house-bound population.

Secondary osteoporosis. Spinal osteoporosis is a recognised feature of Cushing's syndrome and a recognised complication of corticosteroid therapy. Again, malabsorption of calcium — apparently a direct effect of corticosteroid-induced osteoporosis (Fig. 12.5) — is implicated, but an additional factor in postmenopausal women on corticosteroid therapy may be their low oestrogen and androgen levels. These are secondary to corticosteroid-induced suppression of the adrenal glands which are virtually the sole source of sex steroids in women after the menopause (Crilly et al 1978).

There have been no major advances in our understanding of other types of secondary osteoporosis such as that associated with hyperthyroidism, alcohol and (possibly) diabetes, except to confirm that these are risk factors for osteoporosis, the mechanisms of which are poorly understood.

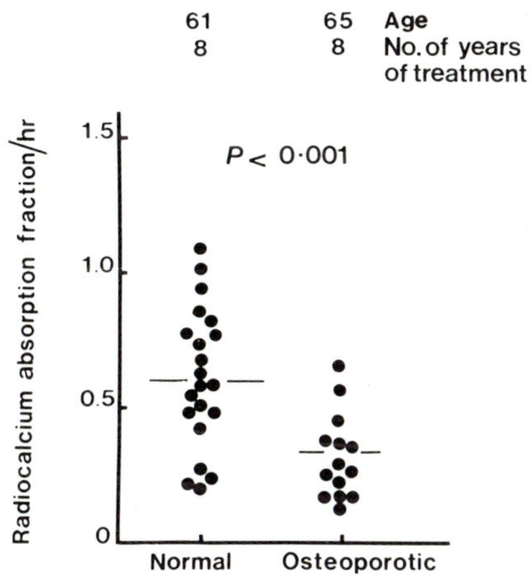

Fig. 12.5 Radiocalcium absorption in corticosteroid-treated subjects with and without spinal crush fractures

Treatment of osteoporosis

Most of the information available is derived from the treatment of postmenopausal osteoporosis monitored by sequential metacarpal morphometry, forearm densitometry or examination of spinal radiographs. Most treatments are designed to prevent further loss of bone, either by protecting it against bone-resorbing agents (with oestrogens and/or progestogens) or by suppressing the secretion of these bone-resorbing agents by the administration of calcium supplements (if calcium absorption is normal) or some form of vitamin D, with or without calcium, if there is malabsorption of calcium. In some patients with calcium malabsorption, oestrogen has been combined with a vitamin D metabolite. The effects of these therapies on peripheral bone loss are shown in Figure 12.6.

Judging by cortical bone loss, the most successful treatment appears to be the combination of 1αOHD (or $1,25(OH)_2D$ in doses of about 1 μg daily with oestrogen therapy in the usual, so-called replacement doses, given cyclically for three weeks out of four. This group appear to gain cortical bone. Oestrogen therapy alone or calcium supplements alone (1–1.5 g daily) also appear to be effective when given to patients with normal calcium absorption. High doses of vitamin D or its metabolite, without calcium or hormones, do not appear to be beneficial and may even be harmful. Assessment of response in terms of vertebral fracture rates yields very similar conclusions (Nordin et al 1980). A possible approach to the management of postmenopausal osteoporosis (as judged by the presence of two or more compressed vertebrae) is therefore as follows. If calcium absorption is normal give 1200 mg calcium in the form of one Sandocal® tablet (calcium lactate gluconate, sodium bicarb. and potassium bicarb.) between meals and one at night. If there is malabsorption of calcium, the oral calcium is supplemented with not more than 10 000 units daily of vitamin D. In patients below the age of 65 years, in whom there is no contraindication to oestrogen therapy, cyclical oestrogens may be used but will be most effective in cases where the initial fasting urinary calcium and hydroxyproline are high, indicating rapid bone resorption. If calcium absorption is low, $1\alpha OHD_3$ or $1,25(OH)_2D_3$ in a dose of 1 μg daily may be added to the oestrogen. The effect of these metabolites on calcium absorption is so powerful that calcium supplements are unnecessary on this regimen, but calcium intake should, of course, be adequate. In

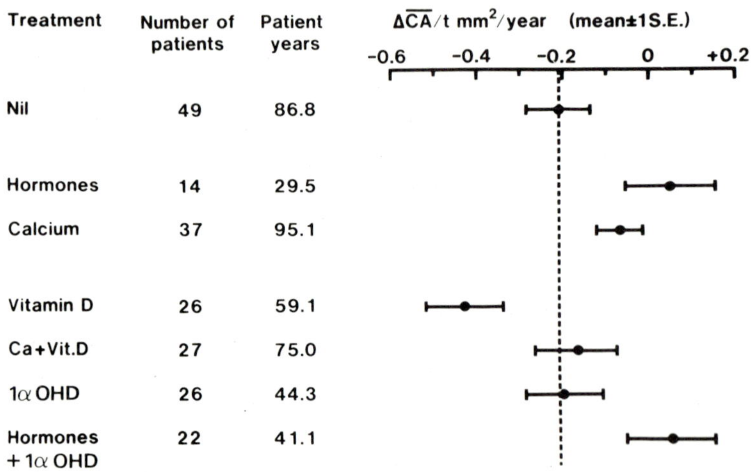

Fig. 12.6 Mean changes in mean metacarpal cortical area in osteoporotic postmenopausal women, untreated and on six different therapies

the present state of knowledge, neither very high-dose vitamin D, nor 1αOHD, nor 1,25$(OH)_2$D, should be given alone to patients with postmenopausal osteoporosis.

Other suggested treatments for spinal osteoporosis include sodium fluoride in doses up to 50 mg daily (usually combined with calcium and vitamin D) (Jowsey 1979) and injections of parathyroid hormone (Reeve et al 1980). Although these therapies may increase trabecular bone volume as judged by iliac crest biopsy, their clinical value is quite uncertain. The same is probably true of therapy with calcitonin and anabolic steroids, although there are reports that both these regimens may increase total body calcium (Chesnut et al 1979).

Osteomalacia

Definition and diagnosis

Osteomalacia is a disease of bone attributable to a delay in the initiation of calcification. Although there are a number of characteristic radiological, biochemical and clinical abnormalities in patients with the fully developed disease, none of these is truly specific and any or all of these features may be absent in the early stages of the condition. The ultimate diagnosis must therefore rest on the results of histological examination, this being the only procedure which permits the direct observation of calcification status. The osteomalacic abnormality is manifest in two ways: first there is a reduction in the calcification fronts; second, because of the delayed onset of calcification, the osteoid seams become wider than normal, the number of bone surfaces covered with osteoid increases and, finally, there is an increase in the total osteoid volume. However, it must be remembered that osteoid tends to increase in any state of high bone turnover, such as hyperparathyroidism or hyperthyroidism; the really specific, early histological feature of osteomalacia is the reduction in the percentage of osteoid seams showing calcification fronts — normally over 60% (Fig. 12.7).

In clinical practice, bone biopsies are not generally obtainable and the diagnosis rests on other features. Advanced cases with Looser zones are easily recognised but earlier stages may present diagnostic problems. In particular, there is a tendency for clinicians to fail to recognise proximal muscle weakness without muscle wasting, especially affecting the hip girdle, which is an important sign of osteomalacia. The patient has difficulty in walking up stairs and rising from a chair and may have a characteristic waddling gait. However, most early cases will present with nothing but a biochemical abnormality, the nature of which varies with the type of osteomalacia. It is therefore necessary to consider the various types of osteomalacia in turn.

Classification

The main forms of osteomalacia are classified in Table 12.1. The disease may be acquired or congenital; the former is the most common and will be dealt with first. The only biochemical abnormalities common to *all* forms of osteomalacia are a raised plasma alkaline phosphatase and a raised urine hydroxyproline (Table 12.2); however, neither of these is specific.

Acquired osteomalacia: a. *Vitamin D deficiency.* The characteristic feature of this type of osteomalacia is the low plasma level of 25OHD; the plasma 1,25$(OH)_2$D level may be normal or low. The plasma calcium is low-normal or low and the plasma

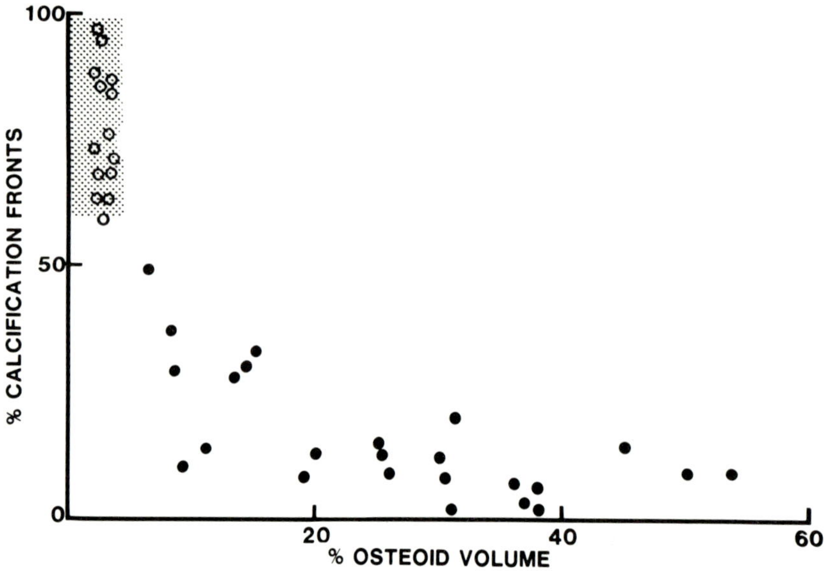

Fig. 12.7 The relation between the percentage volume of osteoid and the percentage of forming surfaces with calcification fronts in iliac crest biopsies from patients with vitamin-D-deficient osteomalacia, either untreated (●) or after treatment with vitamin D (○). The normal range is indicated by the stippled area

phosphate tends to be low because of malabsorption of phosphate and secondary hyperparathyroidism. Calcium absorption is generally reduced, but may be normal. Although all patients with this type of osteomalacia have low plasma 25OHD levels, all subjects with low 25OHD levels do not have osteomalacia. However, where

Table 12.1 Classification of the osteomalacias

Type	Pathogenesis
1. *Acquired*	
a. Vitamin D deficiency (Asian, senile, gastrointestinal)	Lack of sunlight Poor diet Malabsorption
b. Failure of $25OHD_3$ synthesis	Drugs Liver disease
c. Failure of $1,25(OH)_2D$ synthesis	Renal disease Idiopathic
d. Hypophosphataemia	Tumours Aluminium hydroxide
e. Miscellaneous	Parenteral feeding Fluoride Diphosphonate Aluminium
2. *Congenital*	
a. Hypophosphataemia (sporadic, familial)	Low tubular reabsorption of phosphate
B. Pseudo-vitamin-D deficiency	25-hydroxylase deficiency 1α-hydroxylase deficiency

Table 12.2. Biochemistry of the osteomalacias

Type	Calcium	Phosphate	Creatinine	PTH	25OHD	$1,25(OH)_2D$	Alkaline phosphatase	Calcium absorption	Fasting urine hydroxyproline
Acquired									
a. Vitamin D deficiency	↓N	↓N	N	↑	↓	↓N	↑	↓N	↑
b. 25OHD failure	↓N	↓N	N	↑	↓	↓N	↑	↓N	↑
c. $1,25(OH)_2D$ failure	↓N↑	↓N↑	↑	↑	N	↓	↑	↓	↑
d. Hypophosphataemia	N↑	↓	N	N	N	↓	↑	↓	↑
e. Others*									
2. *Congenital*									
a. Pseudo-D-deficiency	↓	↓	N	↑	↓	↓	↑	↓	↑
b. Hypophosphataemia	N	↓	N	N	N	↓N	↑N	↓	↑N

N = normal; ↑ = increased; ↓ = decreased

*There are no characteristic biochemical features in the osteomalacias associated with fluoride, diphosphonate and aluminium vitamin D deficiency is sufficiently severe and prolonged, secondary hyperparathyroidism develops and, at this stage, osteomalacia is usually present (Fig. 12.8).

This form of osteomalacia is often described as nutritional, which implies that the deficiency is dietary in origin, but this is misleading. The main source of vitamin D for normal subjects, even in the United Kingdom, is exposure of the skin to sunlight, which is why the plasma 25OHD level is subject to seasonal variation (Stamp & Round 1974).

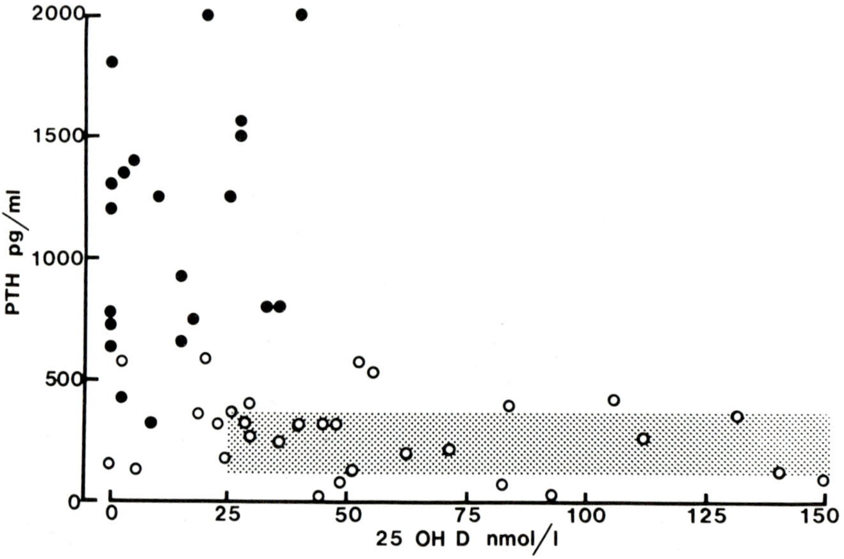

Fig. 12.8 The relation between plasma PTH and plasma 25 OH vitamin D in osteomalacic (●) and non-osteomalacic subjects (○) as defined histologically. The normal range is indicated by the stippled area

Certain groups in the population are at special risk of developing vitamin D-deficient osteomalacia. The elderly comprise the largest group: their plasma 25OHD concentrations are significantly reduced (Fig. 12.9), mainly because of inadequate exposure to sunlight. Osteomalacia is particularly common in patients with femoral-neck fractures, because they are drawn from a relatively house-bound elderly population (Baker et al 1979). In ambulant elderly subjects the plasma 25OHD level is a function of exposure to sunlight and unrelated to the dietary intake of vitamin D. In house-bound subjects, the plasma 25OHD level is a function of dietary vitamin D intake which (in Britain) comes mainly from fortified margarine and amounts to 100–200 I.U. (2.5–5.0 μg) daily.

Another large group at risk comprises Asian immigrants, whose plasma 25OHD levels tend to be low. Early rickets, late rickets and osteomalacia are distressingly common in this community (Dunnigan et al 1981) probably from a combination of factors. Their skin pigmentation and traditional clothing reduce the effectiveness of sunlight, and the women among them tend to keep to their homes. Their traditional diet tends to be low in vitamin D and there is a suggestion that chapatti flour may actually interfere with vitamin D absorption (Dent et al 1973). Pregnant women are

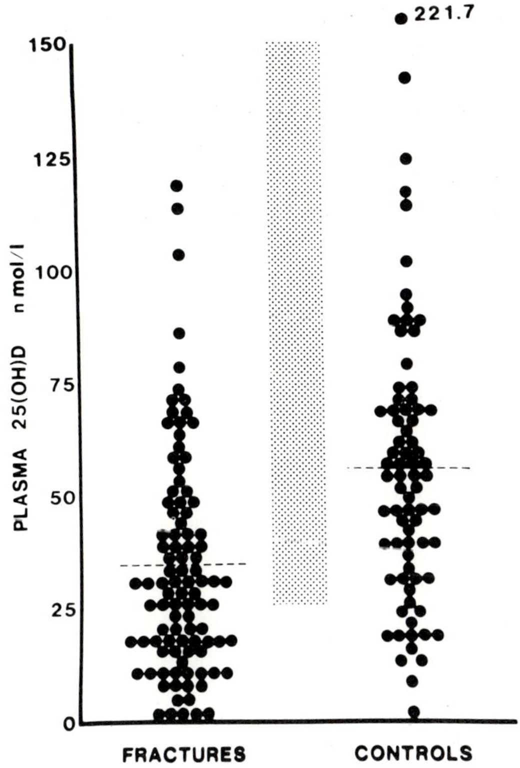

Fig. 12.9 Plasma 25 OH vitamin D in female patients with fractured neck of femur and age-matched female controls. The normal range is shown by the stippled area ($P < 0.001$) (Baker et al 1979 British Medical Journal 1: 589)

particularly vulnerable. The cord blood at delivery may contain little or no measurable 25OHD (Heckmatt et al 1979).

In patients with small-bowel disease and malabsorption, failure to absorb vitamin D, or its loss into the bowel through the enterohepatic circulation, may contribute to vitamin D deficiency but, again, such patients will be more at risk if their exposure to sunlight is inadequate. However, the incidence of osteomalacia in patients with small-bowel disease (Compston et al 1978) is so high that it appears that more is involved than a simple failure to absorb dietary vitamin D.

A low plasma 25OHD level of 'nutritional' origin may also be found in many chronic diseases and this may aggravate or precipitate an osteomalacia which is primarily due to other causes such as renal or hepatic disease.

All forms of 'nutritional' osteomalacia should respond to treatment with 1000–2000 I.U. of vitamin D (25–50 μg) daily, but larger doses may be required in cases of malabsorption.

b. *Failure of 25OHD*$_3$ *synthesis.* Failure of the enzyme 25-hydroxylase, which is present mainly in the liver, leads to a low plasma 25OHD level. This is likely to be one reason why low levels are found in patients with chronic liver disease (Long et al 1978), but how many of these are actually caused by failure of 25-hydroxylation and how many by lack of vitamin D because of poor sunlight exposure or malabsorption is not clear. Low plasma 25OHD levels are also found in patients on enzyme-inducing drugs such as the anticonvulsants (Hahn et al 1972) but in many of these patients the plasma 25OHD can be restored with 'physiological' doses of vitamin D.

It is therefore probable that increased enzyme induction is only one of several factors leading to the low plasma 25OHD levels in patients with epilepsy. The biochemical abnormalities in this form of osteomalacia are the same as in the 'nutritional' type. The optimum treatment is likely to be with $25OHD_3$ but, failing that, oral vitamin D can be given in rather larger doses than in nutritional osteomalacia.

c. *Failure of $1,25(OH)_2D_3$ synthesis.* Renal disease is the commonest cause of a low plasma $1,25(OH)_2D$ level in the presence of a normal plasma level of 25OHD, and is the main cause of the osteomalacia frequently seen in patients with chronic renal failure. This failure of 1-hydroxylation may be a very early manifestation of renal failure and it accounts for the malabsorption of calcium which is almost invariably present when glomerular filtration rates are below about 60 ml/min or plasma creatinine values over about 100 μmol/l (Figs 12.10 and 12.11). Although the malabsorption of calcium and osteomalacia of the elderly is generally 'nutritional' in origin and attributable to low 25OHD levels, a component in some elderly people is undoubtedly low $1,25(OH)_2D$ levels from mild renal failure. Other forms of 1-hydroxylase failure are considered with the congenital osteomalacias (see below).

The treatment of this form of osteomalacia is with 1αOHD or $1,25(OH)_2D$ in doses of about 1 μg daily.

d. *Hypophosphataemia.* The osteomalacia of severe hypophosphataemia is generally congenital (see below) but may present in adult life. In many of these cases

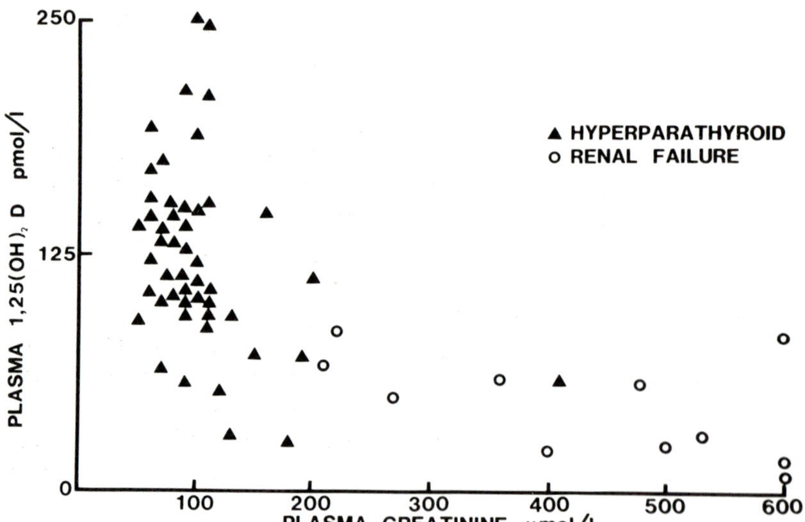

Fig. 12.10 The relation between plasma $1,25(OH)_2D$ and plasma creatinine in patients with primary hyperparathyroidism (▲) and in patients with renal failure (○) (Nordin et al 1980 Clinics in Endocrinology and Metabolism 9: 177

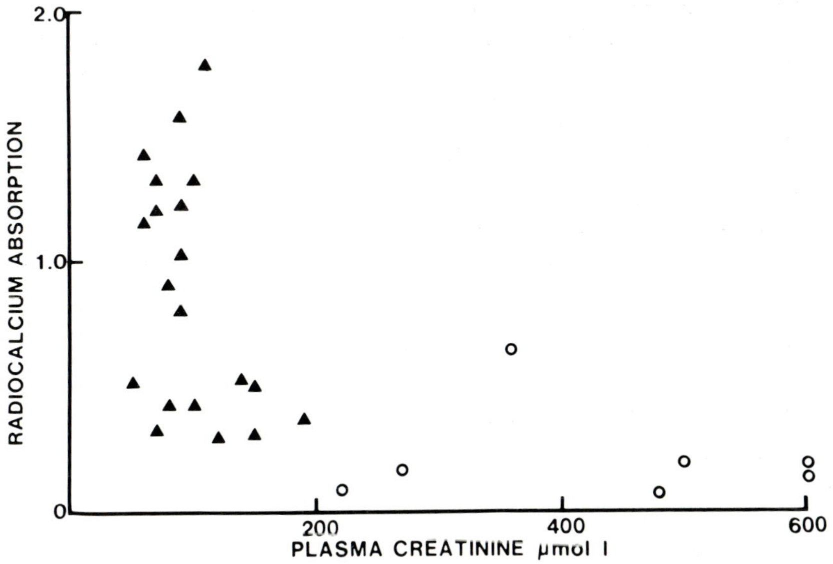

Fig. 12.11 The relationship between radiocalcium absorption and plasma creatinine in patients with primary hyperparathyroidism (▲) and in patients with renal failure (○)

no cause can be found, but some are associated with certain mesenchymal tumours — notably angiomata. Patients may present with bone pain, myopathy and all the other features of severe osteomalacia, and when a tumour can be identified may respond to its removal (Prader et al 1959, Daniels & Weisenfeld 1979). The hypophosphataemia is caused by a low tubular reabsorption of phosphate despite a normal plasma calcium and normal parathyroid activity. The plasma 25OHD is normal but the plasma $1,25(OH)_2D$ level has been reported to be low or normal (Haussler & McCain 1977, Peacock et al 1979b) whereas, in the presence of hypophosphataemia, it would be expected to be high. The implication appears to be that a compound secreted by the tumour inhibits tubular reabsorption of phosphate and $1,25(OH)_2D$ production. A similar mechanism may well be operative in other cases, presenting in adult life, which at the moment must be classified as idiopathic. The treatment of this form of osteomalacia (unless of course the offending tumour can be identified and removed) is with 1αOHD or $1,25(OH)_2D_3$ in large doses (up to 5 μg daily) initially and lower doses (about 1 μg) for maintenance (Peacock et al 1979b). Phosphate supplements (about 1.5 g daily) are generally given as well (Fig. 12.12).

Excessive use of phosphate-binding agents (notably aluminium hydroxide) may also cause hypophosphataemic osteomalacia (Bloom & Flincham 1960) and it is possible that their use in renal failure, to prevent hyperphosphataemia, may occasionally contribute to renal osteomalacia. This is a particularly interesting form of osteomalacia because no abnormality of vitamin D intake or metabolism appears to be involved.

e. *Parenteral feeding.* A severe form of osteomalacia has been described, which affects patients receiving parenteral nutrition (Klein et al 1980). Its cause is completely unknown and no biochemical abnormality has been described, apart from hypercalciuria.

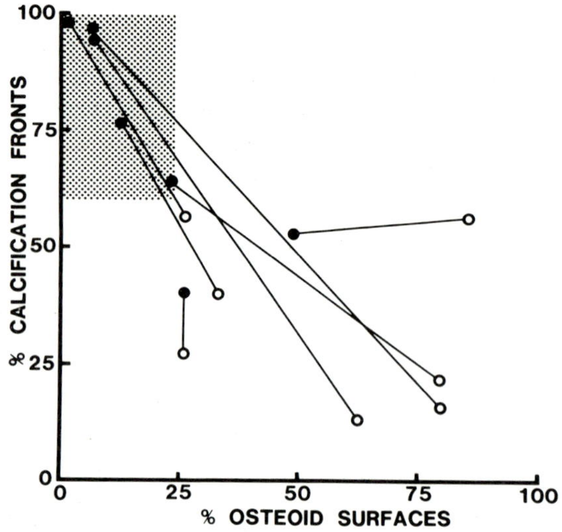

Fig. 12.12 The relationship between the percentage of forming surfaces and the percentage of those with calcification fronts in iliac crest biopsies from patients with hypophosphataemic osteomalacia before (○) and after treatment with 1α or 1,25$(OH)_2$ vitamin D (●). The normal range is shown by the stippled area. (Nordin et al 1980, Clinics in Endocrinology and Metabolism 9: 177

f. *Other forms of acquired osteomalacia.* A histological appearance resembling osteomalacia may be associated with disphosphonate treatment (Russell et al 1974), fluorosis and fluoride therapy for osteoporosis (Meunier et al 1978) and aluminium intoxication caused by prolonged haemodialysis with tap water of high aluminium content (Ward et al 1978). These may all be due to a 'poisoning' of the calcification front comparable to that seen in experimental 'strontium rickets' and 'beryllium rickets'.

Congenital osteomalacia a. *Hypophosphataemia.* This type of congenital osteomalacia (previously known as 'vitamin-D-resistance') may be familial or sporadic, generally (but not always) presenting as rickets in childhood. The essential abnormality is the 'tubular leak' of phosphate. Plasma calcium and PTH levels are normal, as is the plasma 25OHD, but low (or inappropriately low) plasma 1,25$(OH)_2$D levels have been reported (Haussler & McCain 1977). Occasionally there are other tubular lesions which give rise to amino-aciduria and/or renal tubular acidosis. These cases used to be treated with heroic doses of vitamin D, with variable success. It is now clear that the best therapy is 1αOHD or 1,25$(OH)_2$D in high doses initially (up to 5 μg daily) followed by a maintenance dose of perhaps 1 μg daily when healing has been established (Fig. 12.12). Phosphate supplements may be helpful. The plasma phosphate rises on this regimen but the histological response is very variable (Peacock et al 1979b).

b. *Pseudo-vitamin D deficiency.* This condition (sometimes called vitamin D dependency) is characterised by an increased requirement for vitamin D. It is probably caused by impaired 25-hydroxylation in the liver (Fraser et al 1973) but it is possible that renal 1-hydroxylation may also be at fault. The condition has all the features of 'nutritional' osteomalacia but requires larger doses of vitamin D for its correction.

Renal bone disease

Renal bone disease is a mixture of osteomalacia (presumably attributable to $1,25(OH)_2D$ deficiency) and osteitis fibrosa (caused by secondary hyperparathyroidism). The histological appearances embrace a spectrum of histological changes with varying proportions of these two abnormalities. The plasma alkaline phosphatase is raised and the plasma calcium is generally low-normal when the osteomalacic component predominates and high-normal when the hyperparathyroid element predominates. The lower plasma calcium values are often associated with low tubular reabsorption of calcium (Cochran & Nordin 1971). The plasma $1,25(OH)_2D$ level is, of course, low but low plasma 25OHD levels have also been reported in many of these patients (Eastwood et al 1979) presumably because of inadequate exposure to sunlight.

The plasma phosphate concentrations are extremely variable. Reduced renal tubular reabsorption of phosphate (caused by secondary hyperparathyroidism) is present from an early stage of renal failure. Plasma phosphate itself may be low, normal or high according to the degree of renal failure and the degree of secondary hyperparathyroidism. In advanced renal failure, when the plasma phosphate is definitely raised, reciprocal depression of plasma calcium concentration may aggravate parathyroid stimulation and also lead to ectopic calcification in soft tissues. Calcification in the skin is thought to be one of the factors in the pruritus of advanced renal failure (Massry et al 1968).

Although the bone disease of renal failure may be associated with any type of renal disease, there is a tendency for the osteomalacia to be more common in the renal failure of chronic pyelonephritis than in other types and it has been suggested that this may be linked with the more severe metabolic acidosis which is a feature of this type of renal disease (Cochran & Nordin 1971).

Whether or not bone disease supervenes in chronic renal failure, malabsorption of calcium due to a low plasma $1,25(OH)_2D$ level becomes apparent at a very early stage of renal insufficiency, and there is an inverse relationship between plasma creatinine on the one hand and calcium absorption and plasma $1,25(OH)_2D$ on the other (Figs 12.10 and 12.11).

In some cases of chronic renal failure with severe secondary hyperparathyroidism, osteitis fibrosa and ectopic soft-tissue calcification, it has been found that parathyroidectomy is the only effective treatment (Stanbury et al 1960). This procedure breaks a vicious circle in which hypocalcaemia stimulates the parathyroid glands, which resorb calcium and phosphate from bone which increases the plasma phosphate concentration and perpetuates the hypocalcaemia. In this situation, parathyroidectomy produces a fall in plasma calcium concentration, which may have to be corrected with vitamin D, but also a fall in plasma phosphate concentration, a consequent fall in the plasma Ca × P, and a reduction in ectopic calcification and amelioration of osteitis fibrosa which may be very dramatic.

Dialysis bone disease

A form of osteomalacia resistant to treatment with vitamin D has been seen during chronic haemodialysis treatment in certain parts of the country – notably Newcastle upon Tyne (Ward et al 1978). This is now thought to be caused by aluminium intoxication, the aluminium preventing the normal process of calcification at the calcification front. In the Leeds area. it has been shown that the severity of renal osteomalacia is related to the aluminium content of the dialysis fluid (Walker et al 1982).

Treatment of renal bone disease

The treatment of the osteomalacia of renal failure has been discussed above. The treatment of the secondary hyperparathyroidism is much more difficult, particularly when the plasma phosphate is high, but it is now clear that oral phosphate binders have a part to play both in the prevention and management of this condition. Great care should be taken to avoid increasing the plasma calcium with vitamin D or one of its metabolites when the plasma phosphate is high; the effect is simply to cause calcium phosphate precipitation in the soft tissues, and pruritus. Although, in theory, increasing the plasma calcium concentration into the high-normal range should reduce the stimulus to the parathyroid glands and correct hyperparathyroid bone disease, in practice it is extremely difficult to achieve this control of plasma calcium concentration without producing hypercalcaemia, and the suppression of hormone secretion by the hyperplastic parathyroid glands present in chronic renal failure may be difficult and slow.

Primary hyperparathyroidism

Prevalence

This condition used to present most commonly as calcium stone disease, and much less commonly as hyperparathyroid bone disease, but with the increasing use of screening tests it is now most commonly diagnosed accidentally by the discovery of hypercalcaemia — usually of mild degree. As a result of this development, the estimated prevalence of asymptomatic hypercalcaemia is now reported as 0.6%. Most of these cases are likely to be due to primary hyperparathyroidism, the prevalence of which is about 1 in 300 (Christensson et al 1977), the group most commonly affected being postmenopausal women (Muller 1969).

Presentation

Primary hyperparathyroidism can present at any age but is most common in postmenopausal females. It may be discovered in at least five ways, the first of which is with asymptomatic hypercalcaemia discovered on routine biochemical screening of hospital patients for other reasons. Some of these patients have conditions associated with hyperparathyroidism, such as peptic ulcer and hypertension, but many others do not. Secondly, there are diseases such as phaeochromocytoma, pituitary adenoma and insulinoma in which the association with hyperparathyroidism is so well recognised that it is discovered by active investigation. (Biochemical screening of affected families may also produce a number of asymptomatic cases.) Thirdly, it may present as renal stones — the commonest abnormality in primary hyperparathyroidism — which is present in 5–10% of all patients with calculi. The fourth presentation is with clinical bone disease — fracture, cyst formation and bone pain — but this is relatively uncommon. Finally, a few patients present with symptomatic hypercalcaemia — polyuria, constipation, weakness and confusion. In these cases the plasma calcium level may be 4 mmol/l or more, and they are usually first seen as medical emergencies.

Diagnosis

The diagnosis of primary hyperparathyroidism is always established biochemically because there are no signs or symptoms which are specific. Hypercalcaemia in the presence of a raised plasma PTH level is required to make a positive diagnosis but false-negative results are not uncommon. It is prudent, therefore, to include other biochemical variables in the biochemical diagnosis. Increased nephrogenous cyclic AMP, hypophosphataemia and reduced tubular reabsorption of phosphate are useful additional pointers. Plasma alkaline phosphatase and urinary hydroxyproline reflect the degree of bone involvement but are often within the normal range (Fig. 12.13).

Other investigations may be helpful. Radiography of the skeleton, for subperiosteal erosions and cysts, detects only the severe forms of the disease. Iliac crest biopsy usually shows an increase in forming and resorbing surfaces, even when the plasma alkaline phosphatase and urinary hydroxyproline are normal. Again, excessive osteoclastic resorption and osteitis fibrosa are present only in severely affected cases. It is possible to make a positive diagnosis in most cases of primary hyperparathyroidism by using these biochemical variables. There remain, however, some diagnostic difficulties. Renal impairment, not an infrequent complication, lowers plasma calcium and $1,25(OH)_2D$ and raises the plasma phosphate, with the result that the diagnosis is not even considered. A similar problem is seen in patients with vitamin D deficiency and primary hyperparathyroidism, in whom the plasma calcium and $1,25(OH)_2D$ may be normal or even low; the severe hypophosphataemia

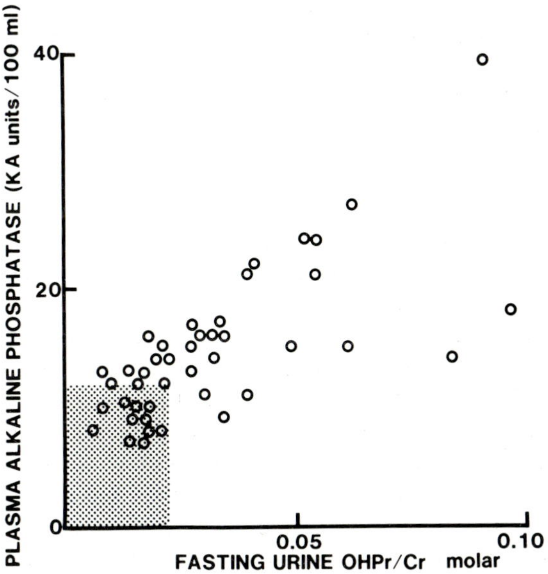

Fig. 12.13 The relationship between plasma alkaline phosphatase and fasting urine hydroxyproline/creatinine ratio in patients with primary hyperparathyroidism. The normal range is indicated by the stippled area

and very high plasma alkaline phosphatase usually ensure, however, that the patient is fully investigated. Probably the most difficult diagnostic area is in differentiating patients with mild hyperparathyroidism from those with idiopathic calcium stone disease. Both diseases have several biochemical abnormalities in common: hypophosphataemia, decreased tubular reabsorption of phosphate, increased plasma $1{,}25(OH)_2D$ levels and hyperabsorption of calcium. Very accurate plasma calcium and PTH levels are therefore essential for differentiating between these two diseases and it may be necessary to measure the relevant variables several times.

In patients with unequivocal hypercalcaemia the differential diagnosis lies between primary hyperparathyroidism, malignant disease (with or without bone secondaries), vitamin D intoxication, hyperthyroidism and sarcoidosis. There is also a familial form of hypercalcaemia attributable to high tubular reabsorption of calcium (Marx 1980). The hypercalcaemia associated with metastases in bone should not present a problem, but the hypercalcaemia of malignant diseases without metastases can cause difficulty. Many such cases have been reported in which excision of the tumour has corrected the hypercalcaemia (Skrabanek et al 1980) but although the condition is often referred to as 'pseudo-hyperparathyroidism' it is doubtful whether it is actually parathyroid hormone which is secreted. In this form of tumour hypercalcaemia, the commonest primaries are in the lung, kidney, oesophagus and ovary, but a similar hypercalcaemia may be seen in various types of lymphoma. Hypercalcaemia is also common in myelomatosis, presumably due to bone resorption, and in sarcoidosis, in which calcium absorption is often high; however, in both these conditions renal failure is often present and contributing to the hypercalcaemia. The single most important measurement distinguishing these forms of hypercalcaemia from primary hyperparathyroidism is the plasma PTH level, which should be unmeasurable or low in the non-hyperparathyroid cases. However, the diagnosis may be very difficult, both because primary hyperparathyroidism may co-exist with any of the other causes of hypercalcaemia, and because some immunoassays detect measurable PTH concentrations even in the absence of PTH secretion.

Treatment

The treatment of choice is parathyroidectomy with removal of all abnormal tissue. Inspection of all four parathyroids at surgery is necessary, because more than one gland is involved in almost 15% of cases. Examination of frozen sections during the operation is desirable. In the absence of symptoms, there is an increasing tendency to leave untreated those cases of mild hyperparathyroidism with plasma calcium below 3 mmol/l but to keep them under observation (Purnell et al 1974); in most of these patients the disease does not appear to progress. However, it seems likely that mild hyperparathyroidism accelerates bone loss in postmenopausal women and this may come to be regarded as an indication for surgery in this group (Graham et al 1980).

Hypoparathyroidism

This condition may be due to trauma to the parathyroids (generally surgical), to parathyroid gland insufficiency (generally congenital), or to end-organ resistance (pseudo-hypoparathyroidism). It usually presents with tetany or even major seizures, but may be discovered fortuitously in milder cases. The diagnosis generally depends on the combination of hypocalcaemia with a normal or low urinary calcium excretion, and hyperphosphataemia with a high tubular reabsorption of phosphate.

Surgical

Surgical hypoparathyroidism is becoming rare with improved surgical techniques and the increasing use of medical management of hyperthyroidism. However, when thyroid surgery is performed for hyperthyroidism, hypocalcaemia is a not uncommon sequel and does not necessarily imply permanent parathyroid insufficiency. There are at least three possible reasons for this postoperative hypocalcaemia. The first is that hyperthyroidism is associated with a tendency to hypercalcaemia (because of increased bone resorption) which tends to suppress the parathyroid glands. The sudden reduction of thyroid activity after surgery leads to a fall in bone resorption, and consequent fall in plasma calcium, to which the relatively atrophic parathyroid glands cannot immediately respond. The second reason is that correction of hyperthyroidism reduces bone resorption before it reduces bone formation, and a period of positive bone balance occurs in which more calcium is going into bone than is coming out. Since the average time-lag between the start of bone resorption and completion of the 'bone metabolic unit' is about 3 months, this period of time may be expected to elapse before reduced bone resorption is accompanied by a corresponding reduction in bone formation. The third reason may be temporary damage to the parathyroids and/or their blood supply. As a result of these interrelated mechanisms, a period of hypocalcaemia and relative parathyroid insufficiency may be anticipated after thyroidectomy in cases where bone turnover is high, and some form of vitamin D or even a calcium infusion may be required during this period. However, every effort should be made to discontinue vitamin D after a few months to establish whether chronic hypoparathyroidism has supervened. Frequently, no further vitamin D is required.

Idiopathic

Idiopathic hypoparathyroidism is generally a congenital disease which presents in childhood (with fits, dental hypoplasia or cataract) but it may also present in adult life when the absence of a relevant history suggests that it may sometimes be acquired. The congenital form may be sporadic or familial, the latter often associated with adrenal insufficiency and/or steatorrhoea and/or moniliasis (Spinner et al 1968).

Pseudo-hypoparathyroidism

This is an apparent hypoparathyroidism which is congenital and associated with moon face, mental retardation, ectopic calcification and (frequently) shortening of one or more metacarpals or metatarsals. As predicted by Albright et al (1942), the condition is not true parathyroid insufficiency but a resistance to the phosphaturic action of parathyroid hormone on the renal tubule and (sometimes) to its bone-resorbing action. It has recently been divided into two types: type 1 in which there is no increase in urinary phosphate or cyclic AMP following parathyroid hormone injection, and type 2 in which urine cyclic AMP rises but phosphate does not (Stogmann & Fischer 1975). Plasma calcium may be normal or low, possibly depending upon plasma $1,25(OH)_2D$ (Drezner & Haussler 1979). Plasma phosphate is raised because of high tubular reabsorption. Occasionally, evidence of secondary hyperparathyroidism is seen in bone X-rays (Kolb & Steinbach 1962); these are presumably the cases with normal or high 1,25$(OH)_2$D levels. Whether there is ever a true 'resistance' to parathyroid hormone in the bone itself is not clear.

Treatment of hypoparathyroidism

Vitamin D and dihydrotachysterol have been the standard treatments of hypoparathyroidism for many years. They have now been largely superseded by $1\alpha25(OH)_2D$ and $1\alpha OHD$ which are extremely effective in doses of about 1 μg daily and offer the enormous advantage of a short half-life with rapid correction of hypercalcaemia, should it occur, when therapy is withdrawn (Kanis & Russell 1977). It is an interesting fact that effective therapy not only raises plasma calcium but also lowers plasma phosphate (Fig. 12.14) by lowering the tubular reabsorption of phosphate.

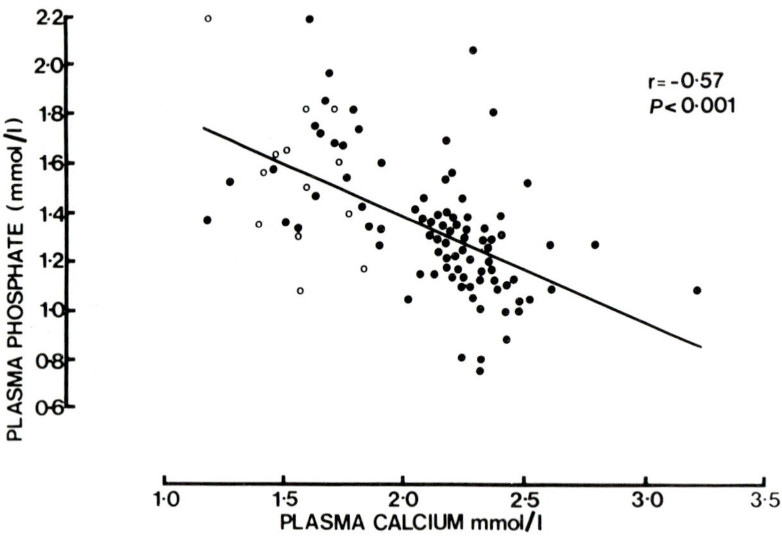

Fig. 12.14 The relationship between plasma phosphate and plasma calcium in hypoparathyroid patients before (●) and on treatment with vitamin D (○). (Heyburn & Peacock 1977 Clinical Endocrinology 7: 209s

Paget's disease

Paget's disease of bone

Paget's disease of bone is a common disorder, affecting some 10% of the population by the age of 80 (Pygott 1957). It may be very disabling and in severe cases produces pain, deformity, fracture and deafness. In a small percentage of cases, it may progress to osteosarcoma. The radiological features are well known. Biochemically, the main features are the raised alkaline phosphatase and urine hydroxyproline. There have been two important advances in respect of this disease. The first is the suggestion, advanced by Rebel et al (1974) that it may be caused by a virus, now thought to be possibly a slow virus related to the measles virus (Rebel et al 1979).

The second development is in respect of treatment. The condition responds in terms of alkaline phosphatase and urinary hydroxyproline to the administration of calcitonin, which may be given as porcine calcitonin 160 units daily or salmon calcitonin (which has a longer half-life) in doses of 50–100 units daily or two or three times a week. Treatment should be reserved for patients with significant disability because it is relatively expensive and it is liable to cause sensitivity reactions in some individuals. The plasma alkaline phosphatase and urinary hydroxyproline decline over a period of about 6 months but seldom return to normal. It is common practice to treat the patients for 3–6 months and then to discontinue treatment for a similar period or until these biochemical variables start to rise again (De Rose et al 1974).

An alternative treatment, which has just become available in the United Kingdom, is based on the administration of a diphosphonate — etidronate disodium — one of a class of compounds which inhibits bone turnover. Since this can be administered by mouth, and appears to be as effective as calcitonin, it may become the treatment of choice. The recommended dose is 200–400 mg/d, and treatment should be continued for about 6 months (Khairi & Johnston 1977).

Renal stone disease

Urinary stone disease affects about 3% of the population in industrialised countries although there are wide geographical variations. There are four main types of stone disease. Cystine and uric acid stone disease are uncommon and account for less than 10% of cases. Infected stone disease is probably decreasing in frequency but still accounts for about 20% of cases. The remainder are due to calcium stone disease. In only a small proportion of these cases is there an underlying disease such as primary hyperparathyroidism, hyperoxaluria, renal tubular acidosis, sarcoidosis, Cushing's disease and steroid treatment. In the majority no underlying disease is diagnosed and these patients are considered to be suffering from idiopathic calcium stone disease

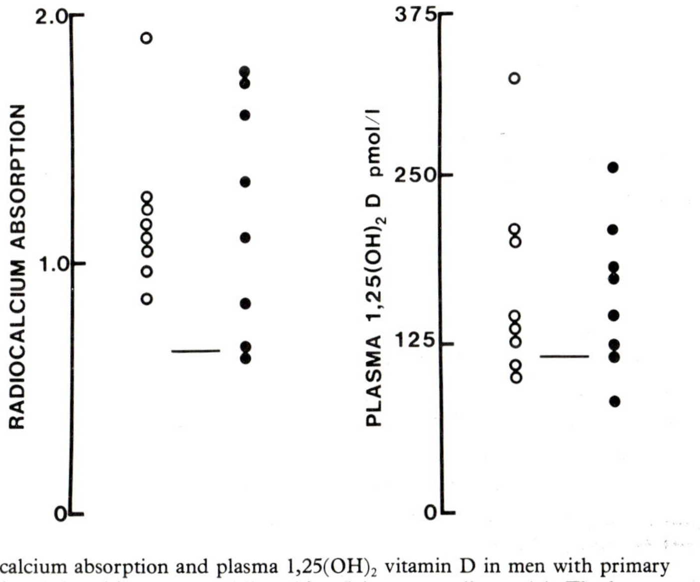

Fig. 12.15 Radiocalcium absorption and plasma 1,25$(OH)_2$ vitamin D in men with primary hyperparathyroidism (○) and in men with idiopathic calcium stone disease (●). The bars indicate the mean values in young normal subjects

(Peacock et al 1979a). In this group of stone-formers, usually men aged 20–60 years, there have been significant advances in the understanding of stone formation. At least five urinary risk factors have been identified — calcium, oxalate, pH and uric acid are positive factors and glycosaminoglycan excretion is a negative risk factor (Robertson et al 1978). The tendency to hypercalciuria in the calcium-stone-forming population is generally agreed to be attributable to increased absorption of calcium associated with a rather high plasma 1,25$(OH)_2D$ level which may be secondary to the mild hypophosphataemia which is a feature of these cases (Haussler & McCain 1977) (Fig. 12.15). The tendency to mild but significant hyperoxaluria (Robertson & Peacock 1980) is due to increased absorption of dietary oxalate secondary to high absorption of calcium, which leaves less calcium in the bowel to trap dietary oxalate. Mild hyperuricosuria is also a feature of calcium-stone-formers and is a risk factor for two possible reasons — firstly because it is able to nucleate calcium oxalate precipitation and secondly because it neutralises the glycosaminoglycan inhibitors in urine which normally inhibit crystal growth and aggregation. Urine pH is a risk factor by virtue of the decreasing solubility of calcium phosphate with increasing pH. The inhibitory activity on crystal formation and growth in urine is related to the excretion of glycosaminoglycan, and calcium-stone-formers tend to have a slightly reduced excretion of these compounds (Robertson et al 1978). Of these five risk factors, oxalate is probably of greatest importance since small changes in its excretion have a marked effect on calcium oxalate crystalluria (Robertson & Peacock 1980). Recently

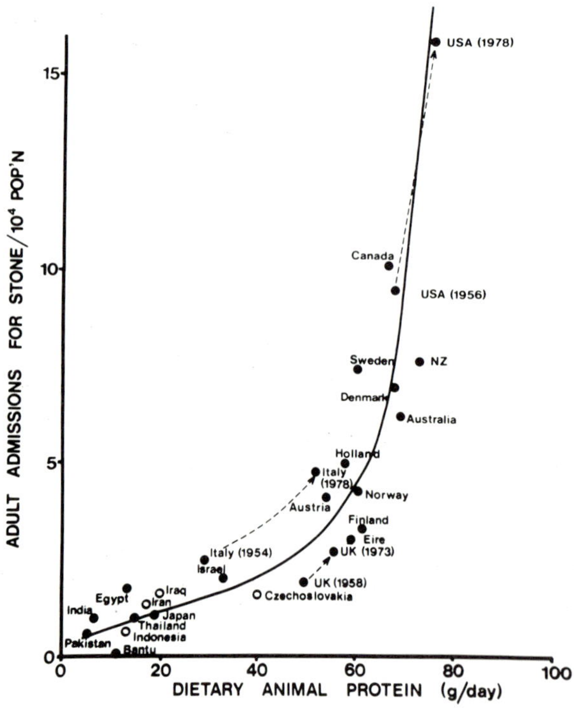

Fig. 12.16 The relation between dietary animal protein and admissions for stone in different countries. The interrupted lines join data from the same countries in different years (supplied by W. G. Robertson)

it has been suggested that calcium stone disease may be related to animal protein intake. Both within and between countries there is a relationship between the prevalence of urinary stone disease and animal protein intake (Robertson et al, 1980) (Fig. 12.16). This is probably because a high protein intake increases three of the five main urinary risk factors — oxalate, calcium and uric acid. If this concept is correct, it illustrates an elegant contrast between the calcium stone disease of the wealthy protein-eating countries and endemic bladder stone disease, which is now confined to poorer countries where the stone formation results from a low urinary phosphate with the excretion of a very acid urine due to lack of protein in the diet (Andersen 1973). The high vegetable intake which goes with the low meat intake produces a high urinary oxalate and the combination of these factors tends to oversaturate the urine with acid ammonium urate and calcium oxalate, the main constituent of bladder stones today as it was in Western Europe in times past (Brockis 1980).

Various treatments designed to correct these risk factors have been shown to be effective in calcium stone disease. These include a diet low in calcium and oxalate (Peacock et al 1979a), thiazide diuretics which lower urinary calcium (Yendt et al 1970), allopurinol which lowers urinary uric acid (Coe & Kavalach 1974) and phosphate supplements which block calcium absorption and lower urinary calcium (Smith 1978) (Fig. 12.17). A low fluid intake and consequent low urinary volume are always a risk factor in the individual and all treatment regimens should include a fluid intake sufficient to produce a 24-h urine volume of not less than 2 litres.

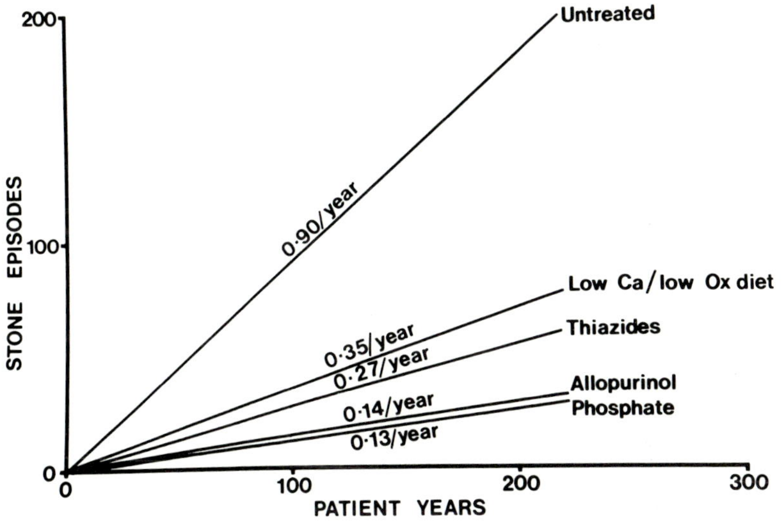

Fig. 12.17 The effect of treatment with a low calcium/low oxalate diet, thiazide diuretics, allopurinol and oral calcium supplements on stone recurrence rate in urinary stone formers. The variables are expressed as cumulative sums on both axes (Peacock et al 1979 Proceedings of EDTA 16: 556

REFERENCES

Aaron J E, Gallagher J C, Anderson J, Stasiak L, Longton E B, Nordin B E C 1974 Frequency of osteomalacia and osteoporosis in fractures of the proximal femur. Lancet 1: 229–233

Albright F, Burnett C H, Smith P H, Parson W 1942 Pseudohypoparathyroidism, an example of 'Sebright-Bantam' syndrome. Endocrinology 30: 922–932
Andersen D A 1973 Environmental factors in the aetiology of urolithiasis. In: Cifuentes Delatte L, Rapado A, Hodgkinson A (eds) Urinary calculi. Karger, Basel, p 130
Baker M R, McDonnell H, Peacock M, Nordin B E C 1979 Plasma 25-hydroxy vitamin D concentrations in patients with fractures of the femoral neck. British Medical Journal 1: 589
Barnett E, Nordin B E C 1960 The radiological diagnosis of osteoporosis. Clinical Radiology 2: 166–174
Bloom W L, Flinchum D 1960 Osteomalacia with pseudofractures caused by ingestion of aluminium hydroxide. Journal of the American Medical Association 174: 1327–1330
Bouillon R, Van Baelen H 1979 The transport of vitamin D. In: Norman A W et al (eds) Vitamin D, basic research and its clinical application. Walter de Gruyter, Berlin/New York, p 137
Brockis J G 1980 Proceedings of the Stone Symposium, Perth
Brockis J G, Bowyer R C, McCulloch R K, Taylor T A, Wisniewski Z S, Kamardi T et al 1981 Physiopathology of endemic bladder stones. In Brockis J G, Finlayson B (eds) Urinary calculus. PSG Publishing Co, Littleton, p 225
Cameron J R, Sorenson J 1963 Measurement of bone mineral in vivo. Science 142: 230–232
Care A D, Bates R F L 1972 Control of secretion of parathyroid hormone and calcitonin in mammals and birds. Journal of Comparative Endocrinology (supplement) 3: 448–458
Chesnut C H, Ivey J L, Nelp W B, Baylink D J 1979 Assessment of anabolic steroids and calcitonin in the treatment of osteoporosis In: Barzel U (ed) Osteoporosis. Grune and Stratton, New York, p 135
Christensson T, Hellstrom K, Wengle B 1977 Hypercalcaemia and hyperparathyroidism. Prevalence in patients receiving thiazides as detected in a health screen. Archives of Internal Medicine 137: 1138–1142
Cochran M, Nordin B E C 1971 The causes of hypocalcaemia in chronic renal failure. Clinical Science 40: 305–315
Coe F L, Kavalach A G 1974 Hypercalciuria and hyperuricosuria in patients with calcium nephrolithiasis. New England Foundation of Medicine 291: 1344–1350
Cohen S L, MacIntyre I, Grahame-Smith D, Walker J G 1973 Alcohol-stimulated calcitonin release in medullary thyroid carcinoma. Lancet 2: 1172–1174
Compston J E, Horton L W L, Ayers A B, Tighe J R, Creamer B 1978 Osteomalacia after small intestinal resection. Lancet 2: 1–4
Coombs R C, Ellison M L, Easty G C, Hillyard C J, James R, Galante L et al 1976 The ectopic secretion of calcitonin by lung and breast carcinomas. Clinical Endocrinology 5: 387–396
Crilly R G, Horsman A, Marshall D H, Nordin B E C Postmenopausal and corticosteroid-induced osteoporosis. Frontiers of Hormone Research 5: 53–75
Crilly R G, Jones M M, Horsman A, Nordin B E C 1980 Rise in plasma alkaline phosphatase at the menopause. Clinical Science 58: 341–342
Daniels R A, Weisenfeld I 1979 Tumorous phosphaturic osteomalacia. American Journal of Medicine 67: 155–159
Dent C E, Round J M, Rowe D J F, Stamp T C B 1973 Effect of chapatties and ultraviolet irradiation on nutritional rickets in Indian immigrants. Lancet 1: 1282–1284
De Rose J, Singer F R, Avramides A, Flores A, Dziadiw R, Baker R K 1974 et al Response of Paget's disease to porcine and salmon calcitonins—effects of long-term treatment. American Journal of Medicine 56: 858–866
Drezner M K, Haussler M R 1979 Normocalcaemic pseudohypoparathyroidism. Association with normal vitamin D metabolism. American Journal of Medicine 66: 503–508
Dunnigan M G et al 1981 Policy for prevention of Asian rickets in Britain: a preliminary assessment of the Glasgow rickets campaign. British Medical Journal 282: 357–360
Eastwood J B, Daly A, Carter G D, Alaghband-Zaheh J, De Wardener H E 1979 Plasma 25-hydroxy vitamin D in normal subjects and patients with terminal renal failure on maintenance haemodialysis. Clinical Science 57: 473–474
Exner G U, Prader A, Elsasser U, Ruegsegger P, Anliker M 1979 Bone densitometry using computed tomography. British Journal of Radiology 52: 14–23
Fraser D, Kooh S W, Kund H P, Hollick M F, Tanaka Y, DeLuca H F 1973 Pathogenesis of hereditary vitamin D-dependent rickets. An inborn error of vitamin D metabolism involving defective conversion of 25-hydroxy vitamin D to 1α 25-dihydroxy vitamin D. New England Journal of Medicine 289: 717–822
Gallagher J C, Riggs B L, Eisman J, Hamstra A, Arnaud S B, DeLuca H G 1979 Intestinal calcium absorption and serum vitamin D metabolites in normal subjects and osteoporotic patients. Journal of Clinical Investigation 64: 729–736

Garn S M 1970 The earlier gain and later loss of cortical bone. In: Nutritional perspectives. Thomas, Springfield, Illinois
Graham J J, Harding P E, Hoare L L, Thomas D W, Wise P H 1980 Asymptomatic hyperparathyroidism: an assessment of operative intervention. British Journal of Surgery 67: 115–118
Hahn T J, Hendin B A, Scharp C R, Haddad J G Jr 1972 Effect of chronic anticonvulsant therapy on serum 25-hydroxy calciferol levels in adults. New England Journal of Medicine 287: 900–904
Haussler M R, McCain T A 1977 Basic and clinical concepts related to vitamin D metabolism and action. New England Journal of Medicine 297: 1041–1050
Heaney R P 1965 A unified concept of osteoporosis. American Journal of Medicine 39: 877–880
Heaney R P, Recker R R, Saville P D 1977 Calcium balance and calcium requirements in middle-aged women. American Journal of Clinical Nutrition 30: 1603–1611
Heckmatt J Z, Peacock M, Davies A, McMurray J, Isherwood D M 1979 Plasma 25-hydroxy vitamin D in pregnant Asian women and their babies. Lancet 2: 546–548
Hillyard C J, Stevenson J C, MacIntyre I 1978 Relative deficiency of plasma calcitonin in normal women. Lancet 1: 961–962
Horsman A, Nordin B E C, Crilly R G 1979 Effect on bone of withdrawal of oestrogen therapy. Lancet 2: 33
Horsman A, Gallagher J C, Simpson M, Nordin B E C 1977 Prospective trial of oestrogen and calcium in postmenopausal women. British Medical Journal 2: 789–792
Horsman A, Nordin B E C, Aaron J, Marshall D H 1981 Cortical and trabecular osteoporosis and their relation to fractures in the elderly. In: DeLuca H F et al (eds) Osteoporosis—recent advances in pathogenesis and treatment. University Park Press, Baltimore, p 175
Hosking D J 1980 Treatment of severe hypercalcaemia with calcitonin. Metabolic Bone Disease and Related Research 2: 207–212
Jasani C, Nordin B E C, Smith D A, Swanson I 1965 Spinal osteoporosis and the menopause. Proceedings of the Royal Society of Medicine 58: 441–444
Jowsey J 1979 The long-term treatment of osteoporosis with fluoride, calcium and vitamin D. In: Barzel U (ed) Osteoporosis. Grune and Stratton, New York, p 123
Kanis J A, Russell R G G 1977 Rate of reversal of hypercalcaemia and hypercalciuria induced by vitamin D and its 1α hydroxylate derivatives. British Medical Journal 1: 78–81
Khairi M R, Johnson C C 1977 Treatment of Paget's disease of bone with sodium etidronate (EHDP). Clinical Orthopaedics and Related Research 127: 94–105
Klein G L, Ament M E, Bluestone R, Norman A, Targoff C M, Sherrard D J et al 1980 Bone disease associated with total parameter nutrition. Lancet 2: 1041–1044
Kolb F O, Steinbach H L 1962 Pseudohypoparathyroidism with secondary hyperparathyroidism and oesteitis fibrosa. Journal of Clinical Endocrinology 22: 59–70
Lindquist O, Bengtsson C, Hansson T, Roos B 1979 Age at menopause and its relation to osteoporosis. Maturitas 1: 175–181
Lindsay R, Hart D M, Forrest C, Baird C 1980 Prevention of spinal osteporosis in oophorectomised women. Lancet 2: 1151–1154
Lindsay R, Hart D M, Maclean A, Clark A C, Kraszewski A, Garwood J 1978 Bone response to termination of oestrogen treatment. Lancet 1: 1325–1327
Long R G, Meinhard E, Skinner R K, Varghese Z, Wills M R, Sherlock S 1978 Clinical, biochemical and histological studies of osteomalacia, osteoporosis and parathyroid function in chronic liver disease. Gut 19: 85–90.
Malluche H H, Henry H, Meyer-Sabellek W, Sherman D, Massry S G, Norman A W 1980 Effects and interactions of 24R, $25(OH)_2D_3$ and $1,25(OH)_2D_3$ on bone. American Journal of Physiology 238: E494–498
Manning R M, Hendry G N, Papapoulos S E, O'Riordan J L H 1980 Development of homologous immunological assays for human parathyroid hormone. Journal of Endocrinology 85: 161–170
Marx S J 1980 Familial hypocalciuric hypercalcaemia. New England Journal of Medicine 303: 810–811
Massry S G, Popvitzer M M, Coburn J W, Mekoff D L, Maxwell M H, Kleeman C R 1968 Intractable pruritus as a manifestation of secondary hyperparathyroidism of uraemia. New England Journal of Medicine 279: 679–700
Meunier P J et al 1978 Radiological and histological evolution of postmenopausal osteoporosis treated with sodium fluoride-vitamin D-calcium. Preliminary results. In: Courvoisier B, Donath A, Baud C A (eds) Fluoride and bone. Huber, Berne, p 263
Muller H 1969 Sex, age and hyperparathyroidism. Lancet 1: 449–450
Nelp W B, Denney J D, Murano R, Hinn G M, Williams J L, Rudd T G et al 1972 Absolute measurement of total body calcium (bone mass) in vivo. Journal of Laboratory and Clinical Medicine 79: 430–438

Newton-John H F, Morgan D B 1968 Osteoporosis: disease or senescence? Lancet 1: 232–233
Nordin B E C (ed) 1976a Calcium, phosphate and magnesium metabolism. Churchill Livingstone, Edinburgh, p 186–216
Nordin B E C (ed) 1976b Calcium, phosphate and magnesium metabolism. Churchill Livingstone, Edinburgh, p. 469–524
Nordin B E C, Marshall D H, Crilly R G 1981a Calcium requirement and osteoporosis. Proceedings of the symposium on Nutrition and Ageing, Talloires, France (in press)
Nordin B E C, Peacock M, Crilly R G, Marshall D H 1979 Calcium absorption and plasma $1,25(OH)_2D_3$ levels in postmenopausal osteoporosis In: Norman A (ed) Vitamin D, basic research and its clinical application. Walter de Gruyter, Berlin, p. 99
Nordin B E C, Horsman A, Crilly R G, Marshall D H, Simpson M 1980 Treatment of spinal osteoporosis in postmenopausal women. British Medical Journal 280: 451–454
Nordin B E C, Peacock M, Crilly R G, Francis R M, Speed R, Barkworth S 1981b Summation of risk factors in osteoporosis. In: DeLuca H F et al (eds) Osteoporosis—recent advances in pathogenesis and treatment. University Park Press, Baltimore, p 359
Parkes C O 1978 The action of vitamin D analogues and metabolites on the chick duodenum in vitro. In: Copp D H, Talmage R V (eds) Endocrinology of calcium metabolism. Excerpta Medica, Amsterdam/Oxford, p 165
Peacock M, Robertson W G, Marshall D H 1979a Disorders associated with renal calcium stone disease In: DeGroot L J et al (eds) Endocrinology. Grune and Stratton, New York, vol 2, p 823
Peacock M, Taylor G A, Norman A W 1977 Actions of vitamin D metabolites and analogues, parathyroid hormone, calcitonin and steroid sex hormones on bone in tissue culture. In:
Peacock M, Heyburn P J, Aaron J E, Taylor G A, Brown W B, Speed R 1979b Osteomalacia treated with 1α hydroxy or 1,25 dihydroxy vitamin D In: Norman A et al (eds) Vitamin D, basic research and its clinical application. Walter de Gruyter, Berlin/New York, p 1177
Norman A W et al (eds) Vitamin D, biochemical, chemical and clinical aspects related to calcium metabolism. Walter de Gruyter, Berlin/New York, p 411
Prader A, Illig R, Urhlinger E, Stalder G 1959 Rachitis infolge Knockentumours. Helvetica Paediatric Acta 14: 554–565
Purnell D C, Scholz D A, Smith L H, Sizemore G W, Black B M, Goldsmith R S et al 1974 Treatment of primary hyperparathyroidism. American Journal of Medicine 56: 800–809
Pygott F 1957 Paget's disease of the bone. Radiological incidence. Lancet 1: 1170–1171
Rebel A, Malkani K, Basle M, Bregon C 1974 Particularités ultrastructurales des osteoclastes de la maladie de Paget. Revue du Rhumatisme et des Maladies Osteoarticulaires 41: 767–771
Rebel A, Pouplard A, Kolyoumdjian S, Filmon R, Lepatezour A 1979 Comptes Rendus Hebdomadaires des Séances de l'Academie des Sciences, Paris D289: 225–228
Recker R R, Saville P D, Heaney R P 1977 Effect of estrogens and calcium carbonate on bone loss in postmenopausal women. Annals of Internal Medicine 87: 649–655
Reeve J, Meunier P J, Parsons J A, Bernat M, Bijvoet O M, Courpron P et al 1980 Anabolic effect of human parathyroid hormone fragment on trabecular bone in involutional osteoporosis: a multicentre trial. British Medical Journal 280: 1340–1344
Robertson W G, Peacock M 1980 The cause of idiopathic calcium stone disease: hypercalciuria or hyperoxaluria? Nephron 26: 105–110
Robertson W G, Peacock M, Heyburn P J, Hanes F A 1980 Epidemiological risk factors in calcium stone disease. Scandinavian Journal of Urology and Nephrology 53: 15–28
Robertson W G, Peacock M, Heyburn P J, Marshall D H, Clark P B 1978 Risk factors in calcium stone disease of the urinary tract. British Journal of Urology 50: 449–454
Russell R G G, Smith R, Preston C, Walton R J, Woods C G 1974 Diphosphonates in Paget's disease. Lancet 1: 894–898
Rutherford W E, Blondin J, Hruska K, Kopelman R, Klahr S, Slatopolsky E 1975 Effect of 25-hydroxycholecalciferol on calcium absorption in chronic renal disease. Kidney International 8: 320–324
Singh M, Nagrath A R, Maini P S 1970 Changes in trabecular pattern of the upper end of the femur as an index of osteoporosis. Journal of Bone and Joint Surgery 5 2-A: 457–467
Skrabanek P, McPartlin J, Powell D 1980 Tumour hypercalcaemia and 'ectopic hyperparathyroidism'. Medicine 59: 262–282
Smith W C 1978 Use of phosphates in patients with calcareous renal calculi. Kidney International 13: 390–396
Spinner M W, Blizzard R M, Childs B 1968 Clinical and genetic heterogeneity in idiopathic Addison's disease and hypoparathyroidism. Journal of Clinical Endocrinology 28: 795–804
Stamp T C B, Round J M 1974 Seasonal changes in human plasma levels of 25-hydroxy vitamin D. Nature 247: 563–564

Stanbury S W, Lumb G A, Nicholson W F 1960 Elective sub-total parathyroidectomy for renal hyperparathyroidism. Lancet 1: 793–798.

Stevenson J C, Hillyard C J, McIntyre I, Cooper H, Whitehead M I 1979 A physiological role for calcitonin: protection of the maternal skeleton. Lancet 2: 769–770

Stogmann W, Fischer J A 1975 Pseudohypoparathyroidismic disappearance of the resistance to parathyroid extract during treatment with vitamin D. American Journal of Medicine 59: 140

Walker G S, Aaron J E, Peacock M, Robinson P J A, Davison A M 1982 Dialysate aluminium concentration and renal bone disease. Kidney International 21: 441–415

Ward M K, Feest T G, Ellis H A 1978 Osteomalacic dialysis osteodystrophy: evidence for a water-borne aetiological agent, probably aluminium. Lancet 1: 841–845

Yendt E R, Guay F G, Garcia D A 1970 The use of thiazades in the prevention of renal calculi. Canadian Medical Association Journal 102: 614–620

Index

Abortion, spontaneous, in patients with systemic lupus erythematosus, 264
ABVD combination chemotherapy in Hodgkin's disease, 180–181
Acanthosis nigricans, 13
Acetazolamide, inducing thrombocytopenia, 144
Acidaemia, lactic, risk with phenformin, 45–46
Acromegaly in GH-secreting adenomas, 4, 5
Acycloguanosine therapy in herpes infections, 132
Acyclovir therapy
  in herpes infections of the brain, 132
  in herpes zoster, 132
Adenosine arabinoside therapy in herpes simplex encephalitis, 132
Adenosine deaminase (ADA) deficiency, 67–68
Adenosylcobalamin
  deficiency, resulting in methylmalonic aciduria, 155
  and vitamin B_{12} deficiency, 154–155
Arednal insufficiency in idiopathic hypoparathyroidism, 307
ß-Adrenergic blocking drugs
  in malignant hypertension, 217
  in myocardial infarction, 93, 94, 95–96
  in periodic migrainous neuralgia, 128
  in portal hypertension, 248
  in renovascular hypertension, 215–217
Adriamycin (doxorubicin)
  combination chemotherapy
    in acute myelogenous leukaemia, 176
    in bladder carcinoma, 170
    in Hodgkin's disease, 180–181
    in ovarian carcinoma, 170
  single agent chemotherapy in small cell bronchogenic carcinoma, 191, 192, 194
Agranulocytosis, produced by chlorpromazine, 157
Airflow obstruction
  chronic diffuse obstruction, 116–120
    asthma, 116
    chronic bronchitis, 116–120
    chronic obstructive lung disease (COLD), 116, 117
  chronic obstruction, 116
    causes, 116
    treatment, 116
  investigative techniques, 114–116
Alcohol
  associated with secondary osteporosis, 293
  stimulates calcitonin secretion, 289
  withdrawal, treatment, 245
Alcoholic liver disease
  mechanisms of liver damage, 243–244
  occurrence, 242
  stages, 242
  susceptibility, 242–243
  treatment, 244–245
Alcohol-induced chronic active hepatitis, 238–239
Allergic granulomatosis
  symptoms, 103, 277
  treatment, 104, 277–278
Allergic reactions in Sjögren's syndrome, 258
Allergic rhinitis, as a receptor-antibody disease, 13
Allergy
  food antigens and the intestinal tract, 71–72
  vs. food intolerance, 72–73
  food reactions in adults, 72–73
  milk allergy, clinical features, 72
Allupurinol therapy for calcium stone disease, 311
Alopecia
  feature of systemic lupus erythematosus, 262
  feature of scleroderma, 270
  side effect of VP16–213, 172
  in type 1B diabetes, 24
Alprenolol therapy after myocardial infarction, 95–96
Aluminium
  cause of dialysis encephalopathy, 206
  cause of dialysis osteomalacia, 205, 302, 303–304
Aluminium hydroxide
  causing adverse effects in high-dose therapy for duodenal ulcer, 224
  causing hypophosphataemic osteomalacia, 301
Alveoli
  bronchoalveolar lavage (investigative technique), 101–102
  therapeutic lavage, 102

Amaurosis fugax and carotid artery disease, 129
Amine precursor uptake and decarboxylation *see* APUD
Amino acid therapy in acute alcoholic hepatitis, 245
Amino aciduria, in Sjögren's syndrome, 258
Aminoglycoside therapy in Legionnaires' disease, 109
Amosite (asbestos), 109
Amphetamine abuse, causing polyarteritis nodosa, 275
Amphiboles (asbestos), 109, 110, 111, 114
Amphotericin therapy of fungal infections in leukaemia patients, 177
Anaemia
  in acute myelogenous leukaemia, 173, 175
  aplastic
    diagnosis, 155
    drug-induced, 157
    idiopathic, 157
    inherited, 158
    immunological aspects, 157, 158
    irradiation-induced, 157
    role of haemopoietic microenvironment, 156
    thrombocytopenia in, 144
    viral involvement, 157
  of chronic disease
    low serum iron in, 151
  Fanconi's, 158
  in giant-cell arteritis, 278
  haemolytic
    due to haemoglobin insolubility, 159
    in sickle-cell disease, 159
    in systemic lupus erythematosus, 263–264
  iron deficiency, 151–152
  megaloblastic, 153–155
    folate deficiency, 152–155
    role of vitamin B_{12}, 154–155
  pernicious
    Addisonian, and loss of intrinsic factor, 155
    juvenile inherited, 155
    in Sjögren's syndrome, 258
  sideroblastic
    haemosiderosis in, 152
  Steel, in mice, 156
  in systemic lupus erythematosus, 264
Anaesthetic, general, and sickle-cell disease, 160
Anaphylactic reactions, side effect of DDP, 170, 171
Angina pectoris
  'cold spot' imaging, 79
  verapamil therapy, 83
Angina, Prinzmetal's, verapamil therapy, 79
Angiography
  investigation of pituitary lesions, 4
  in transient ischaemic attacks, 130
  in polyarteritis nodosa, 276
  radionuclide, 80–81
Angiomata and hypophosphataemic osteomalacia, 301
Angiotensin antagonist therapy in renovascular hypertension, 215, 216–217
Angiotensin-converting enzyme (ACE), high serum levels, 107
Animal protein intake and calcium stone disease, 310–311
Antacid therapy in duodenal ulcer, 224, 225
Anthophyllite (asbestos), 109
Antibiotic therapy
  infective endocarditis, 84
  legionnaires' disease, 109
Antibodies, monoclonal, 62–64
  advantages, 63
  disadvantages, 63
  future possibilities, 63–64
  and lymphocyte function and dysfunction, 63, 64, 65–66
  treatment of cancer, 64
Antibody demonstration tests for systemic lupus erythematosus, 264–265
Anticancer drugs
  DDP, 169–171
  human tumour stem cell assay, 166–169
  VP-16-213, 171–172
  see also combination chemotherapy
Anticoagulant, circulating, in systemic lupus erythematosus, 264
Anticoagulant therapy
  in cardiac valve replacement, 85
  secondary prevention after myocardial infarction, 94–95
Anti-inflammatory drug therapy
  in scleroderma, 273
  in systemic lupus erythematosus, 266
Antilymphocyte globulin (ALG), 208
Antimalarial agent therapy in systemic lupus erythematosus, 266
Antithrombin III, reduced, in tendency to thrombosis, 146
Antithyroid therapy in Graves' disease, prediction of relapse after, 14
α_1-antitrypsin deficiency, involvement in chronic active hepatitis, 239
Aortic regurgitation, acute vasodilator therapy, 87
Aortic arch (Takayasu's) arteritis, 280
Aortic valve endocarditis, 84
Aortitis, giant-cell, 279
Aplasia
  bone marrow *see* anaemia, aplastic
  pure red cell, 157–158
    autoimmune aetiology, 158
    Diamond-Blackfan syndrome, 158
    drug-induced, 157
Aplastic crises in sickle-cell disease, 160
Apnoea, sleep
  in chronic airflow obstruction, 118
  in diabetic autonomic neuropathy, 50
Apronal, inducing thrombocytopenia, 144
APUD system tumours, 10–12
Arabinoside therapy in herpes simplex encephalitis, 132
Argon laser photocoagulation, 227
Arteriography in renovascular hypertension, 212

Arteriolar dilator therapy in cardiac failure, 85–87
Arteritis
  Takayasu's, 280
  temporal (giant cell), 274, 279–280
Arthralgia
  in pure polymyositis and dermatomyositis, 267
  in vasculitis, 276
Arthropathy, in primary idiopathic haemochromatosis, 152
Asbestos
  effects of inhalation, 111
  properties, 109–110
  uses, 110
Asbestos-induced diseases, 109–114
  asbestosis, 109, 114
  diffuse pleural thickening, 112
  mesothelioma, 112–114
  pleural effusions, 112
  pleural plaques, 111–112
Asbestosis
  clinical features and treatment, 114
  definition, 109
  symptoms, 111
L-asparaginase combination chemotherapy in acute myelogenous leukaemia, 176
Aspirin therapy
  after myocardial infarction, 95
  contraindicated in systemic lupus erythematosus, 266
  in transient ischaemic attacks, 130–131
Asthma
  differentiation from chronic bronchitis, 116–117
  as a receptor-antibody disease, 13
  therapeutic lavage, 102
  in vasculitis, 276
Atenolol therapy
  for renovascular hypertension in patients with impaired renal function, 215
  in threatened myocardial infarction, 93
Atheroma
  cause of renal artery stenosis, 211
  complication of diabetes, 204
Atherosclerosis
  immunological aspects, 69–71
  and transplantation, 70–71
Autoantibodies, in systemic lupus erythematosus, 259–261
Auto-immune chronic active hepatitis, 237–238
Auto-immune diseases and type 1B diabetes, 24–28
Auto-immune mechanisms
  and Bell's palsy, 123
  and bone marrow aplasia, 158
Auto-immune phenomena developed as a consequence of PNP deficiency and defective T-cell function, 68
Auto-immune thrombocytopenic purpura, 142–144
  classification, 143
  clinical features, 143
  treatment, 143–144
Autonomic facial neuralgia *see* neuralgia, periodic migrainous
Autonomic neuropathy, complication of diabetes, 49–50
Autoplex preparations
  risks of, 148
  treatment of haemophilia A in patients with inhibitors, 148–149
Azathioprine therapy
  in autoimmune chronic active hepatitis, 237–238
  in autoimmune thrombocytopenic purpura, 143
  induces neutropenia in systemic lupus erythematosus, 264
  in lupus nephritis, 201, 263
  in primary biliary cirrhosis, 241
  in polymyositis, 268
  produces pure red cell aplasia, 157
  in renal transplantation, 208, 209
  in vasculitis, 277–278

BACOP combination chemotherapy in stage III and IV diffuse histiocytic lymphomas, 182
Bacterial infections provoke relapse in Wegener's granulomatosis, 104
Bacteriuria, asymptomatic, 197–198
Balloon dilation for correction of renal artery stenosis, 214
Balloon-pumping, intra-aortic, treatment of shock after acute myocardial infarction, 92
BCNU therapy in small cell bronchogenic carcinoma, 191
Bell's palsy, 122–124
Benzene, causing acute myelogenous leukaemia, 172
Bernard-Soulier giant platelet syndrome, 145
Bicarbonate therapy in diabetic ketoacidaemia, 48
Bile acid treatment for gallstones, 229
Biliburin, abnormal, indicating liver metastases in small cell bronchogenic carcinoma, 190
Biostator (artificial pancreas), 52
Bjork-Shiley valve, 85
Bladder cancer therapy with DDP and adriamycin, 170
Bleomycin combination chemotherapy
  in head and neck carcinoma, 170
  in Hodgkin's disease, 180–181
  in testicular teratomas, 188
ß-blocking drugs *see* ß-adrenergic blocking drugs
Blood coagulation disorders, 147–149
Blood glucose monitoring and regulation, 37–41
Blood transfusion
  followed by thrombocytopenia, 144
  multiple, followed by haemosiderosis, 152
  prior to renal transplantation, 207–208

Blood transfusion *(Contd.)*
in ß thalassaemia major, 161–162
'hypertransfusion', 161
'supertransfusion', 161–162
Bone
fracture risks in the elderly, 290–293, 298
infarction, in sickle-cell disease, 159
involvement in sarcoidosis, 105–106
marrow
aplasia *see* anaemia, aplastic
iron storage pool, 150
involvement in diffuse histiocytic lymphomas, 182–183
involvement in small cell bronchogenic carcinoma, 190–191
irradiation, in experimental animals, 156
and normal haemopoiesis, 155–156
suppression, consequence of anti-leukaemic therapy, 175
transplantation
in acute myelogenous leukaemia, 177–178
cyclosporin A therapy, 74
scleroderma-like condition following, 270
see also leukaemia
metabolism
and calcium physiology, 287–289
clinical disorders, 290–311
Bowel
involvement in scleroderma, 271
small
biopsy, in milk allergy, 72
malabsorption, and osteomalacia, 299
mucosal damage and milk allergy, 72
resection, and vitamin B_{12} malabsorption, 155
Brain
biopsy, in diagnosis of acute nectrotic encephalitis, 132
death, 135–138
confirmatory tests, 137–138
diagnostic criteria, 136–137
recommendations, 138
effect of iron deficiency on, 152
imaging techniques, 133–135
computer axial tomography, 133
digital radiography, 133–134
emission tomography, 133
nuclear magnetic resonance, 134–135
irradiation, prophylactic, to prevent c.n.s. relapse in small cell carcinoma, 192
scans, abnormal metabolic, in cerebral lupus, 263
Breast cancer, associated with myositis, 266
Brittle diabetes, 35–36
Bromocriptine therapy
in GH-secreting adenomas, 5
in prolactinomas, 7–8
side effects, 8
Bronchitis, chronic, 116, 117–120
differentiation from asthma, 116
Bronchitis sicca, in Sjogren's syndrome, 258
Bronchogenic carcinoma, small cell, 189–194
Bronchopulmonary lavage, 102
in sarcoidosis, 105
Bronchoscopy
in chronic airflow obstruction, 100–102
fibreoptic techniques, 100–102
in sarcoidosis, 105
Bumetanide, 216

Calcification, of skin and subcutaneous tissues, in scleroderma, 270
Calcitonin
increased
in pregnancy, 289
in stomatostatinomas, 12
therapy
in hypercalcaemias, 289
in osteoporosis, 295
in Paget's disease, 309
Calcium
antagonists, 82–84
nifedipine, 83
side effects, 83–84
verapamil, 83
side effects, 83
metabolism, 287–289
abnormal, in sarcoidosis, 106
calcitonin, 289
disorders, 289–311
diagnostic procedures, 289
and the menopause, 290–292
parathyroid hormone, 288
plasma calcium homeostasis, 287–288
vitamin D, 288–289
stone disease, 309–311
clinical features, 309–311
treatment, 311
supplement therapy
to delay or prevent bone loss, 292
in osteoporosis, 294, 295
Calcium-containing antacid therapy for duodenal ulcer, 224
side effects, 224
Cancer
anticancer drugs, 165–172
medical management
of acute myelogenous leukaemia, 172–178
of the lymphomas, 178–183
of ovarian cancer, 183–185
of small cell bronchogenic carcinoma, 189–194
of teratomas, 185–189
Medical Oncology Units, 166
specialisation in medical oncology, 165–166
Captopril therapy
in heart failure, 85–87
in renovascular hypertension, 215, 216–217
in scleroderma kidney, 272
side effects, 217
Carbamazepine therapy
inducing thrombocytopenia, 144
in trigeminal neuralgia, 126

Carcinomata, associated with hypersensitivity vasculitis, 278
Cardiac
arrhythmia
after myocardial infarction, 94, 97
detection by long-term electrocardiographic monitoring, 81–82
therapy to prevent ventricular fibrillation, 90–91, 97
failure
arteriolar dilator therapy, 85–87
complication of malignant hypertension, 217
cause of death in infective endocarditis, 84
in scleroderma, 272
venodilator therapy, 85–87
involvement in polymyositis, 267
involvement in scleroderma, 272
scintigraphy, 79–81
valve replacement, 85
Cardiomyopathy, post-infectious, 68–69
triggered by virus, 68
Cardiovascular disease, causing death in diabetes, 52–54
Carotid
angiography in transient ischaemic attacks, 130, 131
artery disease
microsurgical anastomosis (ECIC), 131
in transient ischaemic attacks, 129, 130–131
endartectomy, 130
stenosis demonstration by digital radiography, 134
Catheters
coronary artery angioplasty, 90
percutaneous transluminal balloon angioplasty, 214
Swan-Ganz, 92
CAV combination chemotherapy in acute myelogenous leukaemia, 176
CCNU therapy in small cell bronchogenic carcinoma, 191
Central nervous system
effect of virus infections on, 131–132
involvement
in non-Hodgkin lymphomas, 182–183
in Sjögren's syndrome, 258
in small cell bronchogenic carcinoma, 190–191, 192
in systemic lupus erythematosus, 263
Centromere antibodies in scleroderma, 270, 273
Cerebral arteriography in diagnosis of hypothalamic disorders, 3
Cerebral lupus, 263
Cerebral oedema in herpes simplex encephalitis, 132
Chagas' disease, and 'infectious-immune' theory, 68
Chelation therapy in ß thalassaemia major, 161
Chenodeoxycholic acid (CDCA) for dissolution of gallstones, 229
Chloramphenicol
producing pancytopenia, 157
producing pure red cell aplasia, 157
Chlorambucil therapy
in non-Hodgkin lymphomas, 181
in polymyositis, 268
and radiotherapy in ovarian carcinoma, 184
in VPP combination chemotherapy in Hodgkin's disease, 180
Chlordiazepoxide therapy for restlessness after alcohol withdrawal, 245
Chlorpromazine, producing agranulocytosis, 157
Chlorpropamide therapy in diabetes, 44, 45
Cholangitis, primary sclerosing, and chronic liver disease, 239
Cholecystectomy, 228–229
and increased risk of colonic carcinoma following, 229
Cholestatic episodes in early alcoholic liver disease, 242
Cholesteatoma and facial palsy, 122
Cholesterol
gallstones, 228–229
dissolution, 229
level reduction, clofibrate therapy trials, 88
Cholestyramine, 242
CHOP combination chemotherapy in stage III and IV diffuse histiocytic lymphomas, 182
Chromosomal abnormalities
in acute myelogenous leukaemia, 173
in Fanconi's anaemia, 158
Chromosome mapping of haemoglobin, 158
Chrysotile (white asbestos), 109, 111, 114
Churg-Strauss vasculitis, 103-104, 274, 277
treatment, 277–278
Cigarette smoking *see* smoking
Ciliary neuralgia *see* neuralgia, periodic migrainous
Cimetidine therapy
in duodenal ulcer, 222–225
in gastrinomas, 11
for gastric erosions in patients with fulminant hepatic failure, 226
side effects, 223
in upper gastrointestinal haemorrhage, 226-227
Cirrhosis
in HBs Ag-associated chronic active hepatitis, 233
in non-A non-B hepatitis, 235
primary biliary, 239–242
aetiology, 240–241
association with hypersensitivity vasculitis, 278
clinical course, 241
occurrence, 239–240
treatment, 241–242
in primary idiopathic haematochromosis, 152
see also Alcoholic liver disease
Cis-diamminedichloroplatinum (cis-platinum) *see* DDP
Clofibrate in cholesterol level reduction trials, 88–89

Clonidine, withdrawal effects, 216
Cluster headache *see* neuralgia, periodic migrainous
C-MOPP combination chemotherapy in stage III and IV diffuse histiocytic lymphomas, 182
COAP combination chemotherapy in acute myelogenous leukaemia, 176
Cobalamins
  deficiency, 155
  and vitamin B_{12} deficiency, 154–155
Coeliac disease
  and type 1B diabetes, 25
  and vitamin B_{12} malabsorption, 155
Coeliac-axis arteriography for diagnosis of gastrinomas, 11
Colchicine in management of scleroderma, 273
COLD (chronic obstructive lung disease), 116, 117–120
Cold agglutinin disease and plasma exchange, 76
'Cold spot' detection using thallium-201
  in angina pectoris, 79–80
  in myocardial infarction, 80
Cold-induced vasospasm in scleroderma, 270
Colitis, ulcerative, association with hypersensitivity vasculitis, 278
Colonic cancer, increased risk following cholecystectomy, 229
Combination chemotherapy
  in acute myelogenous leukaemia, 176, 177
  in Hodgkin's disease, 180–181
  in non-Hodgkin lymphomas, 182–183
  in ovarian carcinoma, 184–185
  in small cell bronchogenic carcinoma, 191–194
  in testicular teratomas, 187–188
COMLA combination chemotherapy in stage III and IV diffuse histiocytic lymphomas, 182
Computerised axial tomography
  bone density measurement, 287
  brain scanning, 133
  diagnosis of prolactinomas, 6
  diagnosis of gastrinomas, 11
  in herpes simplex encephalitis, 132
  in hypothalamic disease, 3
  investigation of pituitary lesions, 4
  staging small cell bronchogenic carcinomas, 190–191
Conjunctivitis
  in Sjögren's syndrome, 258
  in vasculitis, 276
Connective tissues disease, association with hypersensitivity vasculitis, 278
Constipation, side effect of bromocriptine, 8
Continuous subcutaneous insulin infusion (CSII), 31–32, 53
  in patients with diabetic nephropathy, 52
Copper accumulation, in primary biliary cirrhosis, 240
Coronary arterial spasm, and calcium antagonist therapy, 83
Coronary artery
  angioplasty, percutaneous transluminal dilation, 90
  bypass surgery, 89–90
    in post-infarction patients, 92, 96–97
    post-operative assessment by thallium scintigraphy, 80
    prognosis, 89
  disease, secondary to corticosteroid therapy in systemic lupus erythematosus, 262
Coronary heart disease *see* heart disease, ischaemic
Corticosteroid therapy
  in asthma, 117
  in autoimmune thrombocytopenic purpura, 142–144
  contraindicated, in primary biliary cirrhosis, 241
  in facial palsy, 124
  in giant-cell arteritis, 279–280
  in granulomatous lung diseases, 104, 106
  and increased risk of infection in s.l.e., 264
  inducing spinal osteoporosis, 293
  for inflammatory myositis, 273
  in 'lupoid' chronic active hepatitis, 234
  in lupus nephritis, 263
  in polymyalgia rheumatica, 280
  post-transplantation, increasing risk of coronary diseases, 71
  in relapsing polychondritis, 280
  in Takayasu's arteritis, 280
  in vasculitis, 277–278
Corticotroph adenomas, 8
Co-trimoxazole, 177
Cow's milk allergy
  clinical features, 72
  protein sensitisation following gastroenteritis, 71–72
Coxiella burnetti, 84
Coxsackie virus infections
  and atherosclerosis, 69
  and congestive cardiomyopathy, 68
  and diabetes mellitus, 26
  and myositis, 266
C-reactive protein (CRP) investigation
  in systemic lupus erythematosus, 265
  in Wegener's granulomatosis, 277
Creatinine/calcium ratios in bone disease diagnosis, 289
'CREST' syndrome, 270, 273
Crithidia luciliae test in systemic lupus erythematosus, 265
Crocidolite (blue asbestos), 109, 114
Cryoglobulinaemia
  associated with hypersensitivity vasculitis, 278
  in Sjögren's syndrome, 258
Cushing's syndrome and spinal osteoporosis, 293
CVP combination chemotherapy in non-Hodgkin's lymphomas, 181–182
Cyclophosphamide therapy
  in acute myelogenous leukaemia, 176
  in Churg-Strauss vasculitis, 277–278

Cyclophosphamide therapy *(Contd.)*
in lupus nephritis, 201, 263
in non-Hodgkin lymphomas, 181–182
in ovarian carcinoma, 170, 185
in polyarteritis nodosa, 277–278
in small cell bronchogenic carcinoma, 191, 192, 194
in Wegener's granulomatosis, 104, 277
Cyclosporin A (CSA), 73–74, 208–209
clinical studies, 74
properties, 73–74, 209
side effects, 74, 209
therapy in primary biliary cirrhosis, 241
use in transplant immunosuppression, 209
Cytogenic analysis in acute myelogenous leukaemia, 173
Cytomegalovirus
reactivation, side effect of CSA therapy, 74
in remission induction in acute myelogenous leukaemia, 176
Cytosine arabinoside therapy
in acute myelogenous leukaemia, 176
in herpes simplex encephalitis, 132
high dose, and reduced risk of c.n.s. involvement in diffuse histiocytic lymphomas, 183
Cytotoxic drug therapy
in aplastic anaemia, 157
in inflammatory myositis, 273
in Sjögren's syndrome, 259
in s.l.e. nephritis, 201
in vasculitis, 277–278
see also specific drugs

Dantrolene, causing chronic liver disease, 239
Daunorubicin combination chemotherapy in acute myelogenous leukaemia, 176
DDP (cis-diamminedichloroplatinum), 169–171
anticancer activity, 170
toxicity, 170–171
Deafness
in diabetes, 18
in Fanconi's anaemia, 158
side effects of DDP, 171
Delirium tremens, after alcohol withdrawal, 245
Dementia
in dialysis patients, 206
in megaloblastic anaemia with defective cobalamin synthesis, 155
and Parkinson's disease, 126–127
Dental caries in Sjögren's syndrome, 258
Dental extraction and infective endocarditis, 84
Dental hypoplasia, feature of idiopathic hypoparathyroidism, 307
Deoxyribonucleic acid *see* DNA
Dermatomyositis *see* polymyositis and dermatomyositis
Desferrioxamine therapy in thalassaemia, 161
Dexamethasone therapy
in facial palsy, 124
in herpes simplex encephalitis, 132
Dextran 40 therapy in acute myocardial infarction, 92
Diabetes
insipidus
in hypothalamic disease, 2
in Sjögren's syndrome, 258
mellitus
classification, 18–19
revised BDA classification, 19
complications
atheroma, 204
autonomic neuropathy, 49–50
blindness, 52, 53, 204
impotence, 50
ketoacidaemia, 46–49
nephropathy, 50–52, 202–204
peripheral vascular disease, 204
diagnostic criteria, 17–18
familial incidence, 20–21
feature of primary idiopathic haemochromatosis, 152
feature of somatostatinomas, 12
fibre-rich diets, 41–43
gestational, 21
impaired glucose tolerance (IGT), 17, 21
and the kidney, 202–204
prospects for prevention of diabetic renal disease, 203
proteinuria, 202–203
structural changes in the kidney, 202
treatment of end stage renal failure
dialysis, 203–204, 207
transplantation, 52, 204
latent, 21
possible association with secondary osteoporosis, 293
potential, 21–22
and pregnancy, 21, 41, 54–55
primary type 1, 19–20
aetiology, 23–28
primary type 2, 20–21
prognosis and prevention, 52–54
secondary to other diseases, 13, 22–23
treatment, 28–46
insulin therapy, 28–37
assessment of control, 37–41
oral hypoglycaemic agents, 43–46
biguanides, 45–46
sulphonylureas, 43–45
Diabetic glomerulosclerosis, 202
Diabetic ketoacidaemia, 46–49
therapy, 47–49
bicarbonate, 49
fluid, 48
general and supportive, 47
phosphate, 48
potassium, 48
Diabetic retinopathy, 52, 53, 204
Dialysis
continuous ambulatory peritoneal (CAPD), 206–207
dementia, 206

Dialysis *(Contd.)*
in diabetics, 203–204
CAPD for diabetics, 52, 204, 207
encephalopathy, 206
intermittant peritoneal (IPD), 206
osteomalacia, 205, 302, 303–304
and renal bone disease, 205–206
see also haemodialysis
Diamond-Blackfan syndrome, 158
Diazoxide therapy
causing tachycardia, 217
in renovascular hypertension, 216
Dibromodulcitol therapy in small cell bronchogenic carcinoma, 191
DIDMOAD syndrome, 18
Dietary treatment
in alcoholic liver disease, 245
in calcium stone disease, 311
in diabetes mellitus, 35, 41–43
Digital radiography for brain imaging, 133–134
Digitalis therapy in acute myocardial infarction, 92, 94
Digitoxin, inducing thrombocytopenia, 144
Dihydrotachysterol therapy in hypopapthyroidism, 308
25-Dihydroxycholecalciferol, overproduction, in sarcoidosis, 106
Diphosphonate therapy in osteoporosis, causing osteomalacia, 302
Diphosphonate-etidronate disodium therapy in Paget's disease, 309
Dipyridamole therapy in transient ischaemic attacks, 130–131
Disseminated intravascular coagulation (DIC), management in acute leukaemia, 175
Diuretic drug therapy in renovascular hypertension, 215–217
DNA synthesis, impaired
in megaloblastic anaemia, 153
and role of vitamin B_{12}, 154–155
L-Dopa therapy in Parkinson's disease, 126–127
Domperidone and diagnosis of prolactinomas, 6
Dopamine
affected by hypothalamic disease, 2
receptor blockade, in diagnosis of prolactinomas, 6
therapy in acute myocardial infarction, 92
Doxorubicin *see* adriamycin
Drug allergy in Sjörgen's syndrome, 258
Drug-induced diseases
agranulocytosis, 157
aplastic anaemia, 157
chronic active hepatitis, 238–239
hypersensitivity vasculitis, 278
myositis, 275
pancytopenia, 157
thrombocytopenia, 144
vasculitis, 275
Drugs, anticancer
DDP, 169–171
selection methods, 165–169
VP16-213, 171–172
see also Combination chemotherapy
'Dry gland' manifestation of primary biliary cirrhosis, 240
Duodenal ulcer
current management recommendations, 224–225
treatments, 222–225
antacids, 224
histamine H_2-receptor antagonists, 222–223
tripotassium dicitrato bismuthate (TDB), 223–224
Dyskeratosis congenita, 158
Dysostosis, metaphyseal, in Shwachman-Diamond syndrome, 158
Dysplasia, fibromuscular, causing renal artery stenosis, 211
Dyspnoea in scleroderma, 271
Dysrhythmia
in scleroderma, 272
see also Cardiac arrhythmia

Echocardiography
in infective endocarditis, 84
in transient ischaemic attack patients, 130
EEG in herpes simplex encephalitis, 131–132
Electrocardiographic monitoring, long-term, 81–82
types of recorder, 82
uses, 81
Electromyography
in myositis, 267
in scleroderma, 270–271
Embolism, cause of death in infective endocarditis, 84
Emission tomography for brain imaging, 133
Emphysema, oxygen therapy, 118–119
Encephalitis, acute necrotic, 131–132
computer axial tomography scan, 132
EEG, 131–132
and herpes simplex virus, 131–132
pathology, 131
treatment, 132
Encephalography, air, 3
Encephalomyocarditis virus, and type 1 diabetes, 26
Encephalopathy, dialysis, 206
Endocardial fibroelastosis (EFE), neonatal, and mumps virus, 69
Endocarditis
infective, 84–85
subacute bacterial, complicated by necrotising vasculitis, 275
Endoscopy and upper gastrointestinal haemorrhage, 226, 246
laser photocoagulation in, 227
Enterococci, causing infectious endocarditis, 84
Enteroviruses, causing injury to central nervous system, 131
Environmental factors affecting insulin absorption, 35

Enzyme activity, impaired, in iron deficiency, 151
Enzyme defects, lymphocytes, and immune deficiency, 67–68
Eosinophilia, in Churg-Strauss vasculitis, 276
Eosinophilic fasciitis, 274
Eosinophilic granuloma, 3
Epilepsy and low plasma 25OHD levels, 300
Epipodophyllotoxins, 171–172
Epstein-Barr virus, cyclosporin A therapy, 74
Ergotamine tartrate therapy in periodic migrainous neuralgia, 128
Erythema nodosa, in Takayasu's arteritis, 280
Erythromycin therapy in legionnaires' disease, 109
Erythropoiesis
  extramedullary, in ß thalassaemia, 161
  ineffective, and haemosiderosis, 152
Ethanol, and liver damage, 243–244
Etoposide *see* VP16-213
Exocrine glands, lymphocytic, and plasma-cell infiltration in Sjögren's syndrome, 257–258
External carotid-internal carotid anastomosis (ECIC) in transient ischaemic attack patients, 131
Eye
  in diabetes, 52, 53, 204
  dryness, in Sjögren's syndrome, 258, 259

Facial movement, involuntary, 124–125
  hemi-facial spasm, and exploration of the posterior fossa, 125
Facial palsy, 122–124
Factor VIII, 147–149
  and Bernard-Soulier syndrome, 145
  inhibitor bypass activity (Feiba) treatment of haemophilia A, 148–149
  relationship to platelets, 142
  and von Willebrand's disease, 145
Factor IX deficiency (haemophilia A), 149
Factor IX preparations, activated, in treatment of haemophilia A, 148–149
Falls and fractures in the elderly, 290–293, 298
Fanconi's anaemia, 158
Fatty liver, first stage of alcoholic liver disease, 242
Feiba preparations
  risks of, 148
  treatment of haemophilia A in patients with inhibitors, 148–149
Ferritin, 149, 150–151
Fetal haemoglobin disorders, 159
Fibreoptic bronchoscopy, 100–102
  bronchoalveolar lavage, 101–102
  complications, 102
  contraindication, 100
  indications, 100–101
  staging small cell bronchogenic carcinoma, 190
  technique, 100
Fibre-rich diets
  in diabetes mellitus, 41–43
  in scleroderma, 271
Fibrinopeptide A, raised in tendency to thrombosis, 146
Fibrosis, in scleroderma, 269, 271
Fits, in idiopathic hypoparathyroidism, 307
Flow-volume loop recording, 115–116
Fluid therapy in diabetic ketoacidaemia, 48
Fluorosis and fluoride therapy in osteoporosis, causing osteomalacia, 302
5-Fluorouracil combination chemotherapy in ovarian carcinoma, 185
Folate deficiency in megaloblastic anaemia, 153–154
Food
  additives, and type 1 diabetes, 26, 27
  allergy, 71–73
    management, 73
    milk allergy, 72
  antigens, and the intestinal tract, 71–72
    reactions in adults, 72–73
  intolerance, non-allergic, 72–73
    differential diagnosis, 72–73
Fossa
  pituitary
    and pituitary adenomas, 3, 4
    and prolactinomas, 6, 7
  posterior, exploration of
    in treatment of hemi-facial spasm, 125
    in treatment of trigeminal neuralgia, 126
Fractures and the elderly, 290–293, 298
Friedrich's ataxia and diabetes mellitus, 18
Frusemide therapy
  in malignant hypertension, 217
  in renovascular hypertension, 216
  vasodilator action, 87, 92
Fungal infections
  complication of remission induction in acute myelogenous leukaemia, 177
  in infective endocarditis, 84

Gallstones, cholesterol, 228–229
  dissolution, 229
  feature of somatostatinomas, 12
Gamma-camera scanning
  in brain imaging, 133
  in renal transplantation, 209–210
Gamma-ray absorptiometry for bone density measurement, 289
Ganglioneuroblastomas, and excessive VIP secretion, 11
Gastrectomy, and loss of intrinsic factor, 155
Gastric cancer, possible side effect of cimetidine, 223
Gastrinomas, 11
Gastroenteritis followed by specific food intolerance, 71
Gastrointestinal
  haemorrhage, upper
    endoscopy, 226

Gastrointestinal *(Contd.)*
mortality rates, 225–226
treatment, 226–227
cimetidine, 226–227
laser photocoagulation, 227
involvement in diffuse histiocytic lymphomas, 182–183
toxicity
side effect of DDP, 170–171
side effect of VP16-213, 172
Gentamycin therapy for granulocytopenia in patients with acute myelogenous leukaemia, 175
Germinomas, 3
GH *see* Growth hormone
Giant-cell arteritis, 279–280
differential diagnosis, 279
management, 279–280
prognosis, 279
Gigantism, feature of GH-secreting adenomas, 4
Glanzmann's disease, 145
Glibenclamide, 44
Glibornuride, 44
Gliclazide, 44–45
Glipizide, 44
Gliquidone, 45
Glomerular nephritis, rapidly progressive, and plasma exchange, 76
Glomerulonephritis, 198–202
diffuse proliferative, in s.l.e., 200–201
focal proliferative in s.l.e., 200
membranous, 198–199
in s.l.e., 200
mesangial, in s.l.e., 200
in Sjögren's syndrome, suggests s.l.e., 258
in Wegener's granulomatosis, 276
Glomerulosclerosis, diabetic, 50, 51, 202, 203
after kidney transplantation, 52
Glossitis in iron deficiency, 151
Glucagon
excess, in diabetic ketoacidaemia, 46
and insulin, treatment of acute alcoholic hepatitis, 245
Glucagonoma syndrome, 11–12
Glucose
monitoring methods
glycosylated haemoglobin, 39–41
home blood glucose, 37–39
tolerance, impaired (IGT), and diabetes, 17, 21
Gluten enteropathy, associated with milk allergy, 72
Glyceryl trinitrate, 85
Glycoprotein receptor deficiency in Glanzmann's disease, 145
Glycosylated haemoglobin method of assessment of long-term glucose monitoring, 39–41
Goitre of Graves' disease as a receptor-antibody disease, 12–13
Gold
allergy, in Sjögren's syndrome, 258
therapy may induce pure red cell aplasia, 157
Gonadotroph adenomas, 9
Gonadotrophin-releasing hormone in diagnosis of GH-secreting adenomas, 5
Goodpasture's syndrome
penicillamine-induced, 275
plasma exchange and immunosuppression, 75, 76, 199
Granulocyte transfusions in remission induction therapy for acute myelogenous leukaemia, 176
Granulocytopenia in acute myelogenous leukaemia, 173, 175
Granuloma, eosinophilic, 3
Granulomatosis
allergic, 103–104, 277
symptoms, 103, 277
treatment, 277–278
lymphomatoid, 278
treatment, 278
Wegener's, 103–104, 177
symptoms, 103–104
treatment, 104, 277–278
Graves' disease
as a receptor-antibody disease, 12–13
relapse of hyperthryoidism after therapy, 14
in Sjögren's syndrome, 258
Growth hormone-release inhibiting hormone (GH-RIH)
in diabetic ketoacidaemia, 46
treatment of peptic ulcer bleeding, 226–227
Growth hormone secreting adenomas, 4–6
diagnosis, 4–5
treatment, 5–6
Guanethidine therapy in scleroderma, 273
Guar, dietary, in treatment of diabetes, 42
Guillain-Barré syndrome and facial palsy, 122
Gum hypertrophy in acute myelogenous leukaemia, 173

Haematuria in lupus nephritis, 200–201
Haemochromatosis, 152–153
primary idiopathic, 152–153
diagnosis and treatment, 153
genetic aspects, 153
secondary, 152
Haemodialysis
vs. CAPD, 206–207
and vaccination against hepatitis B virus infection, 234–235
see also Dialysis
Haemoglobin
disorders, 158–160
fetal, 158, 159
glycosylated, in diabetes, 39–41
variants, 159
and sickle-cell disease, 159–160
and the thalassaemias, 160–162
Haemolysis in systemic lupus erythematosus, 264
Haemolytic anaemia
drug-induced, 144
and HbA_1 level, 40

Haemolytic crises in sickle-cell disease, 160
Haemophilia A
approaches to patients with antibodies
factor VIII inhibitor bypass activity (Feiba) preparations, 146
high dose factor VIII, 146
development of antibodies to administered factor VIII, 146
factor VIII treatment, 145–146
Haemophilia B, 149
Haemopoiesis and aplastic anaemia, 155–158
role of the haemopoietic microenvironment, 156
Haemoptysis in vasculitis, 276
Haemorrhage, upper gastrointestinal, 225–227
Haemorrhage, variceal, 245–248
Haemosiderin, 149, 150–151
Haemosiderosis, 152
after multiple blood transfusions, 152
Hamburger and Salmon human tumour stem cell assay, 166–169
Hearing loss, side effect of DDP, 171
Heart attack, acute coronary *see* myocardial infarction
Heart disease, ischaemic, 87–89
epidemiology and prevention, 87–89
controlled intervention trials, 88
drug therapy to lower lipids, 88
mortality trends, 87–88
see also myocardial infarction
Heart failure *see* Cardiac failure
Hemi-facial spasm, 125
exploration of posterior fossa, 125
Heminevrin, to prevent delirium tremens, 245
Henoch-Schoenlein purpura, associated with hypersensitivity vasculitis, 278
Heparin
inducing thrombocytopenia, 144
for management of disseminated intravascular coagulation (DIC), 175
Hepatic failure, fulminant, complicating hepatitis B infection, 232
Hepatitis A (infectious hepatitis)
and aplastic anaemia, 157
clinical illness, 230
diagnosis, 230
side effect of plasma exchange, 75
side effect of transfusion, 235–236
Hepatitis, alcoholic *see* alcoholic liver disease
Hepatitis B (serum hepatitis), 230–235
antigenaemia, 231–234
association with hypersensitivity vasculitis, 274
association with polyarteritis nodosa, 104, 274
carriers of HBsAg, 232–234
and remission induction in acute myelogenous leukaemia, 176
risk with large doses of factor VIII, 148
risk with prothrombin complex concentrates, 148
spectrum of clinical illness following HBV infection, 232–234
treatment of chronic HBsAg-associated disease, 234
vaccination against HBV infection, 234–235
Hepatitis, chronic, associated with hypersensitivy vasculitis, 278
Hepatitis, chronic active, 236–239
classification of causes, 237
definition, 236
diagnostic categories, 236–239
treatment of viral CAH, 234, 236–237
Hepatitis, chronic persistant, 233, 234, 236, 238
Hepatitis, non-A, non-B, 235–236
clinical course, 235–236
natural history, 235
Hepatocellular carcinoma, primary, and HBsAg carriers, 233–234
Hepatosplenomegaly, in ß thalassaemia, 161
Hepatotoxicity, side effect of cyclosporin A therapy, 74
Hereditary persistance of fetal haemoglobin (HPFH) disorders, 159, 160
Hermansky-Pudlak syndrome, 145
Herpes virus
and atherosclerosis, in chickens, 69
and remission induction in acute myelogenous leukaemia, 177
(simplex) encephalitis, 131–132
computer axial tomography, 132
EEG, 131–132
pathology, 131
treatment, 132
(zoster)
acyclovir therapy, 132
facial nerve involvement, 122
libility to, with cyclosporin A therapy, 74
HexaCAF combination chemotherapy in ovarian carcinoma, 185
Hexamethylmelamine
combination chemotherapy in ovarian carcinoma, 185
single agent therapy in small cell bronchogenic carcinoma, 191
Hip, aseptic necrosis, in systemic lupus erythematosus, 262
Hirsutism
side effect of cyclosporin A, 74
side effect of minoxidil, 216
side effect of prolactinomas, 6
Histamine headache *see* neuralgia, periodic migrainous
Histamine H_2-receptor antagonists in treatment of duodenal ulcer, 222–223, 224–225
Histocompatability locus antigens *see* HLA
HLA typing
and asbestosis, 111
and diabetes mellitus, 18, 19, 23–28
and relapse of hyperthyroidism in Graves' disease, 14
and renal transplantation, 208
and sarcoidosis, 107

Hodgkin's disease
classification, 178
management, 179–181
response to VP16–213 therapy, 172
serum ferritin raised in, 151
Homocystinuria in megaloblastic anaemia, 155
HOP combination chemotherapy in stage III and IV diffuse histiocytic lymphomas, 182
Horton's cephalgia *see* neuralgia, periodic migrainous
'Hot spot' detection using $^{99}Tc^{m}$ in myocardial infarction, 80
HPFH disorders, 159, 160
Human leucocyte antigens *see* HLA
Human leucocyte interferon therapy in HBV chronic active hepatitis, 234
Human tumour stem cell assay, 166–169
Hydrallazine therapy
in cardiac failure, 85–87
in myocardial infarction, 92
in renovascular hypertension, 216
side effects, 86–87, 217, 275
Hydrochlorothiazide, inducing thrombocytopenia, 144
Hydroxocobalamin
therapy in congenital deficiency of transcobalamin II, 155
and vitamin B_{12} deficiency, 154–155
4-Hydroxy-3-methoxy mandelic acid (HMMA) in screening for phaeochromocytomas, 10
Hypercalcaemia
calcitonin therapy for, 289
feature of primary hyperparathyroidism, 304
in renal osteitis fibrosa, 205
in sarcoidosis, 105–106
Hypercalciuria
in parenteral nutrition osteomalacia, 301
in renal stone disease, 310
Hyperglobulinaemia in sarcoidosis, 105
Hyperglucagonaemia in diabetic ketoacidosis, 46
Hyperkalaemia in acute myelogenous leukaemia, 175
Hypernatraemia in hypothalamic disease, 2
Hyperoxaluria in renal stone disease, 310
Hyperparathyroidism
coincidental, in sarcoidosis, 106
and diagnosis of MEA type 1 syndrome, 9–10
primary, 304–306
diagnosis, 305–306
presentation, 304–305
prevalence, 304
treatment, 306
and renal osteitis fibrosa, 205
secondary
in renal bone disease, 303
treatment, 304
in vitamin D deficiency, 296–298
Hyperphospaturia in acute myelogenous leukaemia, 175
Hyperpigmentation, in Fanconi's anaemia, 158
Hyperprolactinaemia
in hypothalamic disease, 2
in prolactin mas, 6–8
causes, 7
Hypersensitivity
side effect of VP16–213, 172
vasculitis, 274, 278
description, 278
disease associations, 278
management, 278
Hypersplenism in thalassaemia, 161
Hypertension
Detection and Follow-up Program, 88
malignant, 217–218
definition, 217
management, 217–218
in polyarteritis nodosa, 276–277
and renal artery stenosis, 210
and renal failure in scleroderma, 272
necessary investigations in all hypertensives, 211
portal
in primary biliary cirrhosis, 240, 241
treatment, 245–248
beta-blockers, 248
endoscopy, 246–247
shunt operations, 247–248
transhepatic venography, 248
in post-infarction patients, 96
in post-renal transplantation patients, 209
pulmonary, in scleroderma, 272
renovascular
assessment of functional significance of renal artery stenosis, 213–214
clinical features, 211
correction of renal artery stenosis, 214
definition, 210
medical treatment, 215–217
pathology, 211
prevalence, 210
screening investigations, 211–212
arteriography, 212
isotope urogram, 212
IVU, 212
Hyperthyroidism
associated with secondary osteoporosis, 292
associated with thyrotroph adenomas, 8
in Graves' disease, 12–13
prediction of relapse of, 14
Hyperuricaemia in acute myelogenous leukaemia, 175
Hyperviscosity syndrome and plasmapheresis, 75
Hypocalcaemia
post-operative, 307
in renal osteitis fibrosa, 205
side effects of plasma exchange, 307
Hypoglycaemic agents, oral, in diabetes mellitus, 43–46
biguanides, 45–46
sulphoylureas, 43–45
Hypogonadism in primary idiopathic haemochromatosis, 152

Hypokalaemia
in acute myelogenous leukaemia, 175
side effect of plasma exchange, 75
Hypolasia of thumbs and radii in Fanconi's anaemia, 158
Hypomagnesaemia, transient, side effect of DDP, 170, 171
Hyponatraemia, in legionnaires' disease, 108
Hypoparathyroidism, 306–308
diagnosis, 306–307
idiopathic, 307
pseudo-parathyroidism, 307–308
surgical, 307
treatment, 308
Hypophosphataemia
and congenital osteomalacia, 302
and osteomalacia in adults, 300–301
Hypophysectomy, trans-sphenoidal
in GH-secreting adenomas, 5
in prolactinomas, 7–8
Hypopituitarism
in GH-secreting adenomas, 5–6
in hypothalamic disease, 1–2
in pituitary tumours, 3
Hypothalamic diseases, 1–3
classification, 1
clinical features, 1–2
diagnosis, 2–3
treatment, 3
Hypothermia in hypothalamic disease, 2
Hypothyroidism, neonatal
clinical features, 14
screening for early diagnosis, 14–15
prevalence, 15
treatment, 15
Hypovolaemia of plasmapheresis, avoided with plasma exchange, 75
Hypoxaemia in chronic bronchitis, 118
Hypoxia
in alocholic liver disease, 244
in chronic bronchitis, 117–118

Idoxuridine therapy in herpes simplex encephalitis, 132
Ifosfamide therapy in small cell bronchogenic carcinoma, 191
IgA, IgE, and food allergy, 71
IgG and diabetes, 24–26
IgG involvement in autoimmune thrombocytopenic purpura, 142, 143, 144
IGT *see* glucose tolerance, impaired
Imerslund-Gräsbeck disease and malabsorption of vitamin B_{12}, 155
Imidazole carboxamide combination chemotherapy in Hodgkin's disease, 180–181
Imipramine, inducing thrombocytopenia, 144
Immune-complexes
deposition, chronic, in post-transplant atherosclerosis, 70–71
diseases and plasma exchange, 76
measurement techniques, 265
and vasculitis, 274–276
Immune deficiency
enzyme defects and lymphocytes, 67–68
secondary, causes of, 67–68
Immune system
and cardiovascular disease, 68–71
and diabetes, 24–26
and food allergy, 71–73
and granulomatous lung diseases, 104
and monoclonal antibodies, 62–67
and sarcoidosis, 105–107
and thrombocytopenia, 142–144
Immunofluorescent techniques
demonstration of factor VIII, 142
diagnosis of acute necrotic encephalitis, 132
diagnosis of systemic lupus erythematosus, 264–265
diagnosis of vasculitis, 274
Immunoglobulin A and food allergy, 71
Immunoglobulin E and food allergy, 71, 72
Immunoglobulin G involvement in autoimmune thrombocytopenic purpura, 142–143, 144
Immunosuppressive therapy
in autoimmune thrombocytopenic purpura, 143
cyclosporin A (CSA), 73–74, 208–209
in granulomatous lung diseases, 104
in lupus nephritis, 263
and plasma exchange, 75–76
in polymyositis, 268
in renal transplant recipients, 208–209
in systemic lupus erythematosus, 266
in viral chronic active hepatitis, 234
Impotence
in diabetes mellitus, 50
in prolactinomas, 6
Indomethacin therapy in periodic migrainous neuralgia, 128
Indoramin therapy in renal hypertension, 216
Infection
association with hypersensitivity vasculitis, 278
chronic, and anaemia, 151
complication of acute myelogenous leukaemia, 173, 175–176
risk in systemic lupus erythematosus, 264
'Infectious-immune' theory, 68
Infective endocarditis, 84–85
Influenza virus and myositis, 267
Insulin
dependence in type 1 primary diabetes, 19–20
and glucagon, therapy in acute alcoholic hepatitis, 245
therapy
in diabetes mellitus, 28–37
assessment of control, 37–41
brittle diabetes, 35–36
control problems, 33–37
insulin types, 28–29
overtreatment, 34, 36
regimens, 29–30
techniques of administration, 30–33

Interferon, human leucocyte, in treatment of
HBV chronic active hepatitis, 234
Intestinal malabsorption of vitamin B_{12}, 155
Intestinal tract and food allergy, 71–73
Intravenous urogram (IVU) screening
for asymptomatic urinary infection in patients with renal scarring, 198
for renovascular hypertension, 212
Iron
basal requirement, 149–150
deficiency
impaired enzyme activity, 151–152
tissue changes in, 151
overload, 152
measurement of serum ferritin, 151
primary idiopathic haemochromatosis, 152–153
in thalassaemia, 161
storage, 150–153
estimation of storage iron, 150–151
Iron-deficiency anaemia and HbA_1 level, 40
Irradiation
and acute myelogenous leukaemia, 172
and aplastic anaemia, 157
Ischaemic attacks, transient (TIA), 128–131
definition, 129
infarction risks, 130, 131
management, 130–131
natural history, 129–130
pathogenesis, 129
Islet cells *see* Pancreatic islet cells
Isoniozid, causing chronic liver disease, 239
Isorbide dinitrate therapy
in cardiac failure, 85, 86
in myocardial infarction, 92
Isotope renogram, 212

Jaundice, cholestatic, feature of primary biliary cirrhosis, 239, 241
Juvenile-onset diabetes mellitus (JOD), 18, 203

Kawasaki disease, 280
Kayser-Fleischer rings, in metabolic chronic active hepatitis, 239
Keratitis
filamentosa, 258
punctate, 258
Keratoconjunctivitis sicca, in Sjögren's syndrome, 257, 258
Ketoacidaemia *see* diabetic ketoacidaemia
Kidd blood group locus, and type 1 diabetes, 24
Kidney and diabetes *see* Diabetes and the kidney
Kidney disease *see under* Renal
Kidney transplantation *see under* Renal
Klinefelter's syndrome, 9
Koilonychia in iron deficiency, 151
Kveim-Siltzbach test for diagnosis of sarcoidosis, 105

Labetalol, 217
Lactose intolerance and secondary milk intolerance, 72
Laser photocoagulation
treatment of bleeding in peptic ulcer disease, 227
in upper gastrointestinal haemorrhage, 227
Laurence Moon Biedl syndrome, 2
Legionnaires' disease, 107–109
epidemiology, 107–108
symptoms, 108
treatment, 109
Lennert-Kiel classification of non-Hodgkin lymphomas, 179
Leucopenia in systemic lupus erythematosus, 264
Leukaemia
acute
in Diamond-Blackfan syndrome, 158
treatment with VP16-213, 172
acute myelogenous, 172–178
aetiology, 172–173
classification, 173
clinical features and diagnosis, 173–174
management, 174–178
remission induction, 174–177
combination chemotherapy, 176, 177
remission maintenance, 177–178
and facial palsy in children, 122
pre-leukaemic condition of Fanconi's anaemia, 158
serum ferritin raised in, 151
Levadopa therapy in Parkinson's disease, 126–127
Lichen planus, penicillamine-induced, 275
Lignocaine therapy for prophylaxis in cardiac arrhythmia, 91
Lip gland biopsy, diagnosis of Sjögren's syndrome, 258–259
Lipid content of diet
clofibrate therapy trials, 88–89
affect on post-infarction patients, 96
public awareness, 87
Lipoatrophy, and highly purified insulins, 28–29
Lipodystrophy, complications of traditional insulins, 28
Lithium carbonate therapy in periodic migrainous neuralgia, 128
Liver cells
necrosis in alcoholic liver disease, 242
parenchymal, and iron storage and overload, 150, 152
Liver disease
alcoholic *see* alcoholic liver disease
chronic, and osteomalacia, 299–300
chronic HBsAg-associated, 234
and osteomalacia, 299–300
cryptogenic chronic, after post-transfusion non-A, non-B hepatitis, 236
in small cell bronchogenic carcinoma, 190
see also Cirrhosis, Hepatitis

Liver membrane lipoprotein(LSP)antibodies present in patients with alcoholic liver disease, 244
Lung
  cancer
    and asbestos-related diseases, 114
    response to DDP therapy, 170
    response to VP16-213 therapy, 172
    small cell (SCBC), 189–194
      staging, 190–191
      treatment, 191–194
Lung diseases
  asbestos-induced, 109–114
  chronic airflow obstruction, 114–120
  granulomatous, 103–107
  Legionnaires' disease, 107–109
  see also under Pulmonary
Lupus band test, 265
Lupus erythematosus, systemic
  autoantibody spectrum, 259–261
  clinical features, 262–264
    cardiovascular system, 262–263
    kidneys, 200–202, 263
      and plasma exchange, 76, 266
    lungs, 262
    musculoskeletal, 262
    nervous system, 263
    reticuloendothelial system and blood, 263–264
    skin, 262
  infection, 264
  laboratory investigations, 264–265
  penicillamine-induced, 275
  pregnancy, 264
  treatment, 265–266
Lupus-like syndrome, side effect of D-penicillamin therapy, 241
Lymphadenectomy, total retroperitoneal, 186–187
Lymphocytes
  B, and monoclonal antibodies, 62–63
  enzyme defects and immune deficiency, 67–68
  myotoxicity test, 267, 268
  T, 63–68
    and bone marrow aplasia, 158
    deficiency of T cells, 67–68
    and monoclonal antibodies, 63–64
    subsets of T cells, 65–67
Lymphocytopenia, in systemic lupus erythematosus, 264
Lymphocytotoxins, in systemic lupus erythematosus, 264
Lymphomagenesis, side effect of cyclosporin A therapy, 74, 209
Lymphomas
  classification, 178–179
  Burkitt, 183
  diffuse histiocytic, 182
    combination chemotherapy, 182
    prognosis, 182–183
    radiotherapy, 182
    reduced risk of c.n.s. involvement, 183
  Hodgkin's *see* Hodgkin's disease
  large cleaved cell, 183
  large non-cleaved cell, 183
  lymphoblastic, 183
  management, 179–183
  non-Hodgkin, 178–179, 181–183
    c.n.s. involvement, 183
    classification, 178–179
      Lennert-Kiel classification, 179
      modified Rappaport classification, 179
    management, 181–183
  response to DDP therapy, 170
  response to VP16-213 therapy, 172
Lymphomatoid granulomatosis, 278
Lymphoproliferative disorders
  associated with immune thrombocytopenia, 144
  in patients with Sjögren's syndrome, 258

Magnesium
  antacids, side effects in duodenal ulcer therapy, 224
  replacement therapy in DDP-induced hypomagnesaemia, 171
Malignancy, 165–194
  and arteritis, 275
  haematological, and hypersensitivity vasculitis, 278
  and high levels of calcitonin, 289
  and myositis, 266
  see also under specific diseases
Malnutrition in alcoholic liver disease, 244
'Marfanoid appearance' in MEA type 2b syndrome, 10
Maturity-onset diabetes mellitus (MOD), 18
  of young people (MODY), 18
MEA syndromes *see* Multiple endocrine adenoma syndromes
Mediastinal teratomas, 185, 188
Medical oncology units, 166
Medical Royal Colleges
  criteria for diagnosis of brain death, 136
  recommendations, 138
  tests for confirming brain death, 137–138
Melphalan combination chemotherapy in ovarian carcinoma, 185
Menopause, and calcium metabolism, 290–292
Menstruation
  and iron requirements, 149
  and storage iron, 150
Mental retardation
  in Fanconi's anaemia, 158
  in pseudo-hypoparathyroidism, 307
Meprobamate, inducing thrombocytopenia, 144
6-mercaptopurine combination chemotherapy in acute myelogenous leukaemia, 176
Mesenchymal tumours and hypophosphataemic osteomalacia, 301
Mesothelioma, 109, 112–114
  clinical features, 112–113
  treatment, 113–114

Metabolic chronic active hepatitis, 239
Metformin therapy in diabetes, 45–46
Methaemoglobinaemia, 159
Methionine synthesis and vitamin B_{12} deficiency, 154–155
Methotrexate therapy
causing impaired DNA synthesis, 154
in diffuse histiocytic lymphomas, 183
in head and neck carcinoma, 170
in ovarian carcinoma, 185
in polymyositis, 268
in small cell bronchogenic carcinoma, 191
Methyl CCNU therapy in small cell bronchogenic carcinoma, 191
Methylcobalamin
deficiency, 155
and vitamin B_{12} deficiency, 154
Methyldopa therapy
causing chronic liver disease, 239
causing thrombocytopenia, 144
in renovascular hypertension, 144
'Methylfolate trap', and megaloblastic anaemia, 154
Methylmalonicaciduria, 155
Methylprednisolone
pulse therapy in lupus nephritis, 201
trials in systemic lupus erythematosus therapy, 266
Methysergide therapy in periodic migrainous neuralgia, 128
Metoclopramide and diagnosis of prolactinomas, 6
Metoprolol therapy for renovascular hypertension in patients with impaired renal function, 215
Metrizamide cisternography
for diagnosis of hypothalamic disease, 3
for investigation of pituitary lesions, 4
Middle ear cleft and facial palsy, 122
Migraine
classification, 127
complications, 127
periodic migrainous neuralgia, 127–128
in systemic lupus erythematosus, 263
Milk allergy, 72
Minoxidil therapy in renovascular hypertension, 216
side affects, 216
Mitochondrial antibodies and cause of primary biliary cirrhosis, 240
Mitral regurgitation, acute, arteriolar vasodilator therapy, 87
Mitral valve endocarditis, 84
Moniliasis
in idiopathic parathyroidism, 307
in remission induction in acute myelogenous leukaemia, 177
Mononeuritis multiplex, in vasculitis, 276
Mononucleiosis, infectious, in remission induction in acute myelogenous leukaemia, 176
Moon face, in pseudohypoparathyroidism, 307
MOPP combination chemotherapy in Hodgkin's disease, 180–181
Morbilliform drug eruption, penicillamine-induced, 275
Morphine therapy
in acute pulmonary oedema, 87
in pulmonary congestion, 92
Mortality rates
in diabetics, 52
in ischaemic heart disease, 87–88
from upper gastrointestinal haemorrhage, 225
Mucocutaneous lymph node syndrome (kawasaki disease), 280
Multiple sclerosis, demonstration with nuclear magnetic resonance, 135
Mumps virus and endocardial fibroelastosis (EFE), 69
Muscle
iron storage, pool, 150
weakness
in osteomalacia, 295
in polymyositis, 267–268
in scleroderma, 270–271
Mustine
combination chemotherapy in Hodgkin's disease, 180
inducing thrombocytopenia, 144
MVPP combination chemotherapy in Hodgkin's disease, 180, 181
Myalgia
in pure poly myositis and dermatomyositis, 267
in vasculitis, 276
Myasthenia
and bilateral facial weakness, 123
gravis
ineffective immunosuppression, 75–76
and plasma exchange, 75–76
as a receptor-antibody disease, 13
in Sjögren's syndrome, 258
penicillamine-induced, 275
Myeloblastic leukaemia, and cyclosporin A therapy after transplantation, 74
Myelomas and plasmapheresis, 75
Myelosuppression
side effect of DDP, 170, 171
side effect of VP16–213, 172
Myocardial abcess in infective endocarditis, 84
Myocardial fibrosis, 68–69
in scleroderma, 272
viral connections, 68–69
Myocardial infarction, 90–97
calcium antagonist therapy, 82–84
detection by nuclear cardiology, 80
in diabetic patients, 43
electrocardiographic monitoring, 81–82
of myocardial ischaemia, 93–94
home v. hospital treatment, 91
and immune-complex damage, 70
management of cardiac failure and shock, 92
pre-hospital coronary care, 91
prognosis after, 93–94
salvaging the ischaemic myocardium, 92–93

Myocardial infarction *(Contd.)*
secondary prevention measures, 94–97
in systemic lupus erythematosus, 262
in vasculitis, 276
Myositis
in scleroderma, 270–271
see also polymyositis and dermatomyositis
Multiple encodrine adenoma (MEA) syndromes, 9–10
familial incidence, 9, 10
mixed syndromes, 10
type 1, 9–10
type 2a, 10
type 2b, 10

Nasal stuffiness, side effect of bromocriptine, 8
Nausea
side effect
of bromocriptine, 8
of DDP, 170, 171
of VP16–213, 172
Neonatal facial palsy, 122
Neonatal hypothyroidism, 14–15
Nephritis
diabetic, 50–52
and facial palsy in children, 122
lupus, 200–202
histological types, 200–201
treatment, 201–202
penicillamine-induced, 275
rapidly progressive 'crescentic', 199, 200
Nephrotic syndrome in lupus nephritis, 201
Neuralgia
periodic migrainous, 127–128
alternative terms, 127
characteristic features, 127–128
treatment, 128
trigeminal, 126
Neurofibromatosis in hypothalamic disorders, 3
Neuropathy in vitamin B_{12} deficiency, 154–155
Neurotoxicity, side effect of DDP, 170, 171
Neutron-activation analysis for whole-body calcium measurement, 289
Neutropenia
azathioprine-induced, 264
in remission induction chemotherapy in acute myelogenous leukaemia, 175–176
in Shwachman-Diamond syndrome, 158
side effect of DDP therapy, 171
side effect of VP16–213, 172
'Newcastle bone disease', 205, 302, 303–304
Nifedipine (calcium antagonist), 83–84
side effects, 83–84
Nitrofurantoin therapy
causing chronic liver disease, 239
in children with vesicouretic reflux, 197
Nitrogen mustard therapy in small cell bronchogenic carcinoma, 191
Nitroprusside, 86, 87, 93
side effects, 86
treatment of hypertension, 217
N-nitroso compounds and type 1 diabetes, 26
Nuclear cardiology, 79–81
demonstration of myocardial perfusion, 79
detection of myocardial infarction, 80
radionuclide angiography, 80–81
Nuclear magnetic resonance (NMR), 134–135
Nystatin mouthwash, 177

Obesity
and cholesterol gallstone disease, 229
and hypothalamic disease, 2
and overtreatment with insulin, 34
and type 2 primary diabetes, 20
Obstructive airways disease (OAD), 116
Oesophageal symptoms
in acute myelogenous leukaemia, 177
in scleroderma, 271
Oesophageal variceal bleeding, 245–248
Oestrogen administration increasing calcitonin, 289
Oestrogen therapy for post-menopausal bone loss, 291–292
OPAL combination chemotherapy in stage III and IV diffuse histiocytic lymphomas 182
Optic atrophy in diabetes, 18
Orchidectomy in testicular teratomas, 186
Osteitis fibrosa renal, 205–206, 303
Osteomalacia, 295–302
biochemistry, 297
classification, 295–302
acquired forms, 295–302
congenital, 302
definition and diagnosis, 295
in dialysis patients, 205, 302, 303–304
in femoral-neck fracture patients, 293
renal, 205
Osteoporosis, 290–295
definition and classification, 290
primary, 290–293
secondary, 293
spinal, 293
treatment, 293–295
Otitis
and facial palsy, 122
and vasculitis, 276, 277
Ototoxicity, side effects of DDP, 170, 171
Ovarian carcinoma, 183–185
alkylating agent therapy, and risk of secondary malignancy, 172
comination chemotherapy, 170, 185
DDP, and DDP with adriamycin and cyclophosphamide, 170
HexaCAF, 185
platinum-based compounds, 185
radiotherapy, 184–185
Ovarian teratomas, 185, 188
Oxygen
increased consumption in alcoholic liver disease, 244
tension, low, and sickle-cell disease, 160

Oxygen (*Contd.*)
therapy, long-term, in chronic airflow obstruction, 118–119
transport disorders, 159
Oxyphenbutazone, producing pancytopenia, 157
Oxyphenisation, causing chronic liver disease, 239

Paget's disease of bone, 308–309
calcitonin and salmon calcitonin therapy, 309
diphosphonate-editronate disodium therapy, 309
viral cause, 308
Pancreas, artificial (biostrator), 52
Pancreatic insufficiency, in Shwachman-Diamond syndrome, 158
Pancreatic islet adenomas, 9
Pancreatic islet cell antibodies (PICA) and diabetes, 18, 25
Pancreatic islet cell hyperplasia and excessive secretion of VIP, 11
Pancreatic polypeptide-producing tumours (PP-omas), 12
Pancreatic transplantation, 33
Pancreatic tumours and excessive secretion of VIP, 11
Pancytopenia
drug-induced, 157
in Shwachman-Diamond syndrome, 158
Paracetamol, inducing thrombocytopenia, 144
Parathyroid adenomas and MEA type 2 syndrome, 10
Parathyroid hormone, 288
injections, for spinal osteoporosis, 295
Parathyroidectomy in renal osteitis fibrosa, 205, 206
Parenteral nutrition, producing osteomalacia, 301
Parkinson's disease, 126–127
L-dopa therapy, 126–127
and progressive dementia, 126–127
surgery, 127
PAS, inducing thrombocytopenia, 144
Pectin, dietary, in treatment of diabetes, 42
Pemphigoid, bullous, and plasma exchange, 76
Pemphigus, penicillamine-induced, 275
D-penicillamine therapy
in primary biliary cirrhosis, 241–242
in scleroderma, 273
side effects, 241, 267, 275
Penicillin
prophylaxis for dental extraction, 84
therapy in legionnaires' disease, 109
Pentagastrin, stimulates calcitonin secretion, 289
Peptide, vasoactive intestinal (VIP), 11
Percutaneous transluminal balloon angioplasty, 211
Perhexilene (calcium antagonist), 83
Pericardial involvement in scleroderma, 272
Pericarditis
side effect of minoxidil, 216
in systemic lupus erythematosus, 262
Peritoneoscopy with liver biopsy, in staging small cell bronchogenic carcinoma, 190
Peritonitis, complication of CAPD, 207
Persantin-aspirin therapy after myocardial infarction, 95
Phaeochromocytomas
and excessive secretion of VIP, 11
and MEA type 2 syndrome, 10
Phenformin therapy in diabetes, 43, 45–46
Phenoxybenzamine for management of scleroderma, 273
Phenylbutazone
inducing pancytopenia, 157
inducing pure red cell aplasia, 157
Phenytoin
inducing thrombocytopenia, 144
inducing pure red cell aplasia, 157
Philadelphia chromosome, diagnosis of acute myelogenous leukaemia, 174
Phosphate therapy
in calcium stone disease, 311
in diabetic ketoacidaemia, 48
Phosphate-binding agents, causing hypophosphataemic osteomalacia, 301
Phosphaturia in Sjögren's syndrome, 258
Phosphorus-31, used in nuclear magnetic resonance, 134
Photocoagulation, endoscopic laser *see* laser photocoagulation
Physiotherapy for scleroderma management, 273
Pitressin, 247, 248
Pituitary adenomas, 3–12
clinical features, 3
pathology, 3
radiological investigation, 4
Pizotifen therapy in periodic migrainous neuralgia, 128
Plasma calcium homeostasis, 287–288
Plasma exchange, 75–76
combined with immunosuppression, 75–76
in Goodpasture's syndrome, 75, 76
in myasthenia gravis, 75–76
in other diseases, 76
lack of controlled trials, 76
role in systemic lupus erythematosus, 266
side effects, 75
Plasma phosphate levels
and osteomalacia, 300, 302, 303
and pseudo-hypoparathyroidism, 307–308
Plasmapheresis, 75
Platelet
active agents, after myocardial infarction, 95
aggregation inhibiting drugs in TIA therapy, 130
transfusions, in remission induction in acute myeogenous leukaemia, 175
Platelets
abnormalities, 142–147
defects of platelet function, 144–147
inherited defects, 145–146
release reaction defects, 145

Platelets (*Contd.*)
thrombocytopenia, 142–144
autoimmune thrombocytopenic purpura, 142–144
drug-induced thrombocytopenia, 144
post-transfusion thrombocytopenia, 144
behaviour, 141–142
modification of platelet function by drugs, 145–146
treatment and prevention of thrombosis, 145–146
Platinum therapy, 169–171, 185, 188
anticancer activity, 169–171
in ovarian carcinoma, 185
in testicular teratomas, 188
toxicity, 170–171
Pleural
effusions, 112
involvement in systemic lupus erythematosus, 262
plaques, 111–112
thickening, diffuse, 112
Pneumocystitis carinii in remission induction in acute myelogenous leukaemia, 177
Podophyllotoxins, 171–172
Poliomyelitis and facial weakness, 123
Polyarteritis nodosa, 103, 104, 274, 275, 276–277
association with hepatitis B antigenaemia, 104
and crescentic nephropathy, 200
treatment, 200, 277–278
Polyarthritis in scleroderma, 271
Polychondritis, relapsing, 280–281
Polycythaemia, congenital, 159
Polyethylene glycol faecal marker for determination of calcium balances, 289
Polymyalgia rheumatica, 279–280
differential diagnosis, 279
management, 279–280
prognosis, 279
in Takayasu's disease, 280
Polymyositis and dermatomyositis, 266–268
classification, 267
clinical features, 267–268
diagnostic criteria, 266
malignancy and myositis, 266
pathogenesis, 267
penicillamine-induced dermatomyositis, 275
prognosis, 268
treatment, 268
Polyunsaturated fats and coronary heart disease, 88, 89
Polyuria, in Sjögren's syndrome, 258
Potassium therapy in diabetic ketoacidaemia, 48
Practolol therapy after myocardial infarction, 95–96
Prader Willi syndrome, 2
Prazosin (vasodilator) 85–86, 92, 216
Prednisolone therapy
in acute myelogenous leukaemia, 176
in chronic active hepatitis, 234, 237, 238
in facial palsy, 124
in giant-cell arteritis, 279–280
increased infection risk with high doses, 264
in lupus nephritis, 201, 263
in non-Hodgkin lymphomas, 181–182
in polymyositis, 268
in renal transplantation immunosuppression, 208, 209
in systemic lupus erythematosus, 266
in vasculitis, 278
in Wegener's granulomatosis, 104, 278
Prednisone therapy
in autoimmune chronic active hepatitis, 237–238
in autoimmune thrombocytopenic purpura, 143
in periodic migrainous neuralgia, 128
in polymyositis, 268
in renal transplantation immunosuppression, 208
Pregnancy
and bromocriptine therapy in prolactinomas, 8
and diabetes, 54–55
gestational diabetes, 21, 55
impaired glucose tolerance, 21, 55
monitoring diabetic control, 37, 41, 54
and facial palsy, 123
and increased calcitonin level, 289
and iron requirements, 149
and iron storage, 150
and post-transfusion thrombocytopenia, 144
and systemic lupus erythematosus, 264
and urinary tract infection, 197
Prenylamine (calcium antagonist), 83
Prinzmetal's angina, 79
verapamil therapy, 83
Procarbazine therapy
risk of sterility, 181
in small cell bronchogenic carcinoma, 191
Procolitis, ulcerative, possible cause of chronic active hepatitis, 239
Prolactin
deficiency in hypothalamic disease, 2
measurement in GH-secreting adenomas, 5
in prolactinomas, 6
Prolactin-secreting pituitary adenomas, 6–8
clinical features, 6
diagnosis, 6–7
treatment, 7–8
Propranolol therapy
after myocardial infarction, 96
for threatened myocardial infarction, 93
in periodic migrainous neuralgia, 128
in portal hypertension, 248
Protein intake and calcium stone disease, 310–311
Proteinosis, alveolar, therapeutic lavage, 102
Proteinuria
complication of diabetes, 50–51, 202–203
complication of systemic lupus erythematosus, 200–201
side effect of D-penicillamine, 241
Prothrombin complex concentrates
risks of, 148

Prothrombin complex concentrates *(Contd.)*
treatment of haemophilia A in patients with inhibitors, 148–149
'L-6' protocol combination chemotherapy in acute myelogenous leukaemia, 176
Pruritis
feature of primary biliary cirrhosis, 239, 241
feature of renal bone disease, 303
treatment, 242
Psychiatric abnormalities in systemic lupus erythematosus, 263
Pulmonary artery pressure increased in scleroderma, 272
Pulmonary disorders *see also under* Lung
Pulmonary emboli in systemic lung erythematosus, 262
Pulmonary fibrosis, diffuse *see* asbestosis
Pulmonary involvement
in Churg-Strauss vasculitis, 276
in polymyositis, 267
in scleroderma, 271–272
in Sjögren's syndrome, 258, 259
in systemic lupus erythematosus, 262
in vasculitis, 276
in Wegener's granulomatosis, 277
Pulmonary oedema, acute, venodilator therapy, 87
Purine nucleoside phosphorylase (PNP) deficiency, 67–68
Purpura, thrombocytopenic
autoimmune, 143–145
and plasma exchange, 76
thrombotic, 147
Pyelonephritis, acute, risk in pregnant women with asymptomatic bacteriuria, 197
Pyrexia, in Takayasu's arteritis, 280
Pyrimethamine, causing impaired DNA synthesis, 154

Quinidine, inducing thrombocytopenia, 144

Radioactive emission tomography, for brain imaging, 133
Radio-allergosorbent test (RAST), 73
Radiography, digital, for brain imaging, 133–134
Radioimmunoassay
of blood platelets, to predict risk from thrombosis, 146
diagnosis of herpes simplex encephalitis, 132
diagnosis of Vipomas, 11
measurement of parathyroid hormone, 288
Radioisotopes in nuclear cardiology, 79, 80
Radionuclide angiography, 80–81
equilibrium studies, 81
first pass studies, 81
of left ventricular function, 81
Radiotherapy
and chemotherapy combined, increase risk of second malignancy, 172, 181
in GH-secreting adenomas, 5
in Hodgkin's disease, 180–181
in non-Hodgkin lymphomas, 181–182
in ovarian carcinoma, 184–185
in prolactinomas, 7–8
in small cell bronchogenic carcinoma, 191, 192–194
in testicular teratomas, 187–188
Ranitide therapy for duodenal ulcer, 222
Rappaport classification of non-Hodgkin lymphomas, 178, 179
Raynaud's phenomenon
management of, 272–273
and oesophageal disease, 271
in pure polymyositis and dermatomyositis, 267
in scleroderma, 270
side effect of bromocriptine therapy, 8
Receptor-antibody diseases, 12–13
Reed-Sternberg cells in Hodgkin's disease, 178
Renal abnormalities
in Fanconi's anaemia, 158
in Sjögren's syndrome, 258, 259
Renal artery stenosis
assessment of functional significance, 213–214
correction of, 214
following renal transplantation, 209
pathology, 211
Renal bone disease, 303–304
treatment, 304
Renal disease
chronic, and thrombocytopenia, 141
diabetic *see* diabetes and the kidney
in legionnaires' disease, 109
in scleroderma, 272
Renal dysfunction during chemotherapy in acute myelogenous leukaemia, 175
Renal failure
chronic, management for avoidance, during DDP therapy, 170
end stage, treatment in diabetics, 203–204
Renal osteitis fibrosa, 205–206
Renal osteomalacia, 205, 300, 301, 303
Renal scarring
intravenous urogram (IVU), 198
and urinary infection, 197–198
Renal stone disease
clinical features, 309–310
treatment, 311
Renal toxicity
side effect of cyclosporin A therapy, 74
side effect of DDP therapy, 170–171
Renal transplantation, 207–210
blood transfusion before, 207–208
in diabetics, 204
gamma camera, 209–210
hypertension after, 209
immunosuppression, 208–209
tissue typing, 208
ultrasonography, 210
Renal tubular acidosis, in Sjögren's syndrome, 258
Reovirus type 3 and type 1 diabetes, 26
Respiratory muscle weakness in polymyositis, 267

'rest angina', nuclear detection of 'cold spots', 79
Reticuloendothelial
  cells, and iron storage, 150
  system abnormalities in systemic lupus erythematosus, 263–264
Retinal haemorrhage in acute myelogenous leukaemia, 173
Retinopathy, diabetic, 52, 53, 204
Rhesus disease and plasma exchange, 75
Rheumatic fever and 'infectious-immune' theory, 68
Rheumatoid arthritis
  anaemia in, 151
  preceptin, in Sjögren's syndrome, 257–258
Rhinitis
  alllergic, as a receptor-antibody disease, 13
  in Wegener's granulomatosis, 277
Rickets
  and congential osteomalacia, 302
  and osteomalacia among Asian immigrants, 298–299
  renal *see* osteitis fibrosa
Rickettsia, 84
Rifampicin therapy
  inducing thrombocytopenia, 144
  in legionnaires' disease, 109
Round heart disease of turkeys, 69

Salivary malfunction in Sjögren's syndrome, 258–259
Salmon calcitonin therapy for Paget's disease, 309
Sarcoidosis, 104–107
  bone involvement, 105–106
  circulating immune-complexes, 105
  high serum ACE, 107
  and HLA-B8, 107
  hypercalcaemia, 105–106
  Kveim-Siltzbach test, 105
  and pulmonary infiltration, 3
Sarcomas, osteogenic, response to DDP therapy, 170
Sarcoplasmic reticulum and calcium release, 83
Scanning *see* Computerised axial tomography; Gamma-camera; Nuclear cardiography; Ultrasonography
Schirmer's test, diagnosis of keratoconjunctivitis, 258
Scintigraphy
  for brain imaging, 133
  for cardiological imaging, 79–81
  salivary, 258
Scleroderma, 269–274
  classification, 269
  clinical features, 270–272
  management, 272–273
  pathology, 269–270
  prognosis, 273
Scleroderma-like conditions, 270, 273–274
Sclerotherapy, injection, for variceal bleeding, 246, 247
Sengstaken-Blakemore tube, 247
Septicaemias associated with vascular illnesses, 275
Serosal, 149, 153
Serum ACE, high, in sarcoidosis, 107
Serum sickness
  and atherosclerosis, 70
  and hypersensitivity vasculitis, 278
  and raised lipid levels, 70
SGOT, abnormal, indicating liver metastases in small cell bronchogenic carcinoma, 190
Sheep red blood cell marker for T cells, 65, 66
Shunts
  distal spleno-renal, 248
  portacaval, 247–248
Shwachman-Diamond syndrome, 158
Sickle-cell disease, 159–160
  heterozygous (sickle-cell trait), 159, 160
  homozygous, 159–160
  test for, 160
Sinusitis in Wegener's granulomatosis, 277
Sjögren's syndrome, 257–259
  clinical features, 258
  diagnosis, 258–259
  immunology, 257–258
  pathology, 257
  treatment, 259
Skeletal deformities in ß thalassaemia, 161
Skin changes
  in primary idiopathic haemochromatosis, 152
  in scleroderma, 269, 270
Skin rash
  in hypersensitivity vasculitis, 276
  in systemic lupus erythematosus, 262
  in vasculitis, 276
Sleep apnoea
  in chronic airflow obstruction, 118
  in diabetic autonomic neuropathy, 50
Sluder's headache *see* neuralgia, periodic migrainous
Small cell bronchogenic carcinoma, 189–194
Smoking
  and asbestos-induced disease, 114
  and chronic bronchitis, 117
  and coronary heart disease, 87, 88
  and diabetic complications, 53, 203
  effect on insulin absorption, 35
  and periodic migrainous neuralgia, 128
  and post-infarction patients, 96
  and scleroderma, 272–273
Somatostatin *see* Growth hormone-release inhibiting hormone
Somatostatinoma syndrome, 12
  clinical features, 12
  diagnosis, 12
  therapy, 12
Somogyi effect, 36
Sphenopalatine neuralgia *see* Neuralgia, periodic migrainous
Spirometer measurement of chronic airflow obstruction, 114–115
Spironolactone, inducing thrombocytopenia, 144

Spleen, iron storage pool, 150
Splenectomy
  in longstanding autoimmune thrombocytopenic purpura, 143
  in ß thalassaemia, 161
Splenomegaly and autosplenectomy in sickle-cell disease, 159
Stagnant loop syndrome and vitamin B_{12} malabsorption, 155
Staphylococci
  and allergic granulmatosis, 103
  causing infective endocarditis, 84
Starr-Edwards silastic ball valve prosthesis, 85
Steatorroea
  in idiopathic hypoparathyroidism, 307
  in primary biliary cirrhosis, 242
Steel anaemia, in mice, 156
Stem cell assay, human tumour, 166–169
Sterility
  risk after total retroperitoneal lymphadenectomy, 187
  side effect of MOPP and similar regimens, 181
Steroid therapy
  in acute alcoholic liver disease, 245
  in HBs–Ag negative chronic active hepatitis, 234, 236
  in herpes simplex encephalitis, 132
  in lupus nephritis, 201, 265
  in osteoporosis, 295
  in periodic migrainous neuralgia, 128
  in polymyositis, 268
  in Sjögren's syndrome, 259
Stomach cancer associated with myositis, 266
Stomatitis, angular, in iron deficiency, 151
Strabismus in Fanconi's anaemia, 158
Streptococci, causing infective endocarditis, 84
Stroke risk, in patients with transient ischaemic attacks, 129, 130
Sulfinpyrazone therapy
  after myocardial infarction, 95
  in transient ischaemic attacks, 130–131
Sulphonamides
  inducing pure red cell aplasia, 157
  inducing thrombocytopenia, 144
  inducing vasculitis, 275
Sulphonylureas
  inducing pure red cell aplasia, 157
  treatment of diabetes, 43–45
Sunlight deprivation and bone disorders, 293, 298, 303
Sun-ray lamp treatment for pruritis, 242
Swan-Ganz balloon-tipped catheter, 92
Syncope
  electrocardiograph monitoring, 81–82
  side effect of bromocriptine, 8
Synovitis
  in polymyalgia rheumatica, 279
  in Takayasu's arteritis, 280

T cells *see* lymphocytes, T
Takayasu's arteritis, 280
Tapeworm infestation causing vitamin B_{12} malabsorption, 155
$^{99}Tc^{m}$
  in detection of myocardial infarction, 80
  in radionuclide angiography, 81
Telangiectases in scleroderma, 270
Temperature control disorders in hypothalamic disease, 2
Tendinitis in systemic lupus erythematosus, 262
Teratomas
  mediastinal, 185, 189
  ovarian, 185, 189
  testicular, 170, 172, 185–189
    assessment and potential uses of AFP and BHCG, 186–187
    DDP therapy, 170
    major areas of debate, 188–189
    response of VP16–213, 172
    staging classification, 186
    treatment regimes
      stage I and minimal stage II, 186–187
      advanced stage II and minimal stage III and IV, 187–188
      bulky stage IV, 188
Tetany in hypoparathyroidism, 306
Thalassaemia, haemosiderosis in, 152
α thalassaemia, 162
ß thalassaemia, 160–162
  clinical classification, 160
  features, 160–161
  geographical distribution, 160
  treatment of thalassaemia major, 161–162
Thallium-201 scintigraphy, 79, 80
Thiazide diuretics in treatment of calcium stone disease, 311
Thiazides causing vasculitis, 275
6–thioguanine combination chemotherapy in acute myelogenous leukaemia, 176
Thrombocytopenia, 142–147
  in acute myelogenous leukaemia, 173, 174
  amegacarocytic, 158
  autoimmune thrombocytopenic purpura, 143–145
  drug-induced, 144, 171, 172, 241
  feature of systemic lupus erythematosus, 263–264
  post-transfusion, 144
  side effect of D-penicillamine, 241
  side effect of DDP therapy, 171
  side effect of VP16–213 therapy, 172
Thrombocytopenic purpura
  autoimmune, 143–145
  and plasma exchange, 76
  thrombotic, 147
Thromboembolism prevention with platelet-modifying drugs, 146
Thrombosis, treatment and prevention with platelet-modifying drugs, 145–146
Thymidylate (dTMP) and DNA synthesis, 153–154
Thymocyte markers for T cells, 65, 66

Thyroid carcinoma
medullary, and MEA type 2 syndrome, 10
response to DDP therapy, 170
Thyrotoxicosis due to LATS, and plasma exchange, 76
Thyrotroph adenomas, 8
Thyrotrophin-releasing hormone (TRH)
and diagnosis of GH-secreting adenomas, 5
and diagnosis of prolactinomas, 6
TIAs (transient ischaemic attacks) *see* ischaemia
Tic douloureux, 126
Timolol therapy after myocardial infarction, 96
Tinnitus, side effect of DDP, 171
Tobacco smoking *see* smoking
Tolbutamide therapy in diabetes, 43, 44
Toxic chronic active hepatitis, 238–239
Toxoplasmosis and 'infectious-immune' theory, 68
Transcobalamin I and III deficiency and low plasma B_{12} without anaemia, 155
Transcobalamin II deficiency and megaloblastic anaemia, 155
Transferrin, 149, 150, 151, 152, 153
Transient ischaemic attacks *see* ischaemia
Transplantation
cyclosporin A therapy, 74
immunological aspects, 70–71
see also Pancreatic transplantation; Renal transplantation
Tremolite (asbestos), 110
Tremors, mild, side effect of cyclosporin A, 74
Trichoderma polysporum, 73
Tricyclic drug therapy in periodic migrainous neuralgia, 128
Trigeminal neuralgia, 126
Trimethaphan therapy in heart failure with malignant hypertension, 217
Trimethoprin, causing impaired DNA synthesis, 154
Trimethoprin-sulphamethoxazole therapy in children with vesicouretic reflux, 197
Tripotassium dicitrato bismuthate(TDB) therapy in duodenal ulcer, 223–224, 225
Tumour
human, stem cell assay, 166–169
markers, 168
Turkey round heart disease, 69
Turner's syndrome, 9

Ulcer, duodenal *see* duodenal
Ultrasonography
diagnosis of gastrinomas, 11
liver scanning, instaging small cell bronchogenic carcinoma, 190
in renal transplantation patients, 210
in transient ischaemic attack patients, 130
Uraemia
and death rate among diabetics, 52
and HBA, levels, 40
with parathormone resistance, as a receptor-antibody disease, 13
Urinary stone disease, 309–311
Urinary tract infection, 197–198
asymptomatic, 197
in non-pregnant women and girls without renal scarring, 197
in older women, 197
in pregnancy, 197
intravenous urogram, 198
need to detect renal scars, 198
treatment in patients with renal scarring, 197–198
adults, 198
children, 197
Ursodeoxycholic acid(UDCA) for dissolution of gallstones, 229

Vaccination against hepatitis B infection, 234–235
Vagina, dryness, in Sjögren's syndrome
Variceal haemorrhage, 245–248
beta-blockers, 248
endoscopy, 246–247
management pathway, 247
shunt operations, 247–248
transhepatic venography, 248
Vasa nervorum vasculitis in polyarteritis nodosa, 276
Vascular abnormalities in scleroderma, 269–270
Vascular disease, peripheral, complicating diabetes, 204
Vascular spasm
cold-induced, in scleroderma, 270
side effect of plasma exchange, 75
Vasculitis, 274–281
aetiology, 275–276
Churg-Strauss, 103–104, 274
clinical features, 276
giant-cell arteritis and polymyalgia rheumatica, 279–280
immunopathology, 274–275
hypersensitivity angiitis, 274, 278
lymphomatoid granulomatosis, 274, 278
mucucutaneous lymph node syndrome, 280
polyarteritis nodosa, 103, 104, 200, 274, 276–277
relapsing polychondritis, 280
Takayasu's arteritis, 280
Wegener's granulomatosis, 103–104, 199, 274, 277–278
Vasoactive intestinal peptide (VIP), 11
Vasodilator therapy
in cardiac failure, 85–87, 93
in renovascular hypertension, 215–217
in scleroderma, 273
Venodilator therapy in cardiac failure, 85–87
Ventricular fibrillation
causing death following heart attack, 90–91
during convalescence from heart attack, 94
Verapamil (calcium antagonist) 83
side effects, 83
Verner-Morrison syndrome, 11

Vesicouretic reflux, 197, 198
Vinblastine combination chemotherapy
in Hodgkin's disease, 180–181
in testicular teratomas, 188
Vincristine therapy
in autoimmune thrombocytopenic purpura, 143
combination, in acute myelogenous leukaemia, 176
combination, in Hodgkin's disease, 180
in small cell bronchogenic carcinoma, 191, 192, 194
Vinyl chloride disease, 273
Vipomas, 11
Viral chronic active hepatitis, 236–237
Viral encephalitis, 131–132
Viral infections
and acute myelogenous leukaemia in animals, 172
and aplastic anaemia, 157
and atherosclerosis, 69–71
and cardiovascular disease, 68
complicating remission induction in acute myelogenous leukaemia, 176–177
and diabetes, 26–27
and facial palsy, 123
and myositis, 267
and Paget's disease, 308
and PNP deficiency and defective T cell function, 68
and relapse in Wegener's granulomatosis, 104
Visual loss in polymyalgia rheumatica, 279
Vitamin B deficiency in megaloblastic anaemia, 153–155
Vitamin D
deficiency
$1,25(OH_2D)$ therapy, 289
causing osteomalacia, 295–299
femoral-neck fracture and sunlight deprivation, 293
hydroxylate derivatives in treatment of hypoparathyroidism, 308
metabolism, 288–289
therapy
in congenital osteomalacia, 302
in osteoporosis, 294–295
in renal failure, using 25OHD, 289
side effects, 205
Vitamin therapy in alcoholic liver disease, 244
Vitamins, fat-soluble, support therapy for primary biliary cirrhosis, 242
Vitiligo
in scleroderma, 270
in type 1B diabetes, 24
Vocal cord paralysis, 116
Vomiting
side effect of bromocriptine, 8
side effect of DDP, 170, 171
VP16–213, 171–172
clinical activity, 172
therapy in small cell bronchogenic carcinoma, 191
toxicity, 172

Waldenström's macroglobulinaemia and plasmapheresis, 75
Water supply
aluminium in
causing dialysis dementia, 206
causing dialysis osteomalacia, 205, 302, 303–304
and possible cause of primary biliary cirrhosis, 240
Wegener's granulomatosis, 103–104, 199, 274, 277
renal failure in, 199
treatment, 104, 199, 274, 277–278
Weight loss in primary biliary cirrhosis, 242
von Willebrand's disease, 145, 147
and factor VIII, 145, 147
Wilson's disease and chronic active hepatitis, 239

X-ray diagnosis
MEA type 1 adenomas, 9
prolactin-secreting adenomas, 6
scleroderma, 272
Xerostomia, in Sjögren's disease, 258, 259
diagnosis, 258
treatment, 259

Yttrium-90 implantation in GH-secreting adenomas, 4–5

Zieve's syndrome, 242
Zollinger-Ellison syndrome, 10, 11